The Healthy Boomer

The Healthy Boomer

*A No-Nonsense Midlife Health Guide
for Women and Men*

Peggy Edwards, Miroslava Lhotsky, M.D.,
and Judy Turner, Ph.D.

Canadian Cataloguing in Publication Data

Edwards, Peggy
    The healthy boomer : a no-nonsense midlife health guide for women and men

Includes bibliographical references and index.
ISBN 0-7710-3050-9

1. Middle aged persons – Health and hygiene.   I. Lhotsky, Miroslava.
II. Turner, Judy.   III. Title.

RA777.5.E38 1999   613´.0434   C99-931856-X

Important Note
This book is not intended to take the place of advice from a health care professional. Readers are advised to consult a physician or other qualified health professional regarding the prevention and treatment of health problems. Neither the publisher nor the authors take any responsibility for any possible consequences from any treatment, action or application of medicine or preparation by any person reading or following the information in this book.

We acknowledge the financial support of the Government of Canada through the Book Publishing Industry Development Program for our publishing activities. Canadä

We further acknowledge the support of the Canada Council for the Arts and the Ontario Arts Council for our publishing program.

Typeset in Minion by M&S, Toronto
Printed and bound in Canada

McClelland & Stewart Inc.
The Canadian Publishers
481 University Avenue
Toronto, Ontario
M5G 2E9

1 2 3 4 5   03 02 01 00 99

In the time of your life, live – so that in that wondrous time, you shall not add to the misery and sorrow of the world, but shall smile to the infinite delight and mystery of it.

– William Saroyan, *The Time of Your Life:*
A Comedy in Three Acts, 1939

CONTENTS

Preface

Our story began in 1991, when we started to offer workshops about menopause and midlife for women we were seeing in our medical and psychotherapy practices. There was just not enough time in an office appointment to deal with the complex physical and emotional issues that concern women in midlife.

The women who came to our workshops said that they felt confused and frustrated by the expanding number of books and articles on menopause and the sometimes conflicting advice they were getting. Many were struggling with an inner conflict – wanting to make their own decisions yet also wanting an expert to tell them what to do. Others were seeking reassurance that they were not alone, that other women and other couples were having a hard time in their supposed "prime of life."

They were also concerned about the changes and stresses their partners and male friends were experiencing. The women wanted clear, straightforward information that they could share with the men in their lives. They wanted advice on how to communicate with men about what each of them was going through. They told us that the men in their lives were changing too, but that they were having trouble talking about it.

We wrote this book for the many women and men in midlife whom we have encountered, as well as for those we will never personally meet. We believe that each of us – men and women – must become our own expert at deciding how to deal with issues of personal health in midlife. We need accurate, comprehensive information about the key aspects of this crucial period of life, as well as encouragement to take charge of our health and take care of ourselves. To be a caring partner and friend, we must also learn as much as we can about how the opposite sex experiences midlife and be open and willing to talk about it. Midlife is an unsettling time for men and women as individuals, and also as couples and friends.

This book is designed to provide you with the information and resources you need to be your own health expert. It summarizes the most current research on midlife health issues, shares the experiences of people we interviewed, and refers you to other reliable resources where you can learn more about a particular topic. Because dealing with emotional concerns, managing stress, and making our relationships work are as important as keeping our blood pressure down, we have tried to provide a balanced view of the physical, psychological, spiritual, and social aspects of well-being.

Why Three Women Are Writing About Men

Our decision to write about the male midlife experience, as well as that of women, was prompted by requests from many of the women (and men) who attended our workshops and seminars. Having made that decision, we undertook a major search of the scientific literature and the popular press for information on the male transition in midlife. We were surprised at how little we found, compared to the extensive amount of material on women. A questionnaire we developed for women had helped us learn about their experiences, so we designed one for men. It was returned to us by sixty men between the ages of forty-five and sixty-five. We followed up this questionnaire by meeting with groups of men and conducting in-depth interviews with individual men. When we offered our first men's workshop at a university in Canada, we were afraid that no one would come. But they did come. They asked candid questions and stayed afterward to talk with us and each other.

The men we interviewed were open and willing to share their experiences – perhaps to some extent because we are women. They talked about their relationships, their sexuality, their fears, and their dreams: things that they often have trouble discussing with other men. What they told us suggests that men's midlife issues are no less complex than women's. However, they are much less acknowledged and understood. Men have fewer sources of information available to them and find it more difficult to raise their concerns with their physicians, partners, and friends.

North American women, encouraged by writers and activists such as Germaine Greer and Janine O'Leary Cobb (who also started a popular self-help newsletter on menopause), have made talk about menopause increasingly acceptable in business and social settings. Menopausal women smile confidently at meetings and parties when they ask, "Is it hot in here or is it me?"

Meanwhile, interest and information on the North American male in middle age have lagged behind until the last year or so. Viagra – the first oral treatment for impotence – has opened the doors to physicians' offices, at least when it comes to discussing erection concerns. Many articles about the male menopause have appeared, and a number of authors have released significant books about men's passages. More and more male baby boomers have discovered how much it helps to communicate in men's groups. Yet most men in midlife are far from eager to discuss their waning sexual drives or their urges to get up several times in the night to go to the bathroom. The silence around men's experience of midlife still remains.

Beyond Viagra

During the time it took us to complete this book, we witnessed and hurried to include information about some major breakthroughs in medicine and drug therapies. The discovery of designer estrogens and other new drugs, as well as changes in how these drugs are prescribed, led us to rewrite the chapters on osteoporosis and hormone replacement therapy (17 and 21) many times. When Viagra hit the market (and 36,000 prescriptions were filled during its first two weeks), we began to ask ourselves if the boomers' quest for eternal youth could be found in chemicals.

We came to the conclusion that, much as we would like to believe in a magic anti-aging pill, chemicals will never be the answer. Well-being will never be simply about the ability to get it up, to stay slim, or to do a hundred push-ups. It is about how we live each day – how we eat, exercise, laugh, and care for each other and for ourselves. And increasingly, as we move through midlife, it is about taking time to go deep inside ourselves, to find meaning in our lives, and make choices for the years ahead.

Sound boring? Not at all. The men and women in midlife we talked with have told us remarkable stories about their experiences and their efforts to stay healthy. Some of these stories are dramatic, some mundane, some funny, some sad. But boring? Never!

On a Personal Note

As we worked together writing this book, we talked through our own differing perspectives on issues such as the pros and cons of using alternative therapies. We believe that this helped to strengthen both our personal decision-making and the balanced approach to health and well-being we have strived to present to you, the reader.

Over the course of the four years that it took to research and write the book, we sometimes felt that what was happening to us and our partners made a better story than the book itself. Among the three of us, we experienced almost every crisis of midlife: death of family members, remarriage, new parenthood, grandparenthood, retirement, career changes, back problems, hormone changes, adolescents in transition, children leaving home, and parents becoming ill. We struggled in our relationships, unwilling to admit that our hormones sometimes made us moody and that our partners were having trouble talking with us about getting older. Working on this book helped us to deal with all of this turmoil, to take charge of our own health, and to strengthen our relationships. It is our hope that it will do the same for you.

The physical and psychological changes explored in this book are common to all women and men. However, concerns specific to gay men, lesbian women, disabled persons, and minority groups are beyond our expertise and the scope of this book. If you have special concerns in midlife that you would like to share, please write to us. (See the Afterword for details on how to contact us.)

How to Use This Book

This book is designed to help midlife men and women take charge of their health, at the same time as they reach out and support each other. The stories which are scattered throughout the text are based on anecdotes we heard from a variety of women and men in midlife. Because we believe that understanding and talking about our differences and similarities will help, quotes, charts, and illustrations that highlight male and female differences and similarities are also interspersed throughout the text. We hope that you will use these to spark conversation with your partner and take time to discuss the parts in this book that are important to each of you.

One of the most gratifying moments for us in the writing of this book was when we gave a draft of the chapter on impotence to a couple who were experiencing problems. Both were concerned about his trouble getting an erection, but they were unable to talk about the problem. After the woman read the chapter, she left it on the bedside table for her partner to read. The result was that they were able to talk about impotence, the probable causes in their particular case, and how they would seek help. We hope this book may serve as a similar "conversation starter" for partners and for male and female friends in midlife.

The book is divided into four parts:

Part I: The Midlife Passage is an introduction to the experience of midlife. It provides a map for the various stages of the journey, as well as the latest information on the new art and science of staying young. It discusses women's experience of menopause, the midlife change that dramatically affects all aspects of women's health and well-being. It also takes on the question of male menopause: Does it exist? Should men – like women – be looking to hormone replacement therapy as an option for improving their health?

Part II: How to Die Young . . . but as Late as Possible is designed to help you take stock and make changes that will improve your physical and emotional well-being. It provides self-assessment tools and practical tips on eating, exercise, weight control, and dealing with stress geared specifically to men and women in midlife. At the same time, it explores the importance of relationships and sexuality in midlife. If you are an action-oriented person looking for some specific lifestyle tips, this may be the most important section for you.

Part III: An Ounce of Prevention Is Worth a Pound of Cure focuses on how to prevent some of the common health problems of midlife, including heart disease, cancer, and osteoporosis. It highlights the differences in the ways men and women experience these problems and provides the latest medical findings on prevention and (in some cases) treatment. This section also deals with physical changes that are gender specific. For men, it gives particular attention to prostate health. For women, there is a decision-making chart to use in deciding whether hormone replacement therapy is for you and a frank discussion about breast health. Finally, this section gives clear direction on how to manage your health care, both through an effective use of the mainstream health-care system and through the use of alternative therapies such as herbal remedies and homeopathic medicine.

Part IV: Looking Ahead reminds us that once we have clear information about the physical changes and emotional and relationship challenges of midlife, it is largely matters of the heart and soul that occupy our thoughts. In Body, Mind, and Soul we look at the search for meaning and spiritual renewal that becomes especially important in midlife. The Conclusion reminds us that the time to act is now.

For More Information

In an effort to keep the length of this book manageable, we have provided a selected number of contacts at the end of each chapter – organizations, websites, and books that provide reliable information on a particular topic. When we first began the project, the number of websites was negligible. By the end, we could not keep up with the changes to existing websites and the new ones emerging every day. So please, while you use the Internet to check out the sites we recommend and to find others, maintain a critical consumer's eye. Except for monitored sites, mounted by credible health organizations, government departments, and universities, the health information you find may not always be totally reliable. More information on how to look for and assess electronic information can be found in Chapter 16, Partners in Health Care.

Acknowledgements

We would like to thank all of the women and men who participated in our seminars, filled out our questionnaires, invited us to their groups, and talked with us one-on-one.

We are grateful to Sari Simkins, a friend, public health nutritionist and registered dietitian in private practice, who joined us without hesitation in the project. Sari is the primary contributor to Chapter 8: *Food for Thought: Healthy Eating in Midlife*. She has also spent many hours reviewing the rest of the book to make sure that the information related to healthy eating is both accurate and practical.

Special thanks to Mary Jane Sterne, who proposed the title and read several versions of the manuscript.

We want to thank our other reviewers, both the experts in their fields and the good friends in midlife who, along with our interview subjects and seminar participants, helped to bring a human face to the myriad of facts:

Charles Ashbach, Ph.D., psychologist, private practice, Philadelphia
B. Norman Barwin, C.M., M.B. M.D., FRCOG; FACOG; FSOG(C), Director of the Midlife and PMS Centre, Ottawa
Estera Bekier, M.D., FRCP(C), staff internist, Mount Sinai Hospital, Toronto
Sue Berlow, expert on osteoporosis, Toronto
Michael Cord, M.D., psychotherapist, private practice, Toronto
Katarina Fiala, D.A.B.D., FRCP(C), staff dermatologist, Wellesley Central Hospital, Toronto

James S. Grotstein, M.D., clinical professor of psychiatry, UCLA School of Medicine, Los Angeles, training and supervising analyst, Los Angeles Psychoanalytic Society/Institute

Jo Hauser, M.D., Director, Riverside Urgent Care Centre, The Ottawa Hospital

Merle Kisby, B.Sc.N., Health Promotion Specialist, Kisby and Colleagues, Toronto

Peter Moran, M.B.B.CH., FRCP(C), staff psychiatrist, Mount Sinai Hospital, Toronto

Frances M. Owen, M.S.W., couples psychotherapist, private practice, Toronto

David B. Posen, M.D., stress expert, private practice, Oakville, Ontario

Marsha R. Werb, M.D., FRCP(C) staff endocrinologist at Sunnybrook Hospital and Women's College Health Science Centre, Toronto

and the following friends:

Brenda Buchanan, Mary Chalmers, Harry Gilles, Madeleine Greey, Anthony Hyde, Patricia Jasper, Barbara Markovits, Sue Merson, Karen Platt, LaDonna Smith, Dorothy Strachan, Paul Tomlinson, Sue Wehrmann.

We would like to thank the Canadian Public Health Association for reviewing and supporting our work, and the following public health professionals who reviewed and commented on the manuscript:

Gerald Dafoe, Chief Executive Officer, Canadian Public Health Association

Bonnie Dinning, R.N., B.Sc.N.Ed., Manager, Adult Health, Public Health Department, Ottawa–Carleton

David Korn, M.D., Visiting Assistant Professor, Harvard University

Edward Ragan, M.D., M.P.H., private practice, specialist in public health, Ottawa

Irving Rootman, Ph.D., Director, Centre for Health Promotion, University of Toronto

Ann Rowe, R.N., M.Ed., community health consultant, Fredericton, New Brunswick

Our thanks to Pat Kennedy, our editor at McClelland & Stewart, to our copy editor, Kathleen Richards, and to our agent, Karen O'Reilly, for their advice and unfailing support; to Heather Ebbs, our indexer; to Judy Field for her assistance in research and typing; to Karly Holmes for her help with finding and verifying helpful Websites; to Tracy Carefoot, who did the illustrations in this book; to Antonin Lhotsky, who kindly took our photographs; to the staff at 90 Medical for their ongoing help with client contact; to Richard Phinney for his encouragement; and to Carl Brett for his advice and support.

Lastly, we would like to thank our partners and families – Jo, Dan, Patty, Julie, and Lisa; Terry and Sarah; Antonin, Lukas, and Karla – for their love, patience, and support.

We dedicate this book to all of the women and men in the throes of midlife, with the hope that *The Healthy Boomer* will smooth and ease the passage.

PART ONE

The Midlife Passage

CHAPTER ONE

The Midlife Journey

Forty is the old age of youth.
Fifty is the youth of old age.
– Old French proverb

What Is Midlife?
Our research with men and women in the middle years suggests that midlife has less to do with your chronological age than it does with your experience of the midlife transition. Sometimes, an early menopause spurs women into midlife at thirty-eight or forty. Some men postpone the journey until their late fifties. And while most of us experience some common upheavals in the middle years, major events, such as the loss of a parent, may occur earlier, when you are in your thirties or forties. So, to a large extent, "midlife" is self-defined. Poet Ogden Nash says it this way: "You know you are middle-aged when it is Saturday night, you're home alone, the phone rings, and you hope it isn't for you."

It is hard to deny that things are changing in the middle years – new aches in our bodies, changes in our sexuality, children leaving home, parents getting older, and a nagging sense of limited time left in life. All of these things suggest that the period from approximately age forty-five to sixty-five is a unique stage of adult development with a discrete set of issues and experiences.

Busy with careers and families, many of us tend to ignore midlife or dismiss it as a period of relative calm compared to the younger years. We think of ourselves as growing in childhood and adolescence, being on a plateau as adults, and declining as seniors. But the experience of adulthood and eventual old age is more like a journey through the rising and falling waves of a turbulent sea than it is like sailing across a tranquil lake.

3

Sometimes, we feel like refusing to board the ship. When we do, we are sure that we will be washed overboard. Whether we like it or not, the midlife journey is an unavoidable and normal part of adult development. By staying informed and taking charge of our health, each of us can grab the wheel, enjoy the voyage, and sail on to the next productive stage of life.[1]

Gender Differences in Midlife

While there are similarities in the way men and women experience the midlife passage, there are also major differences. Menopause – which we refer to as a continuum that includes the period leading up to the cessation of menses (the perimenopause) as well as some time after – is a dramatic biological transition. Yet only recently have women begun to talk and write openly about how menopause affects their sexuality, well-being, and feelings of purpose. Men do not experience a dramatic biological change, yet most men we talked with believe that there is a male menopause. They describe experiences remarkably similar to those of women, including declines in their physical energy, sex drive, and mental sharpness, as well as increased feelings of irritability, anxiety, and fatigue.

Midlife storms can be hard on relationships. Buffeted by hormones, stress, and fatigue, many midlife women find it harder and harder to be the caring partners that they used to be. Upset by changes in their sexuality, career ambitions, and physical well-being, midlife men may withdraw from their partners and deny that they are aging. Some studies show that middle-aged marriages are less happy, fulfilling, and affectionate than younger marriages, even though both partners may be at the height of their careers and powers.[2] Ironically, this dissatisfaction may reflect the enormous potential for change and growth in the midlife transition. Partners struggle to grow with each other as they grow within themselves. In the process, they sometimes grow apart.

In his popular book *Men Are from Mars, Women Are from Venus*, author John Gray suggests that, when it comes to communication, men and women are from two different planets.[3] Understanding how life on these two planets has shaped us can help us avoid the mistakes we often make in relating to each other. Men unwittingly invalidate women's feelings by offering solutions; women mistakenly offer sympathy when men want to figure out what to do. As we have experienced in our workshops and talks with men and women, Martians tend to pull away and silently consider their concerns, while Venusians instinctively need to talk. Gray suggests that only when men and women are able to respect and accept their differences does love have a chance to blossom.

This book is designed to help you understand and discuss what you and your partner are going through in the midlife transition. Having someone understand why we feel and act the way we do in the midst of a surging sea can be the lifeboat we need to move ahead in our journey. There are four steps in successfully navigating midlife as individuals and as partners:

- The first step is acknowledging that you are in a transition period.
- The second step is taking some quiet time, both individually and as a couple, to reflect on this time in your life.
- The third step is recognizing your differences and understanding what you and your partner are going through.
- The fourth step is action – taking charge of your well-being by acting in ways that will strengthen your health and your relationships at the same time.

The Baby Boomer's Birthright

Approximately one-third of North Americans belong to the baby-boom generation. In 1996, some 86 million Canadian and American women and men were entering or in midlife.[4] Growing up in the 1960s and 1970s led us to believe that a long, healthy, affluent, and youthful life was our birthright. Midlife is a shock. Suddenly, the generation whose motto was "Never trust anyone over 30" is brooding about unfulfilled dreams, the risk of heart attacks, and why their hair is turning grey (or mysteriously migrating from the top of their heads to their ears).

We have reacted to the urgent ticking of the biological clock in a number of ways. We smoke less, exercise more, and eat less fat and more vegetables. Incredibly, in 1998, over 50 per cent of the runners in the Boston Marathon (53 per cent of men and 35 per cent of women) were over forty years of age.[5] Interest in antioxidants, alternative therapies, hormone replacement therapy, hair tonics, cosmetic surgery, and skin ointments has dramatically increased. Television talk shows, magazines, and newspapers across North America feature stories about the latest age-reversal techniques. Headlines around the world announced that an Italian woman gave birth at age sixty-two after eggs fertilized with her new husband's sperm were implanted in her uterus. We work out with Jane Fonda or go to concerts by the Rolling Stones and Bob Dylan – aging boomers who still have what it takes, although they have sensibly substituted vegetarian diets for pot or LSD.

Boomer men are just as likely as boomer women to engage in the frantic search for the fountain of youth. In *Dave Barry Turns 40*, the author describes a man in midlife crisis as someone who will "destroy a successful practice as a certified accountant to take up hang gliding and wear designer fragrances."[6] Male boomers, like their female counterparts, will go to great lengths to try to avoid the realities of aging.

There are positives and negatives to the boomer's approach to midlife. On the positive side, healthier lifestyles and medical advances mean that we will live longer, healthier lives than the previous generation. Access to education and economic prosperity mean that we have, for the most part, developed the skills and resources that we need to handle change and take advantage of midlife's potential for personal growth. At the same time, however, the boomer's self-preoccupation and denial of aging conflict with certain realities of midlife – such as the needs to find enduring meaning and purpose, to be realistic about the physical and psychological changes in midlife, and to prepare for what lies ahead.

DID YOU KNOW?

In 1776, a child born in North America lived on average to 35 years of age. One century later, life expectancy was 40. In 1996, life expectancy was 73 years of age for American men and 79 years of age for women. In Canada, a newborn male could expect to live to 76 and a girl to age 81.[7]

Midlife Is a Time of Reckoning: The Journey Begins

Like adolescence, midlife is a necessary stage in the development of a unique sense of self. It is a time to come to terms with the limitations that aging imposes, and the successes and disappointments we have experienced in our work, family, and social life up to this time. It is a time for re-assessing priorities and moving on.

We see the journey of midlife consisting of three phases:

- the beginning is initiated by an experience of loss, and focuses on letting go of the known, predictable past;
- the middle period of turmoil and uncertainty is when you question your purpose in life and re-assess your priorities. You may feel like a trapeze artist, caught in the moment when you have let go of one bar and not yet grasped the next one;
- the regeneration is an emergence out of the "dark night of the soul" of the middle period into a time of renewed energy.

The journey is a spiral. We do not return to the place where we started. Instead, we find ourselves inescapably altered, at the frontier of a new time in our lives.

The Beginning Is a Loss

Paradoxically, most new adventures in life begin with a sense of loss for what has gone before. Critical events such as a fiftieth birthday or a daughter's wedding can abruptly and sometimes painfully bring the midlife storm into focus. Suddenly it hits you. Clothing manufacturers seem to be making size 34 pants smaller than they used to. The gas station attendant calls you Ma'am instead of Miss. Your best friend has a heart attack or develops breast cancer. You stop thinking in terms of growing up and start thinking about growing old.

During midlife, we undergo a variety of annoying and sometimes threatening physical changes. The most visible signs show up in our mirrors every day. Others are happening inside our bodies. Our arteries become less elastic and our muscle strength declines. Chronic health problems such as high blood pressure, arthritis, and heart disease can become a real threat.

Midlife makes us more aware of our mortality and of the limitations on the time we have left. While women experience this shift biologically, men seem to be affected more by external events, such as the loss of a parent or the death of a peer. One man we interviewed was dramatically confronted with the loss of his sense of invincibility when he suffered a heart attack at age fifty-four. The event forced him to recognize his mortality and to make changes in his lifestyle to prevent another attack. Other men encounter less dramatic but equally unsettling events, such as being passed over for a promotion in favour of a younger man or admitting that a son has become stronger and faster on the tennis court.

For a generation of women that has had considerable control over reproduction, the inevitability and finality of menopause can be a bit of a shock. The meaning that each of us attributes to the end of our child-bearing years will depend on our particular circumstances. Most women who have children are happy to be free of birth control and periods. Others who have chosen to never have children may find themselves facing feel-ings of intense regret. Other women express concerns about losing the expected monthly rhythm that has been their companion for more than thirty years. One forty-five-year-old woman said that she felt surprisingly and inexplicably sad the first time her expected menstrual cycle did not arrive. Another woman said in a half-joking, half-serious way, "I don't know how to think about things any more. Every event in my life used to be defined as being before, during, or after my period."

Whether the losses you feel in midlife relate to mortality, fertility, health, or a youthful appearance, it is important to acknowledge your feel-ings. Sometimes our inner grief comes out as pervasive and baffling feel-ings of disappointment, sadness, anger, frustration, or anxiety. One forty-nine-year-old woman told us, "I can't explain why, but on my last birthday I had an overwhelming urge to just sit by myself and cry."

Women are generally more able than men to acknowledge their feelings and share them with female friends. Men are socialized to deny these kinds of feelings and to tell themselves to "act strong" and "get on with it." As one man said, "Society does not allow us to cry over vague feelings or to talk to male friends about them." Men still help each other in different ways, such as spending time together playing tennis, fishing, golfing, or enjoying other activities. One man said, "We don't talk about our feelings, but there is a kind of code between men friends; just being together is an acknowledge-ment of support."

What can you do when you're feeling caught in the first transitional stage of loss?
- Take stock. Ask yourself what has changed as a result of aging and the passage of time. How does it make you feel?
- Mourn your losses. By acknowledging your feelings, you can move on.

- Talk with your partner and with friends about what you are feeling. Listen carefully when the other person speaks of his or her feelings and refrain from providing advice or solutions.

The Middle Stage Is Turbulent

It is the experience of loss that propels us into the second stage of the midlife transition. This is a time of uncertainty and disequilibrium: what was is gone or going, and what will be is not fully formed. In the midst of this turmoil, we experience confusing and conflicting emotions. During this stage, we are likely to critically re-examine familiar relationships, values, and life choices.

For women, this stage is inextricably linked to the ebb and flow (and sometimes overflow) of the hormonal tides in their bodies. Mood fluctuations, unexpected eruptions of anger or tears, and changes in sexual desire may make you question who you are. When increases in family and work pressures are added to this mix, you can easily become despondent or exhausted.

Some women find themselves confronting unrealized youthful aspirations, low self-esteem, buried childhood traumas, and earlier unmourned losses. Issues that we put aside in the busy times of raising a family and building a career resurface with great intensity. In the book *Women of the 14th Moon*, it is summed up well: "Hormones slap you up against the doors of your unfinished business."[8]

For both men and women the physical indignities of aging are hard to deny – hair loss, wrinkled skin, excess pounds, skin tags (those little bits of skin that suddenly appear around your eyes), bent toenails that become impossible to cut, age spots on your hands, and migrating hairs that suddenly show up on women's chins and in men's ears. These daily reminders of change force us to re-assess and confront the aging process.

As mentioned earlier in this chapter, men do not have the intense hormonal flux or biological deadline that menopause provides for women. Yet many describe themselves as feeling more irritable and moody, negative or edgy at this time. One man said, "My emotions seem to be ranging far more," while another said, "I know I feel more moody, anxious, and lonely than I ever felt before."

During this time, many men confront their concerns about unrealized dreams and past relationships. A number of men spoke to us about their unfulfilled wish for a greater connection with their fathers. Men in midlife who are facing retirement or career changes often need to confront feelings of diminished self-worth and importance. This anxiety is exacerbated by fears about future income security. Secure employment that leads to a gold watch and a comfortable retirement is a thing of the past. From 1973 to 1991, the average wage for nonsupervisory workers fell steadily. Meanwhile, Fortune 500 companies shed more than one-quarter of their jobs and increased their assets by 2.3 times.[9] Corporate downsizing has become the order of the day.

In this period of searching, both men and women struggle with negative myths and stereotypes about male and female roles. In *The Middle Passage* James Hollis writes that "men's lives are as much governed by role expectations as women's and they have horrendous fears of not measuring up."[10] During difficult economic times, when layoffs are common, the limitations of roles assigned to men become painfully oppressive. A man who has grown up believing that his strength and identity rest primarily in his career may experience enormous stress in midlife. One man said, "I hate being Hercules holding up the world. I am frustrated. I am tired. I want out."

While the stereotype of our mothers' generation tended to describe the middle-aged woman as hysterical, distraught, over the hill, and barely functional, the 1990s myth may be even more destructive to women's well-being. This myth promotes the image of the superwoman – juggling the demands of career, children, relationships, aging parents, and hot flashes with ease and wondering what is wrong with her when she feels irritable and exhausted.

For both men and women, the negative or dark side of the middle passage seems to take two forms. One occurs when you feel stagnant and believe yourself too old to begin new things. Here, the danger is that a transitory period of uncertainty can become entrenched as a way of living dominated by depression and anxiety. The other danger is the tendency to deny change through compulsive activity. This can take the form of professionally taking on more and more, compulsive exercising, or, in some cases, seeking younger sexual partners to counter fears of lessened attractiveness or potency. This is when the midlife journey turns into the stereotypical midlife crisis with its relentless, ultimately futile, search for eternal youth.

In the face of midlife turbulence, the challenge is to find ways to move on creatively. Erik Erikson, who studied normal adult development, described the challenge in terms of finding new ways to renew or regenerate ourselves. Otherwise, we risk lapsing into stagnation where we become unwilling to change.[11]

How can you negotiate your way through the turbulent second stage of midlife?

- For both men and women, it seems that time alone (however difficult that may be to achieve) is critical for the successful navigation of the midlife passage. The conventional advice in our culture during times of stress is often to keep busy and not dwell on issues. On the contrary, the men and women we talked with came to value an approach that says, "Be still, take time, and go inside." Give yourself time to reflect on what you have experienced in the first part of your life and how you want the next part to be.

- Talk with your partner about the changes you are going through and tell him or her how they can best support you. One woman told us, "I want my partner to hold me and listen to me, not judge me, pity me, or dismiss me as hormonal."

- Talk with same-sex friends who are going through similar experiences. This helps you keep things in perspective and feel less alone. Same-sex friends can be an enormous source of support and encouragement. Several of the people we interviewed told us how they and several friends had celebrated their fiftieth birthdays by having an adventure or a weekend of sharing at a quiet getaway.

- Consider how the difficulties and regrets you have can be a catalyst for growth. Learn how to rediscover or rechannel your creativity in new directions. One fifty-eight-year-old male choreographer said, "Men must learn to be more creative in order to deal with the inevitability of change."

- Goof off and laugh. Many of the men and women we interviewed told us that maintaining a sense of humour about the indignities of aging and the hormonal roller-coaster was enormously helpful.

The Regeneration

The midlife journey, which begins with loss and moves through a time of turmoil and self-reflection, eventually emerges into a phase of regeneration and revitalization. Some people find their true calling at this stage. Others find themselves letting go of a familiar way of being and taking on characteristics that are most often associated with the opposite sex. Men often become more nurturing in the middle years; some women find satisfaction in assuming positions of greater authority and control.

The regeneration offers us a chance to break with the social conditioning that insists that, above all else, men must be strong and women must be nurturing. It gives us an opportunity to find a new balance between the yin and the yang in each of us.

Several men told us of their efforts to establish a new balance between their work and home lives. One man talked of "letting go of his male armour," his need to be strong and always in control. He allowed the musician in him to resurface and began to take pleasure in emphasizing his nurturing roles as a father and as a mentor to a younger man in his business. This is not an easy thing to do. One self-described workaholic admitted that it was harder than quitting smoking to close the door to his office at a reasonable hour and make time for relationships and leisure pursuits.

Many women described how difficult it is to shed their self-definition as the eternal caregiver and to claim more time for themselves. One woman said her change of life happened when she decided never again to pick up a dirty sock that wasn't hers. She added that this decision had nothing to do with whether or not her ovaries were producing eggs.

The regeneration process does not happen overnight. In our interviews with both men and women, two factors emerged as essential for moving on to the regeneration stage:
- a conscious acknowledgement that this is a significant time of change in one's life;
- claiming time for self-reflection, alone, in a group, or with a therapist.

In our seminars and workshops, women tell us that the love and support of female friends, improving their understanding of what is happening to them, and a supportive partner have helped them move on into a period of renewed vigour and peace with themselves. Men tell us that rebalancing work with more time for family and friends and a supportive partner have helped them to feel revitalized for the next stage of life.

As we look ahead, we may wonder with some trepidation what the next stage of adulthood will be like. In a culture that devalues old age and worships youthful energy, it is often difficult to look ahead with optimism. Will we really achieve a sense of renewal?

The women and men we interviewed who knew a vigorous older person seemed much more confident about moving on. As one woman said, "My grandmother taught me that there are no patterns to show us what to do. So, the territory is wide open and new at each moment. Now that's exciting!"

By remaining open to growth and wisdom, each of us has the opportunity to experience regeneration. In *Women of the 14th Moon*, Ursula Le Guin tells a wonderful story of aliens from another planet who search for one wise and exemplary person from whom they can learn. They pick an "ordinary" sixty-year-old woman who has wit, patience, common sense, and experiential shrewdness. She is reluctant to volunteer, suggesting that a scientist or Dr. Kissinger or a shaman would better represent humanity. But the aliens are steadfast. They know that only a person who has "experienced, accepted and acted the entire human condition – the essential quality of which is change – can fairly represent humanity."[12]

After you . . . our spaceship awaits!

THE BOTTOM LINE

While each of us experiences it differently, the midlife period (from approximately age forty-five to sixty-five) inevitably involves feelings of loss and turbulence. By making this period an opportunity for reflection and growth, we can move on to a time of renewal and regeneration.

Contacts and Further Information

Books

- *Crossing to Avalon: A Woman's Midlife Pilgrimage* by Jean Shinoda Bolen. New York: HarperCollins, 1994.

- *Fortysomething: Claiming the Power and Passion of Your Midlife Years* by Ross Goldstein and Diana Landau. Los Angeles: Jeremy P. Tarcher, 1990.
- *Journey Through Menopause: A Personal Rite of Passage* by Christine Downing. New York: Crossroad, 1987.
- *The Middle Passage: From Misery to Meaning in Midlife* by James Hollis. Toronto: Inner City Books, 1993.
- *New Passages: Mapping Your Life Across Time* by Gail Sheehy. New York: Random House, 1995.
- *On Women Turning 50: Celebrating Mid-Life Discoveries* by Cathleen Roundtree. New York: HarperCollins, 1993.
- *Once Upon a Midlife: Classic Stories and Mythic Tales to Illuminate the Middle Years* by Allan B. Chinen. New York: Jeremy P. Tarcher, 1992.
- *Transitions: Making Sense of Life's Changes* by William Bridges. Reading, MA: Addison Wesley, 1980.

CHAPTER TWO

Understanding the Female Menopause

Menopause is not a stage to hasten through, let alone obscure or deny. On these years depends the rest of your life, a life that may be as long as the life you have already lived.

> – Germaine Greer in *The Change: Women, Aging, and the Menopause*[1]

Menopause signals the end of the child-bearing years. It is a normal biological event that occurs in all women; it is *not* a disease. As one of the most significant events in midlife, it is a time for taking stock as well as for physical, psychological, and spiritual change. Families are in transition, careers are in flux, and relationships may need revitalizing. We urge you to view menopause within the context of the larger life transition discussed throughout this book.

In our workshops, we have found that women's first concern is about the physical changes of menopause. Once they have that information, the discussion usually changes its focus toward the emotional and psychological changes in midlife. This chapter follows the same sequence: it begins with managing the physiology of menopause, then moves to the cultural and historical perspective of menopause, and then to the psychological and emotional changes associated with menopause.

What Is Menopause?

Women's bodies are genetically programmed to reduce their estrogen and progesterone secretions over time and eventually to stop releasing eggs. Technically, menopause occurs when a woman has ceased to have menstrual periods for twelve consecutive months. The perimenopause occurs in the years leading up to the cessation of menses. This is the time when many women experience the common complaints described in this chapter. After the cessation of her periods, a woman is referred to as postmenopausal.

Because each woman experiences these stages in a unique way, we prefer to see the menopause as a process or continuum during which women experience both physical and psychological changes. Viewed this way, the entire process of menopause can begin as early as ten years before the end of menstruation and continue for several years after.

For North American women, the age range for period cessation is generally forty-eight to fifty-five years, although some women stop menstruating in their early forties while others continue to menstruate into their late fifties.[2] Women who smoke can expect an earlier menopause – about one and half years earlier than the average.[3] When women have a hysterectomy (removal of the uterus), their periods stop, but the ovaries continue to secrete estrogen and progesterone until natural menopause occurs. Sometimes women who have had a hysterectomy have an earlier menopause than women who have intact uteruses. Women who have hysterectomies with oophorectomies (removal of the ovaries) have quite a different experience of menopause. Because of the removal of their ovaries, they become suddenly and dramatically menopausal.

Each Woman's Experience Is Unique

At age forty-nine, **Alexa** had been experiencing irregular periods for about three years. She had an occasional hot flash and sometimes had difficulty concentrating, but she coped well with these minor complaints. The last of her children left home the past summer and she was happy to have some time for herself again. While she missed the kids, the idea of travelling and having some time to go back to watercolour painting in her leisure time was both appealing and exciting. Two weeks before her fiftieth birthday, Alexa realized that she had not had a period for sixty days. "Can that be it?" she wondered. "It all seemed so easy."

Barb had tried to ignore the complaints of menopause but fatigue did her in. Her hot flashes and night sweats were severe. She woke up soaking wet at least once a night and slept fitfully in between. She knew that lack of sleep was a factor in her irritability and her declining interest in sex. Her gynaecologist prescribed short-term hormone replacement therapy to deal with the problem.

Ivy had always been known as a "superwoman," balancing a high-stress career, two children, aging parents, and volunteer work. Now at age forty-eight, she felt like "superwimp." Every twenty-two days she experienced painful, heavy periods that kept her from going out for the first two days. Her once-a-month migraines now occurred three to four times a month. Her joints ached when she climbed the stairs, and her mood was increasingly blue. She had gained twenty pounds and felt constantly bloated. Nothing (including dieting and sporadic exercise) seemed to help her lose weight. Her family suffered with her in silence as she struggled to put on a happy face for the outside world. By the time she got to her doctor, she was at the end of her rope. Ivy's physician suggested that she was suffering from depression and high stress as well as some common menopausal symptoms. He prescribed the low-dose birth-control pill to relieve her heavy periods and referred her for treatment for depression.

Alexa, Barb, and Ivy demonstrate the varying degrees to which the menopause process affects us. Like Alexa, about 15 to 20 per cent of North American women will sail through with only minor complaints. Like Barb, about 60 to 70 per cent of women may be sufficiently bothered by symptoms to seek help. These most commonly relate to hot flashes, night sweats, and insomnia. Sleep deprivation brought on by insomnia and night sweats can be the start of grinding fatigue and a host of other health problems at the very time of life that women are particularly busy with careers and family obligations. Ivy's experience is typical for another 15 to 20 per cent of women. These women have a very difficult time in the menopause period. Ivy's despair is an outcome of the build-up of serious physical and emotional problems that she had tried to ignore.

The Physical Experience of Menopause

While each of us experiences menopause in a unique way, there are some common complaints and long-term health risks of estrogen withdrawal that affect most of us.

Common Complaints

- menstrual irregularities, such as heavy bleeding with flooding; spotting; and irregular periods;
- hot flashes, night sweats, or both;

- sleep disturbances;
- blue or irritable moods and mood swings;
- difficulty dealing with stress;
- vaginal dryness or itching, pain during intercourse;
- bladder problems, such as an increased need to urinate, recurring bladder infections, and reduced bladder control, especially when coughing or running;
- decreased interest in sex;
- bloating and breast tenderness;
- weight gain and waist thickening.

Other reported problems include headaches, light-headedness, lack of energy, forgetfulness, heart palpitations, constipation or diarrhea, aching muscles and joints, tingling and numbness in the fingers, dry skin, the appearance of new facial hair, and a crawling sensation on the skin.

Sound terrible? Take heart! There are three good reasons you should not let this long list of problems get you down:

- It is highly unlikely you will experience all of these problems. Even if you do have some of them, your symptoms may not be severe enough to require a trip to your physician. In the Massachusetts Women's Health Study (a large, comprehensive longitudinal study of middle-aged women), most women dealt with minor complaints themselves and expressed neutral or positive feelings about menopause.[4] Women aged forty-five to sixty who were surveyed in 1997 by the North American Menopause Society were even more optimistic. Eight in ten women expressed relief about the stopping of their menstrual periods and only 11 per cent of the women who had already passed menopause described the experience negatively.[5]
- There are positive things you can do to decrease your discomfort. For example, regular, enjoyable physical activity can reduce the severity of hot flashes, help you sleep, improve your moods, and help you manage your weight. Alternative therapies also offer symptom relief. Many of the women we talked with said that taking time to have fun with friends helped. Others said that getting into a creative activity such as painting or writing was an enormous comfort in difficult times.
- Once you are through the menopausal period, you will feel more

energetic and healthy (as long as you take care of yourself and lead a healthy lifestyle).

Long-Term Health Risks

Over the long term, aging and low levels of estrogen are associated with increased risk for two serious health problems: osteoporosis and heart disease.

Osteoporosis refers to the gradual thinning of bones and loss of bone density that come with aging. While both men and women lose bone mass, the loss is much more pronounced in women and accelerates immediately after menopause. Women may lose as much as 15 to 50 per cent of their bone mass during the first ten years following menopause.[6] Excessive bone loss can lead to a gradual reduction in height, the appearance of a hump on the upper back, and a greater risk for bone fractures. Eighty-five per cent of hip fractures occur in postmenopausal women, and complications owing to bone fractures can lead to disability or death.[7]

Until menopause, fewer women than men suffer heart disease or stroke.[8] Thereafter, women catch up with men and face the same risk for cardiovascular disease. Women who suffer a stroke or live with heart disease have a reduced quality of life and may be seriously disabled. Heart disease and stroke are the top two causes of death for women over age fifty.[9, 10]

Chapters 17 and 20 provide specific tools to help you assess your risk for osteoporosis and heart disease, as well as practical tips for preventing these serious problems.

Common Menopausal Concerns

One of the best ways to understand the changes you are going through is to record them in a daily journal. The easiest way to do this is to write down your main problems the day they occur right in your daybook. Take this when you see your physician; it will be extremely helpful in your discussion.

You may find yourself experiencing any of the following common complaints associated with the menopausal period:

Menstrual Irregularities

As you approach menopause, fluctuating hormone levels may make your periods irregular or heavy. The cessation of ovulation, combined with relatively high levels of estrogen, thicken the monthly lining of the uterus more than usual. As it is shed, you often have heavier bleeding as a result. Talk with your physician if you experience heavy or frequent bleeding. She will help you establish whether or not any steps are required to control it (for example, very heavy periods may make you anemic). If you have breakthrough bleeding after your periods have stopped for twelve months (and you are not taking hormones), see your doctor immediately. Bleeding after the cessation of menses is a signal that something may be wrong.

Sleep Disturbances

Light sleeping and chronically disrupted sleep associated with hot flashes and night sweats (discussed later) are common in menopause. For occasional sleep problems, improve your sleep hygiene by getting more exercise, using herbal remedies, avoiding caffeine late in the day, and establishing a regular sleeping schedule. If significant sleep disruption continues for longer than two weeks, see your doctor. It is important to determine whether fluctuating hormone levels are the cause (in which case hormone replacement therapy may help), or whether there are other reasons. Clinical depression also causes sleep disturbances, especially difficulty falling asleep and early-morning waking. (See Chapter 15 for more information on sleep and insomnia.)

Emotional Distress

Hormone fluctuations may make you feel blue or irritable. Regular exercise, stress-management techniques, talking with trusted friends, and honest communication with family members can support you through these difficult times. Remember, hormonal changes are only one cause of emotional distress. See your family physician and consider psychotherapy if feelings of anxiety or depression persist or worsen. (See Chapter 15.) Many women find psychotherapy useful at this time, not only to deal with serious mood disturbances, but also as a way to re-assess and set priorities in the middle years.

Vaginal Dryness and Itching

The thinning of the vaginal wall that accompanies decreased estrogen levels may result in vaginal itching or dryness. You may feel a burning sensation during urination and pain during intercourse. Talk with your doctor about ways to alleviate this problem. Some women find that vitamin E creams help (these are not applied to the vagina during intercourse). Vaginal estrogen creams or the slow-release estrogen ring have proved effective for treating the problem.[11] One of the best ways to keep vaginal walls healthy and prevent hormone-related dryness is to stay sexually active. Sexual activity (including self-stimulation) increases lubrication and blood flow to the vagina. There are a number of lubricating and moisturizing products that can be used during intercourse.

Incontinence

As you age, the muscles that hold urine in the bladder get weaker and thinner, especially if you have had several pregnancies. This can be one of the causes of incontinence – an involuntary loss of urine. Urinary incontinence is a pervasive problem that many women are ashamed or embarrassed to talk about. Although it is estimated that it affects 30 to 40 per cent of North American women over age forty, many women do not even mention it to their physicians. They see it as part of aging and having children, as something "you have to put up with." And even though there are effective ways to deal with most incontinence problems, the indignity that we feel about this change in our bodily functions is particularly troubling.

Many women told us stories about having to quit an aerobics class because of bladder leaks, of feeling embarrassed because they have to cross their legs hastily every time they cough, or of being afraid to leave a meeting with a full bladder in case they don't make it to the washroom in time. One woman who had returned to studies at a local university said, "I love being back with all the young people at the university, but my bladder keeps reminding me that I am not twenty-one any more."

INCONTINENCE: TYPES AND SYMPTOMS[12]

Types of Incontinence	Symptoms and Causes
Stress incontinence	Caused by sudden, increased pressure in the abdomen when you sneeze, cough, laugh, lift, or jump. A few drops to one tablespoon of urine are lost.

Unstable bladder	Urge incontinence is caused by an uncontrollable spasm of the bladder that triggers an urgent and sudden need to urinate. Needing to go often (frequency) is another symptom of this type, often provoked by stimuli such as running water or cold temperatures. Urine loss can range between a tablespoon and one cup.
Irritative abnormality in urethra or bladder	With this type of incontinence, frequent urination is induced by discomfort or pain caused by the inability to empty a full bladder completely. Night urination and burning during urination are also symptoms.
Mixed	Some women experience a combination of the above symptoms.

The early stage of incontinence can be prevented and controlled by maintaining a healthy weight and practising Kegel exercises. These exercises strengthen the pelvic-floor muscles that have weakened with age, because we so rarely use them. Once you have incontinence, there are some common-sense things you can try, based on the kind of incontinence you have.

- For urinary frequency and urgency: Reduce your twenty-four-hour fluid intake to five to six cups, avoid or reduce caffeine and alcohol, void at least every two hours (whether or not you feel as if you have to go).
- For night urination: Reduce your twenty-four-hour fluid intake to five to six cups, do not drink after dinner, avoid or reduce caffeine and alcohol, and try to eliminate other unnecessary sleep disruptions.
- For stress incontinence: Void every two hours to keep your bladder volume low; void before any vigorous activity.

If these strategies don't work, see your physician. There are effective treatments for incontinence, including:

- bladder drill – a process of training your bladder to gradually prolong the times between visits to the toilet (for example, start by voiding every two hours, then work toward four-hour intervals, and eventually to sleeping through the night without getting up to go to the toilet);
- medication to increase the tone of the urethral muscles or to relax the bladder;
- biofeedback – the use of a vaginal probe to monitor and teach a woman how to effectively do Kegel exercises (see below);
- functional electrical stimulation, used to strengthen bladder muscle functioning in cases of stress incontinence;
- temporary mechanical devices for supporting or obstructing the urethra, such as plugs or pessaries;
- surgical treatment.

When it comes to incontinence, remember FRED – Fluid Restriction, Exercise, and bladder Drill.

HOW TO DO KEGEL EXERCISES

Kegel exercises, which were named after the physician who invented them, involve repeatedly tightening and relaxing a certain group of muscles around your urethra. To locate these muscles, try stopping your flow of urine midstream until you know which muscles make this happen. Then tighten them (three seconds) and relax them (three seconds). To be effective, you need to make Kegeling a daily habit. Work up to doing 100 Kegels twice a day during routine activities such as lying in bed, doing dishes, driving to work, or standing at the bus stop.

Weight Gain and Waistline Thickening

This is one of the most common and frustrating complaints women talk about in the menopausal period. As we grow older, our metabolism slows down. Unless we eat less and exercise more, we inevitably gain weight and body fat. Hormonal fluctuations may also increase feelings of bloating (caused by retained fluids). One woman remarked, "The weight gain has been really hard on my self-esteem. It was a difficult time in my career and my marriage. I needed to feel good about myself and I didn't."

Many of the women we talked with spoke about how they seemed to gain weight "overnight" after age forty-four or forty-five. Flat tummies become rounded and clothes with tailored waistlines are suddenly uncomfortably snug and unflattering. While the effect of hormonal changes on weight gain is still controversial, there does appear to be some connection. Historically, women gain weight in the three periods of their lives when their hormones are most active: puberty, pregnancy, and menopause.

Recent studies suggest why women may be more susceptible to weight gain during and after menopause. First, the slowdown in metabolism that accompanies aging often leads to increases in body fat. These increases raise estrogen levels, which in turn increase one's tendency to accumulate fat. Second, there is some evidence that the release of progesterone during the menstrual cycle increases calorie burning. When women stop ovulating, they lose this production of progesterone and, therefore, may gain weight. While this requires much more study, adding progesterone to your hormone regimen may be shown in the future to help decrease your risk for weight gain and diabetes.[13]

Losing weight in menopause requires the same behaviours that other periods of your life do – exercising more and eating less. However, menopausal women repeatedly report that it is harder to lose weight than it was when they were younger. Chapters 7 and 8 provide some specific advice on how to maintain a healthy weight and lose excess body fat.

While weight management is important for health in midlife, an obsession with youthful slimness may be equally hard on your well-being and the quality of your life. Many midlife women learn to accept a ten-pound weight gain with grace, realizing that there are more important things to think about. In fact, a slight weight gain in menopause may be a good thing. Since estrogen is stored in body fat, women with a little extra weight have fewer hot flashes and are somewhat protected from osteoporosis.

Hot Flashes and Night Sweats

"Is it hot in here, or is it me?" Women who suffer hot flashes and night sweats frequently ask this question. These vasomotor symptoms are two of the most common signs of menopause. The blood vessels dilate, which leads to a rise in body temperature, sweating, and an increase in heart rate. Most hot flashes last from three to five minutes; the flashes can also come in sequence, giving you the feeling of an extended hot flash that can last as long as one hour. Flashes may be followed by shivering and chills, as the blood vessels constrict and the body cools itself down.

Approximately three-quarters of North American women experience hot flashes at menopause.[14] There is no way to predict who will get hot flashes, although we know that women who undergo a surgical menopause are particularly prone to severe flashing. Most often, hot flashes begin in the early stages of menopause, peak at the time your period ends, and then gradually taper off. Hot flashes come and go in no apparent pattern. The flash does not raise blood pressure or act as a response to stress, although stress may exacerbate flashing.

What causes hot flashes? Although there are a number of theories, we still do not know the exact biochemical cause of hot flashes. We do know that the hypothalamus, our temperature regulator, goes awry. While many people assume that a decline in estrogen is solely responsible for hot flashes, women born with no ovaries (and hence no estrogen production) do not get flashes until after they have taken estrogen therapy that is later stopped.[15] Hot flashes are more likely a result of a number of things, including a drop in estrogen levels (not continuously low levels) and unexplained surges of adrenalin.

Interestingly, women outside North America are much less likely to report hot flashes. In one study, only 20 per cent of Japanese women compared to 60 per cent of Canadian women reported hot flashes.[16] It is not clear why such a variation was reported. Diet is likely an important factor – the Japanese eat many foods that contain natural estrogens, such as tofu, tempeh, soy milk, miso soup. Cultural traditions and positive attitudes toward aging in Japan may also help to explain the differences.

Fortunately, women today feel much more comfortable discussing hot flashes than they did in our mothers' time. We are no longer embarrassed to ask our partners and children to put on a sweater so we can turn down the heat. One women joked, "You are looking at the only woman in the world who has jumped into the frozen-peas section at the grocery store." Others try to find some benefits in hot flashes. One woman said, "When I get a hot flash, I pretend I am being kissed by an angel. This inevitably makes me smile and I forget about the flash. Sometimes I even think about how valuable a hot flash can be in the middle of our Canadian winter!"

How can you manage your hot flashes?

- Keep a record of your flashes. Try to identify triggers such as stress, alcohol, hot drinks, spicy foods, or caffeine. Then make an effort to avoid these triggers.
- Determine how severe your hot flashes are. Are they an annoyance you can live with or are they compromising your sleep and quality of life? If the latter is the case, see your physician. Hormone replacement therapy can reduce the frequency of hot flashes by more than 90 per cent.[17] Many women find that alternative therapies help.
- Wear soft materials that absorb moisture. Dress in layers, so that you can take off some clothes when a hot flash strikes.
- Exercise regularly. Physically active women report fewer and less-severe hot flashes than women who are inactive.
- Sip cool water when a hot flash starts. If you have night sweats, keep a jug of cool water by your bed.
- Eat soy products that are rich in dietary phytoestrogens (such as miso soup, tofu, and soy milk).
- Try nonprescription remedies, such as evening primrose oil and vitamin E (discussed later in this chapter).
- Use an elegant hand-held fan.
- Share your concerns with your partner and friends. They can help you keep your home and work environments cool.

DID YOU KNOW?

Some men get hot flashes when they experience a sudden withdrawal of the male sex hormone testosterone, usually as a result of testicular insufficiency or removal of the testicles to treat prostate cancer.

Changing Sexual Desire

From the time **Rena** decided to go ahead with the hysterectomy, she felt sure it was the right thing to do. She and Ben had two healthy children, and she would consider it a relief to be rid of the pain and heavy bleeding that was the outcome of a serious case of endometriosis. But three months later, she felt a terrible loss. Her interest in sex had deteriorated to the point that she never initiated lovemaking. And when Ben did, she felt a much-diminished sensation in her breasts and during intercourse. Rena missed the anticipation, excitement, and satisfaction of the sex life she used to share with Ben. She knew that Ben was upset about it, too.

When Rena had a hysterectomy and her ovaries removed at age forty, menopause had been dramatically thrust upon her. Estrogen replacement therapy had helped her deal with severe hot flashes after the surgery and she had recovered well. So she was totally unprepared for this other common complaint in menopause – a reduction in sexual desire.

Menopause does not mean the end of an active sex life. Indeed, once free from birth control, PMS, and periods, many women report enhanced sexuality in their postmenopausal years.[18, 19] Nonetheless, some women experience a noticeable decrease in sexual desire during this period.[20] Changes in sexuality can likely be explained by a number of causes, including how you see yourself as a woman, your lifestyle, your health, and your partner's health and attitude, as well as the hormonal changes of menopause.[21] Other reasons include depression, embarrassment about urinary incontinence, and the effect of certain medications.

Women like Rena who have a surgical menopause may have additional concerns. For some women, the removal of the cervix and the uterus may change their sexual response. The loss of pressure on the cervix and the rhythmic contractions of the uterus may reduce the quality of their orgasms.[22]

Chapter 11 provides more information on sexuality in the middle years. If waning sexual desire is part of your experience of menopause, reassure your partner that these changes are not because of a change in your interest in him. Talk with your physician about what you can do. Sometimes when troubling symptoms of menopause are treated with hormone replacement therapy, sexual satisfaction also returns.

What about Hormone Replacement Therapy (HRT)?

The most common question we receive in our clinics and seminars is whether or not to take hormone replacement therapy. Despite claims about the many advantages of HRT, many boomer women who have lived through thalidomide, high-dose oral contraceptives, and Dalkon Shields are afraid that HRT is just another part of medicine's grand experiment with their bodies. Others are afraid of the long-term consequences of taking hormones, or say they are unwilling to medicalize a natural process.

Hardly a week goes by that the media does not alert menopausal women to some new development or twist on the benefits or dangers of HRT. Some women in our seminars express confusion about this overload of conflicting information. Others tell us that they know more than their physicians and feel patronized when a physician writes a prescription without involving them in the decision.

The decision to use or not use HRT is a complex one. You need clear and reliable information to make a rational, healthy decision. Chapter 21 reviews the pros and cons of HRT and provides clear guidelines for making your own decision about its use. Essentially, there are three main reasons to try HRT:

- The first is to **relieve menopausal complaints** – including hot flashes and night sweats, dry vagina, bladder problems, mood swings, and irregular bleeding. A decision to use HRT to alleviate these complaints is short term and safe. However, it should still be made carefully in consultation with your physician, because there are contra-indications for some women.

- The second reason to use HRT is to **prevent heart disease and osteoporosis**, if you are at risk for either of these problems. Using HRT to prevent these illnesses requires you to take hormones for a longer period of time (sometimes for ten to fifteen years), with regular re-evaluations of need and effects. Deciding to use HRT in the long term is more critical and requires even more careful consideration because of some studies linking long-term use to an increased risk for breast cancer.

- The third reason to use HRT is to **treat osteoporosis**. This may require a long-term commitment or one that is balanced with lifestyle modifications and the use of other drugs. Again, this is a decision that must be carefully thought out.

Please read Chapter 21 and share it with your physician if you are wondering whether to use HRT.

Managing Menopause without HRT

A recent survey of 750 randomly selected women aged forty-five to fifty-five, carried out by the North American Menopause Society (NAMS), showed that some 46 per cent of women have taken or are taking hormone replacement therapy (HRT) to ease the physical changes associated with menopause. Other strategies women use instead of – or in addition to – HRT to manage the short-term complaints and prevent the long-term consequences of menopause are shown in the chart below.[23] Another study of more than 14,000 midlife women conducted by *Prevention* magazine showed that 62 per cent were using some kind of alternative therapy, including 16 per cent who were using herbal preparations for menopausal complaints.[24]

STRATEGIES WOMEN USE TO MANAGE MENOPAUSAL COMPLAINTS

(instead of, or in addition to, HRT)

Healthy eating	85%
Maintaining a healthy weight	77%
Regular exercise	75%
Vitamins	70%
Calcium supplements	58%
Smoking cessation	28%
Relaxation techniques or yoga	25%
Vaginal lubricants	22%
Plant estrogens	10%

Source: The NAMS 1997 Menopause Survey

Here are some of the ways you can ease the menopausal transition without the use of HRT:

Exercise. Daily walking burns calories, promotes sleep, and helps you handle stress. Many women find that regular exercise reduces the number and severity of hot flashes. Physical activity also deals with the long-term concerns of menopause. Aerobic exercise that makes you puff a bit – brisk walking, jogging, swimming, cycling – protects your heart, and strength training – lifting weights and calisthenics – protects and strengthens your bones. See Chapters 7, 17, and 20 for more detailed information.

Enjoy soy foods and drinks, such as tofu, tempeh, miso soup, and soy milk or mix soy powders with other foods. Soy contains phytoestrogens, which mimic the effects of estrogen and can help balance declines in estrogen levels. Other food sources that contain phytoestrogens include licorice root, papaya, corn, and almonds. Foods such as flaxseed, seaweed, lentils, asparagus, wheat, squash, and garlic contain natural estrogens called lignans. See Chapter 8 for more detailed information.

Limit your intake of caffeine and alcohol. Caffeine may interfere with sleep and increase breast tenderness, and alcohol may cause more headaches. Restricting your intake of caffeine and alcohol, and **not smoking** will also protect your bones.

Boost your vitamin and mineral intake with a healthy, well-chosen diet rich in calcium and vitamin D, iron (only if you are bleeding heavily), vitamin E (an antioxidant that protects against heart disease and can help reduce hot flashes and breast tenderness), vitamin C (helps the body absorb iron), and carotenoids (antioxidants that may protect against cancer).

Manage stress by improving your skills in time management and active relaxation. Activities such as meditation, yoga, and tai chi may be especially helpful.

Consider the use of alternative and complementary therapies, such as naturopathy, homeopathy, and chiropractic or therapeutic massage to deal with aching joints and muscles, and other complaints.

Consider the use of herbal remedies, described below.

Herbs and Menopause[25]
Many women find that a variety of herbal remedies ease their menopausal

symptoms. Remember that herbs are potent medicines that must be treated with respect. If you use herbal remedies, follow these guidelines:

- Always tell your family physician which herbal remedies you are using. Similarly, if you are seeing an alternative practitioner, let him or her know about all of the drugs you are using (prescription, over-the-counter, and herbal). The interaction between herbal remedies and other medications can be dangerous.
- Buy herbal remedies from a reputable source and make sure that the ingredients, instructions for use, contra-indications, and side-effects are described.
- Discontinue use of the remedy if you experience troublesome side-effects or you see no improvements in six months.
- Avoid self-medicating with herbs and plant foods that are natural sources of estrogen if you have a history of breast cancer or heavy bleeding.

There is much anecdotal evidence about the usefulness of various herbal remedies. This is shared among women and attested to by million-dollar sales. Many of these have long traditions of medicinal value in indigenous and Eastern cultures; yet only recently are these herbs being studied in Western double-blind, controlled tests. More research is needed to clarify the uses and dosages of various remedies as well as the usefulness or lack thereof of different herbs.

Here are some of the most popular herbs used in menopause:

Black Cohosh 250–500 mg/day	First used by Native American women. Studies in Germany have demonstrated effectiveness in dealing with PMS, nervousness, and hot flashes. May cause dizziness, headaches, and visual disturbances if used in high doses. The German product Remifemin appears to be superior to a placebo in relieving hot flashes and improving mood.[26] *Women who have a history of breast cancer or heavy bleeding should not use it without consulting a physician.*[27]

Chaste Tree Berry 30–40 mg/day	Used in the Middle Ages by monks to suppress the libido. Believed to raise estrogen and progesterone levels. Slow-acting: needs to be used daily for two months to see effect. May cause an itchy rash in some people. May be useful in managing breast pain.
Don Quai 10–20 drops/day 1–2 capsules, 2 to 3 times/day	Used in traditional Chinese medicine to balance high and low estrogen levels and to deal with hot flashes, cramps, and other menstrual symptoms. May worsen PMS in some women and cause a rash if taken in large doses. A 1997 study showed no difference in menopausal symptoms after six months among women taking don quai and women taking a placebo. Since many women use don quai in combination with other Chinese herbs, studies looking at combinations are needed.[28]
Wild Yam Root ½ tsp/day	Traditionally used to ease menstrual cramps and bloating because of its diuretic effect. Wild yam contains diosgenin, but there is no evidence that the body can convert it to progesterone. Thus, most progesterone creams made from wild yam and sold in Canada and the United States have progesterone added to them in various strengths. They are therefore sold only by prescription.
Motherworth 15–25 drops, 1–3 times/day	Used to deal with hot flashes, insomnia, and nervousness in menopause. Has estrogenic effect and *should not be used by women who have a history of breast cancer or heavy bleeding.*
Ginseng (dosages vary)	Siberian ginseng may alleviate depressed mood and improve your general sense of well-being, but

there is no evidence that it provides relief for hot flashes.[29]

Evening Primrose Oil 1.5–2 g/day	This oil is successfully used by many women during the menopausal period for relief of hot flashes, insomnia, mood swings, and painful breasts; however, a 1994 study showed no improvement in hot flashes over women taking a placebo.[30] It contains gamma-linoleic acid (GLA), which may block prostaglandins responsible for menstrual cramps and fluid retention. It is sometimes taken in combination with vitamin E.

Historical and Cultural Perspectives on Menopause

It is only in the last ten years or so that menopause has been talked about openly and knowledgeably. Our grandmothers and most of our mothers suffered in silence or spoke only in hushed tones about "the change." Despite the fact that menopausal women run major corporations and live complex and capable lives, society's view of the aging woman is still deeply affected by old negative myths and stereotypes – the image of the menopausal woman as hysterical, unstable, dried up, and over the hill.

If you had been a wealthy woman living in London in the 1850s, you would have been treated for menopause by having your arm bled. This was a widely recommended procedure in the nineteenth century, and one seen to be an "imitation of nature."[31] You might well have been described, as Sigmund Freud put it, as "quarrelsome and obstinate, petty and stingy."[32] Even today, some of these antiquated attitudes persist, negatively affecting how we see ourselves.

As recently as 1966, Robert Wilson wrote in his popular book, *Feminine Forever,* "The sensitive doctor must help to keep his female patient glowing through the dismal years of her middle age."[33] In 1971, physician-writer Dr. Gifford-Jones praised the estrogen pill as "one of the early steps in medicine's attempt to produce a wife who doesn't wear out." He went on to say that "it will give women a tremendous psychological boost knowing they finally have something other than the artificial support of make-up to help them keep up with their husbands."[34]

Rather than viewing menopause as a natural event, these writers perpetuate the belief that menopause signifies something wrong that must be righted, a deficit that must be filled.

Many women oppose the medicalization of menopause and insist that it is a natural process that should be dealt with in a natural way. Certainly some women have a difficult time in the menopausal period. Yet some assert that the mood swings and fatigue associated with menopause are related more to cultural attitudes and social expectations than they are to shifts in hormones. Like men, the women we talked with said that concerns about job security and future finances were at the top of their minds. Those caught in the sandwich generation, with aging, sick parents and teens still at home, spoke of the enormous fatigue brought on by these dual responsibilities.

A small number of fascinating cross-cultural studies show that, when women are valued for the wisdom they have accumulated as they age, they seem to show much less menopausal distress.[35] For example, postmenopausal women from certain indigenous cultures, such as women in the Tongan and Papuan traditions, discover increased freedom and power after menopause and seem less bothered by physical symptoms than Western women are.[36]

Jungian analyst and physician Jean Shinoda Bolen tells a story of the ancient blood mysteries. According to these, menstruating women were understood to mysteriously retain their blood for nine months to make a baby. At the end of her child-bearing years, a woman was seen to retain her blood again – this time not to make a baby but to make wisdom. Our culture, Bolen says, does not honour this time.[37]

As we reflect on our own experiences of menopause, it is important to remember that we are influenced by the cultural context in which we live. We are bombarded by Western medicine's focus on treating symptoms and by society's negative messages: getting old is so undesirable and so meaningless that it must be stalled at all costs. We can hardly imagine living in a society where we would look forward in the postmenopausal years to honour, dignity, and an esteemed place in our families, communities, workplaces, and governing councils. Too often in North American culture, aging is not accepted as a natural phenomenon that results in an accumulation of wisdom and power; it is seen as a failure to remain young.

From PMS to PMZ

The emotional and psychological experience of the menopausal period is just as powerful as the physical changes that accompany this transition. As described in Chapter 1, the midlife journey begins with a loss, which is for women both dramatic and undeniable. We stop having our periods and we can no longer bear children. Whether or not this "pause" is a welcome relief or leaves us feeling sad and wistful, the realization that we are aging, and that there is no turning back, plunges many women into a time of great uncertainty and self-doubt.

Who am I now? What does it mean to be an "older woman" in this youth-obsessed society? Am I still a sexual being? Am I still attractive? These are some of the questions that commonly accompany the hormonal storms of the menopausal period. Long-buried dreams and previously unmourned losses tend to resurface and demand our attention with nagging persistence. We sometimes feel uncontrollably sad or angry. We may wonder if we are going crazy. If we are to successfully move out of this tumultuous phase and into the uncharted waters of the next phase of life, as mentioned earlier, we need to take time for ourselves and seek out the support of family members and friends.

An increasing number of women are writing about and describing the renewed sense of vitality, freedom, and well-being they are experiencing in the postmenopausal years. Their accomplishments fly in the face of negative stereotypes. Writer and poet Maya Angelou was asked to create a poem for the inauguration of President Bill Clinton when she was sixty-five years old. Marian Anderson was the first African American to sing at the Metropolitan Opera Company in 1955 – when she was fifty-three years old. Golda Meir served as the prime minister of Israel from the age of seventy-one to seventy-six. Kim Campbell became Canada's first woman prime minister at age forty-six. Joni Mitchell still tours in her fifties. Hillary Clinton and Elizabeth Dole are emerging as strong political contenders in their own rights. At age fifty-two, Helen Thayer skied to the magnetic

North Pole (a distance of 555 km or 345 miles) with her dog, pulling a 73-kg or 160-pound sled for twenty-seven days.

Then there are the (not-so) ordinary older heroines in our lives. Many of the women we interviewed identified an aunt, a grandmother, a teacher, or a neighbour who inspired them with her energy, wit, and wisdom. Anthropologist Margaret Mead expressed this best when she said that the most creative force in the world is the woman who possesses "post-menopausal zest (PMZ)."

One of the goals of this book is to help you move along the road toward PMZ. Here are a few ideas to assist you along the way:

- Make time for yourself. Whether you choose a walk in the woods, a bubble bath, or a weekend retreat, quiet and solitude are essential for reflection. Nurture all aspects of your well-being. Remember that you exist and function in a subtle interplay of psychological, physical, social, and spiritual dimensions.
- Take charge of your health and health care now – whether you are just beginning to experience menopausal complaints or you have stopped menstruating. This means becoming well informed about midlife health issues and health-care options so you can make the best decisions about your own health in the next few years. Become an astute consumer of medical care and alternative therapies. Find a physician who takes the time to listen and learn to communicate well with her or him. Keep a menopause diary.
- As the old adage says, "This above all: to thine own self be true." Trust yourself to decide which approach is right for you. At the same time, stay flexible and ready to change directions when you need to.
- Allow your creativity to move in new directions. Many midlife women find pleasure in new leisure-time endeavours, such as studying a new language, taking up painting or pottery, or reviving an old love for the piano or guitar.
- Think positively. Troublesome aspects of menopause always get better with time. Indeed, in the 1997 Menopause Survey by the North American Menopause Society 52 per cent of American women aged forty-five to sixty-five said that they view menopause as the beginning of a new and fulfilling stage of life. Almost 80 per cent said that

they would advise other women to approach menopause with a positive attitude.[38]

- Enjoy a healthy lifestyle. Part II of this book provides information and practical tips on healthy eating, active living, managing stress, and building healthy relationships. Invest in prevention. Many of the serious health problems that are common in older age can be prevented or delayed through healthful living.

- Use the first three chapters of this book to start discussions with your partner. Share what is going on with you and find out what he is experiencing. Read the chapters on men's health and encourage him to talk about midlife issues that are bothering him. Take time to share your reflections together.

- Make time for your women friends. Cherish and enjoy them. Consider joining a self-help or support group. As women, we have helped each other get through many challenging life experiences. We survived PMS – we can reach PMZ!

- Create your own ritual or have a women's celebration to mark this time. Go on a kayak trip or a spa weekend. Betty Friedan marked her sixtieth birthday by going on a trip with Outward Bound. Each spring, Jean Shinoda Bolen takes a group of postmenopausal women on a trek to an underground cave where each speaks in turn of what she has learned in reaching this stage of life.

- Get serious about laughter. Humour and laughter create PMA (positive mental attitude) by teaching us not to "sweat the small stuff." Many women spoke of the de-stressing value of humour at home, in the workplace, and with female friends. As Ann Shakeshaft says in the hilarious book *The Noisy Passage: Baby Boomers Do Menopause*, "as estro-boomers glide toward 50, we need to look for creative ways to make 'pausin' more glamorous and humorous."[39]

- Compile your own list of women who inspire you.

Feminist author Carolyn Heilbrun, who describes herself as "an older women with pizzazz," speaks of the delicious freedom gained from successfully navigating the midlife rite of passage. She writes: "I have passed through the magic circle of invisibility into the land of new accomplishment and new passion. . . . And I am still trying to discover how I got here. What I want to say to you is . . . come on in. The water's fine."[40]

THE BOTTOM LINE

Menopause is an important life transition. Make sure you understand the physical and psychological changes you are going through. Pay attention to what keeps you well and happy. Take your health seriously and yourself lightly. Our interviewees told us that, after menopause, they felt greater wisdom, freedom, and independence. As one woman said, "I now have a solid sense of who I am. I know what I want and I can go after it."

Contacts and Further Information

Organizations

- American Menopause Foundation Inc., 350 Fifth Ave., Suite 2822, New York, NY 10118. Tel.: (212) 714–2398.
- The Canadian Continence Foundation, P.O Box 66524, Cavendish Mall, Côté St. Luc, QC H4W 3J6. Tel.: (514) 932–3535; (800) 265–9575 (Canada); Fax: (514) 932–3533.
- National Action Forum for Midlife and Older Women (NAFOW), P.O. Box 816, Stony Brook, NY 11790. A clearinghouse of information for women at midlife and beyond; newsletter called *Hot Flash*.
- North American Menopause Society (NAMS), c/o Department of OB/GYN, University Hospitals of Cleveland, 11100 Euclid Ave., Cleveland, OH 44106. Tel.: (216) 844–8748; Fax: (216) 844–8708; E-mail: nams@atk.et.

Websites

- A Friend Indeed Website (sponsored by Manitoba Women's Health Centre): http://www.afriendindeed.ca
- *Menopause: The Journal of the North American Menopause Society*: http://www.menopause.org/journal.htm
- Menopause and aging through an artist's eyes (Helen Redman, artist): http://www.birthingthecrone.com/
- National Kidney and Urologic Diseases Information Clearinghouse (information on urinary incontinence):

http://www.niddk.nih.gov/health/kidney/nkudic.htm
- North American Menopause Society: http://www.menopause.org
- OBGYN.net: The Universe of Women's Health by David Ashley Hill, M.D. (various sponsors):
http://www.obgyn.net.woman.woman.htm

Newsletters

- *A Friend Indeed*, 419 Graham Ave., Suite 203, Winnipeg, MB R3C 0M3 or, in the U.S., P.O. Box 260, Pembina, ND 58271. U.S. Tel.: (204) 989-8028; E-mail: afi@panagea.ca; U.S. Fax: (204) 989-8029. Website listed above.
- *Hotflash: Newsletter for Midlife and Older Women*, Box 816, Stony Brook, NY 11790.
- *MenoTimes: Alternative Choices to Menopause and Osteoporosis*, c/o The Menopause Center, 118 Irwin St., San Rafael, CA 94901. Tel.: (415) 459–5430; E-mail: mtimes@nbn.com (newsletter on complementary approaches)
- *Midlife Woman*, published by the Midlife Women's Network, 5129 Logan Ave., Minneapolis, MN 55419–1019.

Books and Booklets

- *The Change: Women, Aging, and the Menopause* by Germaine Greer. London, England: Hamish Hamilton Ltd., 1991.
- *The Complete Book of Menopause: Every Woman's Guide to Good Health* by Carol Landau, Michelle G. Cyr, and Anne Moulton. New York: Grosset/Putnam, 1994.
- *Getting Over Getting Older* by Letty Cottin Pogrebin. New York: Berkeley Books, 1997.
- *Holistic Menopause: A New Approach to Midlife Change* by Judy Hall and Robert Jacobs. Edinburgh, Scotland: Findhorn Press, 1998.
- *The Menopause Guidebook* from The North American Menopause Society (NAMS), P.O. Box 94527, Cleveland, OH 44101 or go to their website, above.
- *Menopause Handbook* by the Montreal Health Press Collective. Montreal Health Press (P.O. Box 1000, Stn. Place du Parc, Montréal QC H2W 2N1), 1997.

- *The Noisy Passage: Baby Boomers Do Menopause* by Marie Evans and Ann Shakeshaft. Bridgeport, CT: Hysteria Publications, 1996.
- *the pause: Positive Approaches to Menopause* by Lonnie Barbach. New York: Dutton/Penguin Books, 1995.
- *The Silent Passage: Menopause* by Gail Sheehy. New York: Random House, 1992.
- *So Many Changes: Women, Health, and Midlife* by Mary J. Breen and Lindsay Hall. Toronto: Lawrence Heights Community Health Centre Press, 1999.
- *Understanding Menopause* by Janine O'Leary Cobb. Revised ed. Toronto: Key Porter, 1993.
- *A Woman's Book of Life* by Joan Borysenko. New York: Riverhead Books, 1996.
- *A Woman's Midlife Companion* by Naomi Lucks and Hélène Smith. Rocklin, CA: Prima Publishing, 1997.
- *Women of the 14th Moon: Writings on Menopause* by Dena Taylor and A. C. Sumrall, eds. Freedom, CA: Crossing Press, 1991.

Related Chapters in This Book

- *Chapter 1: The Midlife Journey* talks about the various stages of the midlife journey that both women and men go through.
- *Chapter 3: Is There a Male Menopause?* discusses the many parallel changes that men go through in midlife. Must reading for all women and men.
- *Chapter 6: Wrinkles, Chin Hairs, and Baldness* gives you more information about the changes in physical appearance that accompany midlife and what you need to do to maintain a positive body image during this time.
- *Chapter 7: The Active Living Solution* explains how physical activity can help in menopause, and provides practical advice on the kinds of exercise you need.
- *Chapter 8: Food for Thought: Healthy Eating in Midlife* provides more information on healthy eating in the menopausal years as well as advice on weight management.
- *Chapter 11: Enjoying Sex in Midlife* gives you more information on

how age affects sexuality as well as some common-sense advice on keeping the spark alive.

- *Chapter 13: Stress-Proofing in Midlife* and *Chapter 15: When Times Are Tough: Depression, Anxiety, and Insomnia* provide guidance on handling stress, and recognizing depression and other serious problems that may occur during the menopausal period.
- *Chapter 16: Partners in Health Care* suggests ways to prepare for visits to your health care providers and what to ask for when you are experiencing menopausal changes.
- *Chapter 17: Keep Your Bones Strong* will help you assess your risk for osteoporosis and how you can prevent it.
- *Chapter 19: Breast Health* will help you determine your risk for breast cancer and tell you how to monitor your breast health in midlife.
- *Chapter 21: Hormone Replacement Therapy (HRT): The Big Decision* presents the advantages and disadvantages of HRT and provides you with a helpful decision-making chart.
- *Chapter 22: Complementary and Alternative Medicine Is Coming on Strong* provides additional information on the use of complementary therapies in midlife.
- *Chapter 23: Body, Mind, and Soul* discusses the spiritual part of the midlife journey.

CHAPTER THREE

Is There a Male Menopause?

Whoever in middle age attempts to realize the wishes and hopes of his early youth, invariably deceives himself. Each ten years of a man's life has its own fortunes, its own hopes, its own desires.

— Goethe[1]

Ivan was under enormous stress. He was anxious about his company being downsized and he felt very distant from his wife of fifteen years. They hadn't made love in a long time. Ivan was not sure which bothered him more: the lack of lovemaking or the fact that he hardly missed it. He was having trouble sleeping and was feeling tired and irritable at home and work. He hated the weight gain and recurring backache that bothered him every time he played squash or took a long business flight. Ivan wondered if he was suffering the so-called male menopause. But he felt too embarrassed to talk with his wife or with his doctor about these annoying concerns. "Better to tough it out; put it aside," he thought to himself. "This stuff is no big deal. Besides, there's no such thing as male menopause, is there?"

Ivan's experience is fairly typical. While most men sense something is happening to their well-being in midlife, it seems easier to deny or downplay a variety of vague problems than to confront the fact that these problems may be symptoms of serious distress.

Until very recently the lack of discussion about male menopause has supported this general denial. When we first began researching this book, there were only a handful of articles on male menopause, and most of these dismissed the idea that such a thing existed. Indeed, one article published in 1992 in the *Journal of the American Medical Association* was titled "Is Male Menopause Real or Is It Just an Excuse?"[2] By the end of 1998, however, the North American Menopause Society had expanded its focus to include men. The American Academy of Anti-Aging Medicine (with more than 4,000 physician members) had made male menopause a priority issue. Book titles such as *Maximizing Manhood: Beating the Male Menopause* were crowding the best-seller list.

From the beginning, most of the men we interviewed told us that they believed the male menopause existed, even if the term itself did not make sense. By 1998, the medical community was beginning to listen to colleagues who specialized in male aging and male menopause. However, as Michael Valpy pointed out in a feature story in Canada's *Globe and Mail*, "there is considerable debate over whether [male menopause] is – or should be – a treatable condition, comparable to the female menopause."[3]

In this chapter, we explore the core of the male menopause debate – the hormonal changes that men undergo in mid- and later life, coupled with the emotional upheavals that seem to often accompany these changes. There are many unanswered questions. One thing *is* clear. It is high time that we talked about the male midlife experience. Finally, what Gail Sheehy calls "the unspeakable passage" is in the open.

Clarifying the Terms

Before we try to answer the question posed in the title of this chapter, some clarification of terms is in order. Since menopause means the end of menstruation, technically, the word cannot be used with men. The term male menopause can also be confused with a number of other expressions. Some medical textbooks use the term "male climacteric," which is generally considered to cover the years between thirty-five and sixty-five. Increasingly, physicians in North America use the term PADAM, which stands for "partial androgen deficiency (in the) aging male." The term "andropause" is also used, especially in Europe.

Dr. Malcolm Carruthers, a British specialist in male menopause, presented evidence that the male menopause is also related to a "sense of hopelessness and helplessness" at an international scientific gathering in Australia in December 1996. He described it as a "crisis of vitality just as much as virility." "All too often," said Carruthers, "men change their jobs or their women – anything to ease the malaise they feel – usually with little relief."[4]

The phrase "male menopause" has found its way into popular language in North America. Gail Sheehy, in her new book *Understanding Men's*

Passages, has even coined a new phrase: manopause. "Call it viropause, andropause, or manopause," says Sheehy. "Men don't stop being fertile, but there is a pause in their vitality and virility."[5]

In this chapter we use "male menopause" to describe the gradual hormonal shifts that men experience in midlife and later, and the way these shifts may affect their well-being. The word "gradual" is what makes men's experience different from that of women, in which estrogen levels plunge sharply in menopause to pre-puberty levels. It is the gradual nature of the male experience that may explain why men like Ivan find it easier to deny their real pain and put off seeking help.

What Is the Male Menopause Like?

In our interviews and surveys with men, most associated male menopause with physical and emotional changes, such as disrupted sleep, feeling moody, irritable, anxious, lonely, and less tolerant, having a lowered sex drive, and experiencing a loss of physical energy, memory, and mental sharpness. One man said, "Male menopause is about the loss of youth and potency, a slower sex drive, and concerns about your hearing, sexual ability, and physical shape."

It is interesting to note the parallels of these complaints to how women experience menopause, and thus to theorize that men go through a similar (if less dramatic) process that is also affected by drops in hormone levels. Indeed, in recent studies, large numbers of midlife men reported irritability, fatigue, headaches, insomnia, dry skin, thinning hair, and weight gain – complaints that are identical to those of women during the menopause period.[6] One of the men we interviewed concurred with these studies when he said, "Beyond plumbing differences, men and women have much in common."

In a 1999 interview with *Maclean's* magazine, Dr. Norman Barwin, director of a male midlife clinic in Ottawa, said, "Much of the time, men don't realize there is such a thing as andropause." Dr. Barwin founded his clinic some ten years ago after hearing menopausal women talk about how their husbands had similar symptoms, including fatigue, moodiness, and hot flashes.[7]

Although many physicians believe that the advent of Viagra – an unobtrusive new oral treatment for impotence – will bring more middle-aged men into their offices, most men are unlikely to appear at their doctors' offices with the vague kind of complaints associated with male menopause. Nor are they likely to talk openly to their friends or partners about what they are feeling. This silence can be a problem for men and their families. When job and family stresses or the problems of a partner's menopause are added to silent misery, there is a danger that aching joints may turn into a full-blown back problem or that feeling low may turn into the more serious problem of clinical depression.

We believe that men, when asked in confidence, are just as eager as women to discuss and deal with these changes. Indeed, in our interviews, men were relieved to talk about what many of them called body-chemistry changes and to learn that other men had similar experiences. They expressed great concerns about sexual libido, noting that they had a lower and slower sex drive than when they were younger.

The Male Menopause and Sexuality

Testosterone levels decline slowly with age. This gradual drop, which all men experience, parallels the changes associated with aging for both men and women: muscle size and strength decline, body fat increases, bones slowly lose density, and sexual performance wanes. Gradual declines in testosterone do not usually cause erectile dysfunction. In fact, testosterone has a minor role in age-related erection problems. The increased incidence of erection difficulties with aging is due to many causes, including decreases in penis sensitivity and erectional response.[8] However, if testosterone levels fall below normal, there may not be enough in circulation to get and maintain an erection. This crisis in male potency is what most midlife men relate to and fear the most. Approximately 20 per cent of men between age sixty and eighty are estimated to have levels below the normal range.[9] See Chapter 12 for more information on erectile function.

When a man is aroused, he pumps twenty times more blood than normal through his penis. One of the consequences of aging may be a less efficient circulatory system, less blood to the penis, and thus more trouble getting and maintaining an erection. Hence, the joke "You know you're middle-aged when a quickie takes forty minutes."

The gradual decline in testosterone levels also leads to a gentle tapering off of sexual desire. In talking about the role of sex and love in midlife, one man said, "Sex was important at age thirty. It was important at age forty. At fifty, it was somewhat important; now, at fifty-eight, love is more important."

Some of these changes can work to both partners' advantage. When an erection takes longer to achieve, a couple can prolong foreplay. Since middle-aged women respond better to prolonged sexual activity, this extra time, combined with a mature man's improved control of ejaculation, can provide both partners with a more satisfying sexual experience.

Interestingly, the Massachusetts Male Aging Study (1986 to 1989) showed a consistent decline with age in sexual desires, thoughts, and dreams, while the desired levels of sexual activity, frequency of intercourse, and levels of satisfaction did not show the same age-related changes. Men in their sixties reported the same level of sexual satisfaction as men in their forties.[10]

The knowledge that sex remains satisfying, and that aging and the male menopause do not threaten sexual ability, is good news for men and women. This is not to say that most men will not experience the occasional difficulty getting or sustaining an erection. It is to say that men who make healthy lifestyle choices and a positive adjustment in the midlife transition can expect to have a satisfying sex life into very old age.

When asked "What do you fear most about getting older?" one of the men we interviewed was candid in his response. "I could give you the standard answer," he said, "about losing my fitness or my memory, but the real truth is this: most guys are terrified that they will lose the ability to get it up."

Men's fear that they may lose sexual functioning is both real and understandable. In a society that worships youth, the ability to get a rock-hard penis any time and any place has become the stereotypical standard of maleness. So when Viagra (an oral medication for impotence) hit the U.S. market, one million prescriptions were written in two months. Before Viagra was approved in Canada, Canadian men flocked to the United States to get the potency pill. One pundit even renamed Niagara Falls, New York, "Viagra Falls," claiming that "at least we can tell the difference now between that city and Niagara Falls, Ontario."

The advent of Viagra and other new impotence drugs is a major bonus for men who suffer from persistent erection problems (see Chapter 12 for more details). But for the majority of men whose experience of impotence is temporary, Viagra is not the answer. It will not increase your libido or give you intimacy in a relationship.

Do Men Need Hormone Replacement Therapy?

Although the effects of male hormone loss are not as dramatic as female menopause, some physicians and researchers now believe that certain men may benefit from hormone (testosterone) replacement therapy.[11, 12] Testosterone is important for the development and maintenance of bone density and muscle mass as well as sexual and prostate functioning. As with women, hormonal changes in men can lead to an increase in bone fractures, a loss of muscle tone, and a tendency to put on weight. It makes sense to conclude that restoring testosterone levels in men who significantly lack the hormone may help prevent osteoporosis, improve physical performance and overall well-being, and decrease body fat.

Recent Canadian recommendations suggest monitoring and treating men who exhibit a combination of several clinical symptoms associated with reduced testosterone availability.[13] Men with a combination of several of the symptoms described in the chart below should consult a physician. A simple blood test measuring bioavailable testosterone can determine if these symptoms are related to low levels of testosterone. Currently, this test is not covered by medical insurance in Canada and costs about $35.

CONCERNS ASSOCIATED WITH ANDROPAUSE

If you have several of these concerns, talk with your physician about andropause.

Vasomotor and nervous symptoms	• hot flashes similar to those of menopause • episodes of sweating • insomnia • nervousness
Mood disorders and cognitive functions	• irritability and lethargy • decreased sense of well-being • lack of motivation • low mental energy • difficulties with short-term memory • depressive symptoms

	• low self-esteem
	• unusual fright
Masculinity/virility	• decreased vigour and physical energy
	• diminished muscle mass and strength
	• loss of sexual body hair
	• abdominal obesity
Sexuality	• decreased interest in or desire for sex
	• reduction of sexual activity
	• poor erectile function
	• limited quality of orgasm
	• weakness of ejaculation
	• reduced volume of ejaculation

Source: R.R. Tremblay and A. Morales, "Canadian Practice Recommendations for Screening, Monitoring and Treating Men Affected by Andropause or Partial Andropause Deficiency," *The Aging Male*, vol. 1, no. 3 (July 1998): 213–18.

Testosterone replacement (like estrogen replacement) is not a panacea for addressing the natural changes men undergo as they get older. And middle-aged men with abnormally low testosterone levels make up only a small percentage of middle-aged men. Some physicians and researchers see testosterone replacement for healthy men with normal testosterone levels as an impractical and expensive attempt to recapture youth. They warn that prolonged testosterone therapy may mean an increased risk of prostate problems and heart disease. While current studies show that testosterone does not cause prostate cancer, it may induce an existing tumour to grow.[14]

In her newsletter *A Friend Indeed* for September 1994, Janine O'Leary Cobb suggests that men may be vulnerable targets for hormone-replacement hype (leading to lucrative sales for pharmaceutical companies) because they have a shorter life expectancy compared to women, they are expected to ignore complaints that might send a woman to the doctor, and they are more likely to suffer diminished self-esteem as a direct result of a reduced sex drive and impotence.[15] Certainly, demographics support the need for increased attention to male menopause. The baby-boom generation will reach age fifty in greater and greater numbers in the next few years. In the United States, the number of men between forty-five and sixty-five is expected to grow by almost 60 per cent during the next twenty years.[16]

Men can learn from women's experience with hormone replacement therapy. After estrogen was first used to deal with female menopause some twenty-five years ago, it was discovered that estrogen without progesterone caused a dramatic increase in endometrial cancer. One can question whether similar serious side-effects could occur if testosterone replacement is used with healthy men. This is why testosterone therapy should be used only after a thorough medical assessment establishes that testosterone deficiency is the cause of the symptoms.

Midlife: Crisis or Opportunity?

Men begin their midlife journey with a less dramatic experience of loss than women have, but one that still affects their lives powerfully. For them, the loss is one of a sense of eternal youth and infallibility. The undeniable evidence of their own aging and mortality through losses in business, play, and friendships tends to plunge them into a tumultuous time of fearful uncertainty and self-doubt. They are then vulnerable to depression and anxiety and to acting out, through the stereotypical midlife crisis, rather than experiencing their feelings. By facing these fears directly and seeking deeper inner meaning, a man can move on with a sense of renewal.

Some of the men in our study talked about their increased awareness of their mortality and their need to re-evaluate their beliefs, values, and loyalties. One said, "Men at this time can feel very threatened with a loss of power, drive, or control, and a change in body image can threaten your sense of worth." He added, "Attitude is key, to make sure that normal changes in physiology are not seen to be pathology."

Erik Erikson described the major challenge of midlife – for both men and women – in terms of finding ways to renew and regenerate oneself by drawing on your inner resources, instead of stagnating in old fixed patterns. This means coming to terms with both successes and disappointments. A fifty-one-year-old man said, "It can be an emotional time, when you realize that you might have to settle for something that is less than you always believed you would have."

The midlife crisis is thought to occur most often in the early part of midlife (early to mid forties) and is associated with men's fears of becoming old, obsolete, and unattractive. These feelings are manifested in a driving need to succeed in both their careers and their sexual performance. Most of us know someone around age forty who left his wife for a younger woman. Nonetheless, this stereotype of the male midlife experience is greatly exaggerated: the risk of divorce actually declines the longer people are married.

At the same time, many of the men we talked with voiced concerns about their sexuality and their careers well into their sixties. For some, expected promotions and power in the latter stages of their careers had failed to materialize in an era of cutbacks and early retirement packages. They talked of feeling disillusioned and anxious about the financial future for themselves and their families. On the other hand, some men welcomed the chance to slow down, take stock, and be less competitive. One man described his need to "learn to be a whole person, not just a slave-driver like my father, who couldn't boil water."

Poet Robert Bly talks about the two halves of a man's life: "A man usually spends the first half of his life triumphing over nature, competing with other men, dominating women, controlling life. Compassion and wonder are not in his field. But somewhere around age 50 the poles of the battery begin to switch. He begins to enter the second arc and feels sympathy with things instead of competition. He becomes open to the beauty of creatures, and to the beauty of art and grief."[17]

George Leonard, former senior editor of *Look* magazine, got hooked on aikido at age forty-seven and became a master sprinter at age fifty. At age seventy, he was still waiting for his midlife crisis. "I am not denying that people have midlife crises, but I think it tends to happen to people who struggle for that $100,000 salary, that corner office. When they get it, they find it's empty. Instead of a vision, they have a material goal. They want a quick fix. That is going to lead inevitably to disillusionment, depression, and crisis."[18]

In his book *Male Menopause*, therapist Jed Diamond suggests that the midlife crisis is a reaction to the perceived changes of male menopause. Says Diamond, "For those who feel that the changes occurring in the second half of life are to be feared and avoided, who try to cling to youthful ways, this period of life will be seen as a crisis. For those who understand that the physical, emotional, and spiritual changes are helpful in preparing us for the second half of life, this time will be seen as an adventure rather than a crisis."[19]

Perhaps the most difficult part of the male menopause question is society's traditional denial of the painful changes that men go through in midlife. Whether or not they are caused by hormone fluctuations, the losses and stresses of midlife can be hurtful and depressing. The partner of a midlife man needs to be sensitive to these experiences, just as men need to understand and be sensitive to what their female partners are experiencing (see previous chapter). Public acknowledgement is also important. As a society we need to become more comfortable discussing the stresses men undergo in middle age and allow men to express their vulnerability and uncertainty. Then, in turn, our male friends and mates may feel more comfortable about going to a physician or psychotherapist, talking with their partners and friends, or joining a male support group.

You Can Overcome the Problems of Male Menopause

If you are troubled by some of the concerns described in this chapter, it is important that you take charge of your health and well-being now. If you have several of the symptoms of andropause described in this chapter, see your family physician.

- *Don't give in to denial.* Most men experience fluctuations and changes in their sexuality during midlife. Denial, pulling away from intimacy and refusing to talk about these changes, will only make the problems worse. Look at this stage as a pause in virility, not a permanent change.
- *Take the pressure off lovemaking and enjoy it more.* In all likelihood your partner will appreciate your need for longer foreplay. Talk, experiment, and explore new options. Enjoy afterplay, that sweet time for cuddling, caressing, massages, or showering together.
- *Pay attention to your mental and emotional well-being.* If you find yourself feeling depressed or anxious, experiencing persistent moodiness or bouts of unexplained anger, or withdrawing from your partner and friends, seek help. While mood fluctuations may

occur more often in midlife, don't dismiss persistent feelings that cause you distress. These may be signs of an underlying problem that can be helped.

- *Seek new roles for yourself and allow your nurturing side to grow.* It can be a relief to find that your role in life is broader than that of a sexual performer and family provider. Become an intimate partner, a caring father, an involved grandfather, a leader in the community, or a mentor to a younger person at work. Be willing to adjust your career and life goals. For men, the successful shift into the next stage of life is usually accompanied by a shift of emphasis from competition and aggression to softer and gentler characteristics.

- *Make healthy choices.* Almost all of the physical complaints men describe in midlife are alleviated by healthy eating, active living, and refraining from smoking and excessive drinking. These positive practices also help prevent serious health problems such as heart disease and diabetes.

- *Talk about it.* Discuss your health concerns with a family physician. Talk about your problems with a friend, family member, your partner, a therapist, or your priest, rabbi, or spiritual leader. Consider participating in a men's group or a mutual-aid group for a specific concern. All of us need support when we undertake a major process of rediscovery.

- *Consider sharing this chapter and the previous one on female menopause* with your partner. Use them (as well as other pertinent chapters) as a starting point for discussing your midlife concerns and hopes.

THE BOTTOM LINE

Most men appear to go through many of the same experiences that women do in the menopausal period. It is important to talk about these physical, psychological, and emotional changes. The transition to life's afternoon is an opportunity for men to let go of the social expectations that have constrained their lives up to now, and to grow beyond them.

Contacts and Further Information

Organizations

- National Institute on Aging: National Institutes of Health, Information Center, P.O. Box 8057, Gaithersburg, MD 20898–8057. Tel.: (800) 222–2225; TDD: (800) 222–4225; Fax: (310) 589–3014; E-mail: niainfo@access.digex.net
- The North American Menopause Society, P.O. Box 94527, Cleveland, OH 44101–4527. Tel.: (216) 844–8748.

Websites

- The Male Health Center (founded by urologist Dr. Kenneth Goldberg in Dallas, Texas, in 1989): http://www.malehealthcenter.com
- Men's Health Resources (sponsored by the U.S. government): http://www.healthfinder.gov (click on "Men" under "Just for You").
- Midlife Passages: The Institute of Endocrinology and Reproductive and Reproductive Medicine in Atlanta, Georgia: http://midlife-passages.com
- Website of Third Age Wellness and Male Menopause (founded by Jed Diamond, author): http://www.thirdagewellness.com/

Books

- *A Circle of Men: The Original Manual for Men's Support Groups* by Bill Kauth. New York: St. Martin's Press, 1992.
- *In a Dark Wood: Personal Essays by Men on Middle Age* by Steven Harvey. Athens, GA: University of Georgia Press, 1996.
- *Male Menopause* by Jed Diamond. Naperville, IL: Sourcebooks Inc., 1997.
- *Male Menopause: Restoring Vitality and Virility* by Malcolm Carruthers. New York: HarperCollins, 1996.
- *Midlife Man* by Art Hister, MD. Vancouver: Greystone Books, 1998.
- *The Middle Passage: From Misery to Meaning in Midlife* by James Hollis. Toronto: Inner City Books, 1993.
- *The Seasons of a Man's Life* by Daniel Levinson. New York: Ballantine Books, 1978.

- *Stiffed: The Betrayal of the American Man* by Susan Faludi. New York: Morrow & Co., 1999.
- *Understanding Men's Passages* by Gail Sheehy. New York: Random House, 1998.

Related Chapters in This Book

- *Chapter 1: The Midlife Journey* describes the psychological and emotional journey of the middle years.
- *Chapter 2: Understanding the Female Menopause* helps you understand what women go through in the menopausal period and reinforces the similarity of many of the experiences both men and women go through in the middle years.
- *Chapter 4: The Search for the Fountain of Youth* describes anti-aging theories and developments.
- *Chapter 6: Wrinkles, Chin Hairs, and Baldness* provides information on the changes in physical appearance that accompany midlife.
- *Chapter 7: The Active Living Solution* describes how physical activity can help to prevent many of the changes men associate with the male menopause.
- *Chapter 8: Food for Thought: Healthy Eating in Midlife* gives you matter-of-fact advice on eating to prevent disease and maintain a highly tuned body as you age.
- *Chapter 11: Enjoying Sex in Midlife* gives you more information on how age affects sexuality as well as some common-sense advice on how to keep the spark alive.
- *Chapter 12: Dealing with Impotence* provides more details on the causes of impotence and how to deal with it.
- *Chapter 18: Prostate Health* helps you determine if you have a prostate problem and provides information on keeping your prostate gland healthy.
- *Chapter 22: Complementary and Alternative Medicine Is Coming on Strong* provides additional information on the use of complementary and alternative therapies such as naturopathy, homeopathy, and herbal medicines in the midlife period.
- *Chapter 23: Body, Mind, and Soul* discusses the spiritual aspect of the midlife journey.

CHAPTER FOUR

The Search for the Fountain of Youth

Age only matters when one is aging. Now that I have arrived at a great age, I might just as well be twenty.

— Pablo Picasso[1]

Ponce de León Must Have Been a Baby Boomer

Despite our conscious intentions to embrace maturity, the desire to stay young has been part of the documented human condition since at least the time of Cleopatra. In North America, most boomers have read in elementary-school history books about the famous Spanish explorer Ponce de León, who sailed to the New World in the 1550s in search of the fountain of youth. He didn't find it, but enthusiasm for the search has never lagged since. Today, the obsession with finding the magic means to recapture youth has never been greater.

As the baby boomers move en masse through the middle stage of life, the Big Generation is taking a serious interest in the art and science of staying young. Concerns about growing older have spawned glossy magazines, shelves full of anti-aging remedies, theories about down-aging, and a resurgence in hair tonics, cosmetic surgery, and cryonics – the cold storage of bodies in hopes of later regeneration.

The human longing to feel and look young has helped us make a powerful discovery. The secret of youth is not likely to be found in magic pills, potions, or fountains. For the most part, it rests in our genes, our cells, and the decisions we make each day – about how we think, eat, drink, exercise, work, cope, rest, relate, worship, and play. Songwriter Eubie Blake, approaching his hundredth birthday, had it right when he said, "If I had known I was going to live so long, I'd have taken better care of myself."

There is no question that improved lifestyles (quitting smoking, healthy eating, managing stress, and enjoying regular physical activity) have been a major reason for an almost 50 per cent decline in premature deaths (before age seventy) from heart disease in the last twenty years.[2] The number of deaths from all cancers has decreased slightly for men since the late 1980s and deaths from cancer among women has remained relatively stable over the same period.[3] This good news, however, may be short-lived. Women have taken up smoking in alarming numbers. As a result, we are seeing declines in lung cancer in men (largely due to reduced smoking) while the incidence of lung cancer in women is increasing. The recent increase in smoking among teenage girls is even more alarming. If young women continue to take up smoking, we may see female advantages in longevity over men disappear in the next thirty years.

Part II of this book provides you with some sound advice about lifestyle choices that can postpone or even reverse many of the so-called natural effects of aging. In this chapter we explore some of the popular potions for staying young, as well the theories of today's lab-coated conquistadors. Led by biologists and gerontologists, our search for the fountain of youth goes on.

The Normal Process of Aging

While every person ages in a unique way, some biomarkers of aging are common to us all. However, it is not always easy to distinguish which changes are caused by natural aging and which are accelerated by disease and negative lifestyle choices.

- *The sense organs.* The progressive loss of taste, smell, vision, and hearing are the natural result of aging of the end cells of the system, such as the taste-bud cells or the cells in the nose that detect smell.
- *The heart.* While reduced cardiovascular endurance is typical of aging, little is known about how the heart ages. Coronary heart disease that results in heart attacks is not caused by aging at all. It is a disease of the arteries that supply the heart muscle. Many older people have a decreased capacity for physical activity because the heart has not been exercised adequately.
- *The muscles and skeleton.* The changes in the muscles and skeleton are another area where disease is often confused with age. Disuse accounts for a great deal of the decrease in muscle size and strength

that is seen in people as they age. There is some loss of muscle fibres, because some of the nerve cells in the spinal cord that control them degenerate with increasing age. Proper exercise can maintain, strengthen, and enlarge the remaining muscle fibres.

Bones do begin to lose their density with age; for women, this is accelerated at menopause. The bones undergo constant changes, with remodelling of the bone architecture. This is a process of regeneration. After age thirty, more bone is lost than is formed, resulting in a gradual decrease in skeletal size and strength.

- *The brain.* Sometimes disuse, not aging, results in decreased mental functions as one gets older. Lifelong learning, maintaining the ability to concentrate, continuing to stimulate your memory with memory tasks, and problem-solving, all help to maintain mental functions. Alzheimer disease is not a result of normal aging.

The New Science of Staying Young

By one estimate, we spend more than $2 billion a year on various nostrums to ward off aging.[4] The most popular of these are hormone therapies, the use of performance enhancers, herbs, vitamin regimens, and mind-body therapies. Here is a summary of what you can expect from a few of the hottest items on the market.

Hormone Therapies

It makes sense to assume that hormones are directly involved in aging. They regulate our growth, development, and sexual characteristics. For women, estrogen replacement therapy has been touted as the answer to eternal youth and protection from the ravages of old age. Why not assume that a shot of testosterone or some other hormone that is yet to be discovered can be the elixir that guarantees men eternal youth?

But wait a minute. Hormones are powerful chemicals. They serve important natural functions and act as key communicators, carrying messages from one organ in the body to another. They should command our respect.

Estrogen, progesterone, and testosterone are the female and male sex hormones. We believe that men can learn a lot from the female experience of hormone replacement therapy (HRT). After twenty years of study, it is clear that, while HRT has many advantages, including protection against osteoporosis and heart disease for women at risk, it won't keep us from aging. Indeed, for women with breast cancer, its use can exacerbate an existing problem. (See Chapters 2, 3, and 21 for more detailed information on the use of estrogen, progesterone, and testosterone.)

These problems do not mean that research into the power of various hormones to prevent disease and decline should be abandoned. It means that regulators should be conservative in their acceptance of hormone therapies until clear evidence of their effects on humans is known. And if hormones are to be sold as supplements, we must clearly understand their potential to interact with other drugs and strictly control the purity and sale of such products. For their part, consumers should be wary of claims that any hormone holds the secret to the fountain of youth.

DHEA (dehydroepiandrosterone) is a hormone manufactured in the adrenal gland. It is sometimes referred to as a "motherlode" hormone, because the body converts it into active hormones such as estrogen and testosterone. The amount of DHEA the body makes declines with increasing age or during a serious illness. By age seventy, women's and men's levels of DHEA have fallen to about 10 per cent of what they were at their peaks. This has led scientists to theorize that replacing DHEA in older people will help to keep them young.[5] Animal studies have shown that mice treated with DHEA have stronger immune systems and healthier hearts and are less likely to become obese, develop breast cancer, and osteoporosis.

Human studies are far less conclusive. A few small studies have shown that older people taking DHEA have improved immunity and feel more energetic. DHEA may also benefit some people who are HIV positive. On the downside, DHEA may interfere with normal insulin levels, lower the amount of good cholesterol, and cause unwanted hair growth in women. The National Institute on Aging has expressed concern about the risk of liver damage and an increased risk of breast cancer in women and about worsening symptoms of prostate cancer in men who take high doses of DHEA.[6] DHEA is sold in the United States as a dietary supplement; it is not available in Canada, even by prescription.

Since DHEA is a natural substance that cannot be patented, drug companies are testing synthetic DHEA against specific diseases, such as lupus and AIDS. Some health-food stores sell an extract of wild yam that is billed as DHEA, but since DHEA does not exist in plants it is unlikely that the body can convert wild yam into usable DHEA. Only a complex manufacturing process can make this conversion, in which case a prescription is required. If you do decide to try DHEA, make sure that your physician knows about it.

Melatonin is a hormone produced in the brain during the night by the pineal gland, which is involved in regulating the sleep-wake cycle. As with DHEA, the body's production of melatonin declines with age. By the age of sixty, we produce about one-third of the melatonin we did at age twenty. Melatonin has been referred to as a miracle compound that combats aging, reduces your risk of cancer and heart disease, helps you get a good night's sleep, and enhances your sex life. Of these claims, the only proven one is melatonin's ability to improve sleep.[7, 8] It appears to resynchronize disruptions in the sleep-wake cycle as insomnia, jet lag, shift work, or other sleep timing problems.

Dr. Russell Reiter at the University of Texas Health Center is a pioneer in melatonin research with animals. He has established a clear link between the hormone and certain cyclical patterns such as reproduction, migration, and hibernation. Whether this has relevance in humans is yet to be seen. For now, his work has led to new research on melatonin as a birth-control agent and as a possible treatment for hormone-dependent cancers. In 1995, two colleagues of Reiter's published a best-seller, *The Melatonin Miracle*, which claims, among other things, that melatonin has potent antioxidant properties.[9]

In the United States, health-food stores can barely keep melatonin products in stock. The French, British, and Canadian governments have banned its sale because there is no clear evidence of its therapeutic effects and nobody can guarantee the purity of what is being sold or how it might interact with other drugs.

Until we know more about its long-term effects and can regulate the product, users should be aware that they are part of a giant, uncontrolled experiment.

THE MELATONIN JET-LAG PRESCRIPTION

While melatonin is still suspect as an anti-aging product, it has been shown to help with changes in the sleep-wake cycle. Here is the melatonin jet-lag prescription.

For eastward flights: take 3 mg per day in the late afternoon before departure and at bedtime for four more days once you arrive at your destination.

For westward flights: take 3 mg before bed for four days once you have arrived at your destination.

Human growth hormone (HGH) is a natural growth hormone that gradually diminishes as we age. In 1990, endocrinologist Dr. Daniel Rudman published a study in the respected *New England Journal of Medicine* on the use of HGH therapy in older men. He hypothesized that the diminished production of HGH that occurs as we age is responsible for the main changes in body composition – a reduction in lean muscle mass and an increase in body fat. In his study, older men (average age of sixty-nine) who had blood levels of HGH below what is normal for healthy younger men were treated with HGH. Those who received the hormone showed a 6 per cent increase in lean body mass and a 16 per cent reduction in body fat.[10] Since then, there have been a number of experimental studies. Some have shown few or no anti-aging benefits with the use of HGH. Others have shown benefits – with costs. The cost of personal HGH treatment is about $20,000 per year in the United States, and side-effects can include breast growth, carpal tunnel syndrome, elevated blood sugars, and an increased risk of diabetes. In addition, it could be argued that regular trips to the gym could accomplish what HGH promises. As with other hormones, the use of HGH therapy must be carefully studied and controlled.

Performance Enhancers
Creatine and Androstenedione.[11] Creatine, a natural amino acid derivative, and androstenedione, a testosterone precursor, are marketed as "dietary supplements" in health-food stores and are widely believed to enhance

athletic performance. Both were "hot" in 1999, because Mark McGwire, the baseball home-run record-setter, said that he takes both.

Creatine is synthesized in the liver, pancreas, and kidneys and supplied in the diet by meat and fish. A summary of thirty-one studies showed that oral creatine supplements may improve performance modestly in short-duration, high-intensity tasks. However, other studies show that creatine supplements provide *no* consistent advantage during aerobic exercise.

Androstenedione ("andro") has been used in Europe as a nasal spray to enhance athletic perfomance and is available in the United States in tablets. It can increase blood testosterone, but its effect on muscle mass and performance, if any, remains to be established. No information is available on long-term safety, and andro may cause adverse reactions similar to testosterone, such as testicle shrinkage, blood clotting disorders, and breast enlargement.

Herbs[12, 13]

Herbal remedies have been used for centuries in Europe, Asia, and many indigenous cultures, both for healing and as tonics to restore balance and increase vigour. Unfortunately, we no longer grow them in our own back-yards, nor do we have the wisdom our ancestors passed down from generation to generation telling us where, when, how much, and with what we should use them.

Many herbs are now widely available in North American health-food stores and even pharmacies. Yet, without detailed knowledge of them, we are left with two major concerns about their use. First, they do not fall under the regulations governing pharmaceuticals (herbs are considered foods, not drugs), so we cannot be sure of what we are getting. Second, herbs are potent medicine that can cause side-effects and may interact negatively with other medications. When you use herbal therapies, always tell your family physician and other health-care providers what and how much you are taking.

Here are three popular substances associated with promoting vitality:

Bee pollen, which is used for its rejuvenating qualities and for dealing with hot flashes in menopause, is certainly nutritious. It contains 30 per cent protein, 55 per cent carbohydrate, 1 to 2 per cent fat, and 3 per cent minerals and vitamins. **Royal jelly** is the food the queen bee produces that allows her to live forty times longer than other bees. It is high in B vitamins, especially pantothenic acid (B vitamins may aid memory), minerals, and anti-stress vitamins. Bee pollen and melbrosia (which combines bee pollen and royal jelly) can cause severe allergic reactions in people with allergies.

Gingko biloba, which is produced from the world's oldest tree, improves blood flow. It has been used in the early treatment of dementias and has been noted for its ability to improve mental clarity and memory retention. However, gingko increases blood fluidity and should not be used by people on blood-thinners. This herb is discussed further in Chapter 14.

Ginseng has been integral to Chinese medicine for 2,000 years. It is said to increase resistance to stress, improve general vitality, and strengthen normal body functions, including sexual potency. Women with menopausal problems use it to boost energy and relieve hot flashes. Siberian ginseng has been reported to increase physical endurance. Some people take Korean ginseng during convalescence to regain energy, as a performance enhancer, and as a mild immunity booster.

Vitamin Regimens

New, wildly acclaimed anti-aging regimens that feature taking large doses of vitamins pop up every year. One of the best known and still popular regimens from the early eighties is Durk Pearson and Sandy Shaw's *Life Extension* and *The Life Extension Companion*.[14] The Pearson-Shaw formula emphasizes antioxidants, but also suggests the use of prescription drugs and large doses of vitamins and other substances. Pearson and Shaw, both now aged fifty-two and in good health, have been following this regimen themselves since 1968.

Today, Pearson and Shaw, both qualified scientists, spend almost all of their time studying anti-aging research, although the bulk of their income derives from designing and licensing supplement formulas. They have made only minor revisions in the dosages of the nutrients they extolled in their original books, and have added some new discoveries to their list of life-extenders.[15] The Life Extension regimen requires a physician willing to prescribe the drugs and frequent medical tests to detect side-effects.

The conclusion? Most mainstream scientists are sceptical about how readily Shaw and Pearson assume that scientific data from animal studies can be applied to humans and to the development of new products. Others believe that Pearson and Shaw are rightfully pushing the medical establishment into new frontiers.

Mind-Body Therapies

The mind-body therapies stress the powerful influence that one's thoughts and feelings have on the functioning of the body. Deepak Chopra, in his popular book *Ageless Body, Timeless Mind: The Quantum Alternative to Growing Old*, applies this principle to aging. He presents a series of mental exercises that he claims dramatically slow down and even reverse the aging process by challenging our unconscious beliefs about growing old.

Chopra believes that our experience of time directly affects our biological clock. For example, if we always feel that we are "running out of time," this negatively affects us. He suggests that having moments of "timeless awareness," found during meditation and quiet time in nature, can counteract the rigid notions of time we get locked into and thus slow our aging.

Current Theories on Aging

Experts agree that the maximum life span of humans (about 115 years) has not increased during recorded history. What has increased is the proportion of the population coming closer to reaching that maximum. Over the last sixty years, life expectancy for men in North America has increased from 61 to 75; for women it has increased from 64 to 81.[16]

In his book *Dave Barry Turns 40*, the humorist asks, "Why do we get older? Why can't we just go on and on, accumulating a potentially infinite number of frequent flyer points?"[17] No one, including Ponce de León, has yet discovered a foolproof way to satisfy Barry's wish. Even so, as we shall see in this section, there are a number of current theories that help us understand why and how we age.

The Genetic Clock Theory suggests that each of us has a genetically programmed life plan.[18] The minutes, days, and years of our lives tick away to the beat of this internal – or should we say infernal – clock. Thus, the changes that come with age – hair thinning, skin losing elasticity, and bones becoming more fragile – are charted in the DNA control centre in the nucleus of each cell.

The clearest example we have of the genetic clock at work is the Pacific salmon. These amazing fish spawn in fresh water, then swim downstream to live in the ocean. In a few years, their inner clock urges them to fight their way back up the rocky river. Once they reach their birthplace, they lay and fertilize their eggs. At this point, the rate of their aging accelerates dramatically, and within minutes their gills turn grey. Then, with their biological purpose achieved, the salmon die.

In humans, genetically planned aging differs from family to family. In some families, members usually die at age fifty or sixty; in others, they have the good fortune to live into their nineties. Family histories of heart disease, breast cancer, colon cancer, and other diseases suggest that genetic programming is involved. Of course, there are always exceptions. Environmental conditions, such as long exposure to toxic chemicals, and lifestyle choices, such as decades of smoking, can alter the best-laid genetic plans.

Whether or not each of our cells has a built-in biological clock, the influence of heredity is hard to deny. As we learn more about genetics, we may discover it is possible to manipulate a person's biological timetable. For example, by keeping the Pacific salmon out at sea, researchers have found that the steroid hormone rush that urges them to fight their way upstream does not occur, and the fish lives longer than it does if it swims upstream to spawn.

The Oxidative Damage Theory is getting a lot of attention these days. It contends that aging is a result of the wear and tear on our bodies caused by the oxidation process.[19, 20]

Because we live in a oxygen-based environment, we are constantly exposed to oxidative damage. Just as a piece of metal rusts or an apple turns brown when exposed to air, so the body is vulnerable to the effects of oxidation. When oxygen is metabolized or burned by the body, the cells release a waste product called free radicals in the body. This is part of the normal chemical process of living cells. Free radicals can also damage the basic structure of the cells, leading to age-related problems such as cataracts and to chronic diseases such as cancer and coronary heart disease. In her book *The Complete Book of Men's Health*, author Sarah Brewer suggests that free radicals, like those in politics, are "highly unstable entities that race around picking fights and causing damage."[21] Aging and exposure to environmental conditions such as radiation, cigarette smoke, or ozone appear to increase our vulnerability to free-radical attacks.

Because of the oxidant-damage theory, antioxidant vitamins – which protect key cells by neutralizing free radicals – have been getting a lot of media attention. There are four main antioxidants: vitamins C and E, beta-carotene, and selenium. Vitamin C is found in many fruits and vegetables, including oranges, grapefruits, strawberries, broccoli, and potatoes. Vitamin E is found in nuts, certain vegetable oils, and leafy greens. Beta-carotene is found in yellow-orange fruits and vegetables such as cantaloupes, peaches, carrots, and sweet potatoes, as well as in dark-green leafy vegetables such as spinach and collard greens. Selenium is found in meat, chicken, seafood, and grains.

Many population health studies have suggested a potential benefit of beta-carotene in preventing certain cancers. Consumers and the medical community were therefore stunned when a large study of Finnish smokers found that smokers who had been taking a beta-carotene supplement demonstrated a risk of lung cancer 18 per cent higher than that of people in the control group who were not taking the supplement.[22] Debate continues about this finding, since the group of men studied were at very high risk for lung cancer and may not represent men in other cultures and situations.

The findings related to antioxidants and heart disease are far less equivocal. Several studies have documented an association between taking vitamin E supplements and a significantly reduced risk of heart disease in men in both Canada and the United States. In one recent study of 40,000 male health professionals, those who took a high dose of supplemental vitamin E had a 39-per-cent risk reduction in coronary heart disease; those with the highest intake of beta-carotene had a 25-per-cent risk reduction.[23]

In the spring of 1997 a major study appeared in the *Journal of the American Medical Association* in which 1,300 people who had been treated for skin cancer were given 200 micrograms of selenium each day for four years. While the selenium supplement did not prevent the recurrence of skin cancer, the selenium group did show a significantly lowered risk of developing prostate, colon, and lung cancer. While it is too soon to recommend regular use of selenium supplements, we can look forward to seeing whether this exciting study can be replicated.[24] Selenium is found in a wide variety of accessible foods, so most North Americans get enough in their regular diet.

The health community is cautiously optimistic about all of these findings. We need more evidence before we can truly understand the potential power of antioxidants to prevent disease, especially cancer. Experts, however, do agree on two important recommendations:

• Eat lots of fruits and vegetables. They are high in antioxidants and fibre.

• Don't rely on antioxidants to protect you from the harmful effects of tobacco. If you smoke, quitting is the only way to improve your chances of escaping cancer and heart disease.[25]

While public health organizations do not yet endorse routine supplements, millions of people take vitamin pills "just in case" their diets may lack needed nutrients. Remember that vitamin supplements do not take the place of fresh food. (See Chapter 8 for more information.) Based on scientific evidence to date, the following measures seem prudent:

• Eat lots of fruits and vegetables that contain vitamin C and beta-carotene (vitamin A). In addition to antioxidants, these foods provide beneficial, disease-fighting phytochemicals, which are not found in supplements.

• Consider taking vitamin E supplements, because it is impossible to get the protective amount you need through a normal diet.

• Take a vitamin C supplement if you do not regularly eat fruits and vegetables high in vitamin C.

• Eat lots of foods high in beta carotenoids and selenium: there is insufficient evidence to support taking supplements for these as yet.

SUGGESTED DAILY INTAKES FOR KEY ANTIOXIDANTS:

Vitamin E:	100 to 800 IU
Vitamin C:	200 to 500 mg
Beta-carotene:	15 mg (3,000 to 6,000 IU)
Selenium:	70 to 100 mg

• Consider taking folic acid, B12, and B6 if you are at risk of heart disease. These vitamins work together to prevent anemia and to reduce homocysteine, a chemical found in the blood which may predict heart attack or stroke (see Chapter 20 on heart health).

SUGGESTED DAILY INTAKES TO PROMOTE HEART HEALTH:

Folic acid:	0.4 mg
Vitamin B6:	50 to 100 mg
Vitamin B12:	250 micrograms

The Chronic Inflammation Theory suggests that chronic inflammation, which often accompanies aging, may damage the brain neurons as well as the joints. The use of anti-inflammatory drugs such as ibuprofen may inhibit the damage to the brain, just as they do for arthritis. There are now twenty published studies from nine different countries supporting this idea.[26]

The Use-It-or-Lose-It Theory suggests that the decline of many of the physical and mental abilities, which gets blamed on aging, can be prevented or delayed by healthy, active living. As Lucille Ball said, "The secret of staying young is to live honestly, eat slowly, and just not think about your age." The use-it-or-lose-it theory is easy to demonstrate. Anyone who has ever had to wear a cast or spend time in bed with a serious illness has witnessed how quickly muscles atrophy when they are not used.

NASA, the National Aeronautics and Space Administration, was one of the first organizations to take a real interest in the use-it-or-lose-it theory. When the first astronauts returned from two weeks in weightless space without physical exercise, their aerobic fitness and muscle strength had declined significantly. On subsequent missions, astronauts were assigned thirty minutes of daily cycling on a stationary bicycle as part of their routine.

Back on earth, NASA and the Aerobic Research Center in Dallas teamed up to study 1,500 male NASA workers ranging in age from twenty-five to seventy. They found that half of the age-related decline in aerobic fitness could not be attributed to age at all, but to decreased levels of physical activity and increased levels of body fat. Older men who had remained active tended to be much leaner and fitter than younger men who were less active or had more body fat.[27] More recently, a study of more than 40,000 women showed that those who report regular physical activity had a significantly reduced risk for early mortality from both cardiovascular disease and respiratory illnesses.[28]

Other researchers have confirmed the anti-aging effects of physical activity. Dr. Roy Shephard, a well-known exercise physiologist and co-author of *Fit after Fifty*, states that active people in their fifties or sixties can function "on a higher plane ... as though exercise had reduced their age by 10 to 20 years."[29]

Most of us do not have the body build, stamina, or interest in training sufficiently to run marathons. Happily, new research shows that regular, moderate exercise, not running marathons, is what is required. Dr. Steven Blair and his colleagues at the Dallas centre have found that the premature death rate among extremely active men and women is only slightly lower than the rate among people who exercise moderately. Premature death rates increase significantly when moderate exercise levels drop to little or no physical activity. "This is good news for those of us who aren't athletes," says Blair. "It means that 20 to 30 minutes of daily brisk walking, yard work, recreational cycling, or participating in sports can all have important health benefits in terms of longevity."[30]

Recently, neurologists have been comparing brain tissue to muscle tissue. A large, emerging body of research shows that engaging in intellectual exercises can meaningfully better the brain's structure and functioning during adulthood and later life.[31]

One more application of the use-it-or-lose-it theory is worth considering. Some people believe that regular sexual activity prolongs life as well as enriching it. One study from Wales of more than 1,200 men found that mortality from all causes was twice as high for men who reported orgasms less frequently than once a month compared to those who reported having orgasms twice a week or more.[32] While additional evidence to support this theory is largely anecdotal, we do know that healthy lifestyles, healthy sex lives, and a robust old age go hand-in-hand. We also know that sexual pleasure does not decline with age. Indeed, it may even increase!

Caloric Restriction. The caloric restriction theory is based on animal studies and some studies with humans which suggest that avoiding overeating and reducing the number of calories one consumes may increase average and maximum lifespans. These studies have been careful to undernourish without malnourishing, so that the diet is 30 per cent restricted relative to a person's body weight, and fortified with the necessary vitamins, minerals, and trace elements.[33]

Why Do Women Live Longer than Men?

In 1900, older men outnumbered older women. Today, the reverse is true. In 1980 there were 45 men for every 100 women over age eighty-five in the United States; in the year 2000 it is predicted that there will be 39 men for every 100 women over age eighty-five.[34]

Why do women live longer than men? No one knows for sure. There are numerous theories:

- Some scientists suggest that estrogen, with its heart-healthy advantages, is the key factor. However, after menopause, women lose this advantage.
- Epidemiologists point to the higher death rates among men caused by violence and injuries. They suggest that the risk-taking and sometimes violent nature of men is a key factor. Others blame tobacco. Men have been smoking longer than women, so women's lung-cancer mortality statistics are only now beginning to catch up with those of men.
- Some people suggest that men die earlier from stress-induced diseases because of their roles in executive-type jobs. At the same time, other studies show that people in low-income, low-control jobs, which are more often held by women, are more likely to die early.[35]
- Some experts suggest that women's practice of confiding in friends and seeking out social support may help explain their longevity. Studies show that loneliness is a greater cause of mortality than high blood pressure and that men are at high risk for dying soon after the death of their wives.[36]
- Marriage may be an anti-aging remedy for men. Studies in Western countries show that married men live longer than their counterparts who are single, divorced, or widowed. This does not hold true for women. In fact, single women have a better chance than their married sisters of celebrating hundredth birthdays.[37]
- Anthropologist Dr. Kristen Hawkes of the University of Utah postulates that the "granny grocery factor" may be part of the reason

women live longer than men. Unlike other primates, ancient humans relied on long-living elder females to forage for food for young mothers and grandchildren, so that younger adults could exploit new habitats and procreate. The extra food granny supplied promoted her grandchildren's survival, and in transmitting her genes to them she also fostered stronger natural selection for longevity.[38]

MAJOR CAUSES OF DEATH AFTER AGE 65 IN CANADA (1991)

Men	Women
1. Coronary heart disease	1. Coronary heart disease
2. Lung cancer	2. Stroke
3. Stroke	3. Lung cancer
4. Respiratory diseases	4. Pneumonia
5. Prostate cancer	5. Breast cancer
6. Pneumonia	6. Colorectal cancer
7. Colorectal cancer	7. Respiratory diseases
8. Diabetes	8. Diabetes
9. Urinary-tract cancers	9. Alzheimer disease, including pre-senile dementia
10. Aortic aneurysm	10. Kidney disease

Coronary heart disease has ranked first among both sexes for forty years, but rates have declined significantly over the last twenty years. Lung cancer and Alzheimer disease have become significantly more prevalent in recent years, especially among women in old age.

Source: Statistics Canada, Bureau of Chronic Diseases, *Major Causes of Death in Men and Women Age 65+* (Ottawa, 1995).

DID YOU KNOW?

The oldest person whose life has been reliably documented – Jeanne Louise Calment – died in 1997 at the age of 122 in Arles, France. She once remarked, "I've only ever had one wrinkle and I am sitting on it. I will die laughing."[39]

Quality Is as Important as Quantity

Most of this chapter has dealt with the human desire to live longer. That same fascination has led to the study of proud centenarians living in the mountains of Russia and South America who claim to be 100 to 120 years of age. How do they live so long in such good health in such basic and difficult living conditions? Four factors seem to be at work. First, they remain physically active all their lives, working in the fields and carrying provisions up steep hillsides. Second, they don't have to deal with urban stress. Third, they eat more carbohydrates than we do but, because they eat less fat and protein they consume fewer calories overall. Last, they have a positive attitude and a meaningful existence. These centenarians are proud to be old because, in their cultures, elders are respected for their wisdom and their ability to continue to contribute to the community.

We live in a very different world. Most of us want to live beyond age seventy-five, but only if we can remain healthy, independent, and energetic, and only if we can look forward to the respect and dignity our youth-oriented society has tended to deny its elders. While all of us dream of immortality, our real interest is in putting more life in our years than years in our lives. The rest of this book is dedicated to just that – by giving you reliable information and practical ideas for taking charge of your health and well-being in the middle years.

THE BOTTOM LINE

In spite of our concerns about the quality of life in our seventies, eighties, and nineties, most of us want to reach those ages. Research increasingly shows that healthful living now can postpone and reduce disability later. We need to celebrate aging as a natural and positive achievement on our journey.

Contacts and Further Information

Organizations
- National Advisory Council on Aging (Canada), 8th Floor, Jeanne Mance Building, Tunney's Pasture, Ottawa, ON K1A 1B4. Tel.: (613) 957–1968; Fax: (613) 957–7627.
- National Institute on Aging, National Institutes of Health, Information Center, P.O. Box 8057, Gaithersburg, MD 20898–8057. Tel.: (800) 222–2225; TDD: (800) 222–4225; Fax: (310) 589–3014; E-mail: niainfo@access.digex.net

Websites
- National Advisory Council on Aging (Canada) (sponsored by Health Canada): http://www.hc-sc.gc.ca/seniors/aines/naca.htm
- National Institute on Aging (U.S.): http://www.nin.gov/nia
- The Third Age (sponsored by Quaker Oats): http://thirdage.com
- World Health Network (the official site of the American Academy of Anti-Aging Medicine): http://www.worldhealth.net

Books
- *Ageless Body, Timeless Mind: The Quantum Alternative to Growing Old* by Deepak Chopra. New York: Three Rivers Press, 1993.
- *The Age Wave* by Ken Dychtwald. Los Angeles: Jeremy P. Tarcher, 1989.
- *The Fountain of Age* by Betty Friedan. New York: Simon & Schuster, 1993.
- *From Age-ing to Sage-ing: A Profound New Vision of Growing Older* by Zalman Schacter-Shalomi and Ronald S. Miller. New York: Warner Books, 1995.
- *The New Ourselves, Growing Older* by Paula B. Doress-Worters and Diana Laskin Siegal, with Boston Women's Health Collective. New York: Simon & Schuster, 1994.
- *New Passages: Mapping Your Life Across Time* by Gail Sheehy. New York: Random House, 1995.

Related Chapters in This Book

- *Chapter 1: The Midlife Journey* describes the journey of midlife in relation to positive aging.
- *Chapter 7: The Active Living Solution* provides more details on physical activity as an aging antidote and describes how you can get active now.
- *Chapter 8: Food for Thought: Healthy Eating in Midlife* gives you more information on antioxidants and practical advice on healthy eating for a long and healthy life.
- *Chapter 16: Partners in Health Care* gives you more information on taking care of yourself and the genetic connection to disease.
- *Chapter 22: Complementary and Alternative Medicine Is Coming on Strong* gives you additional information on the role of complementary and alternative medicine (such as homeopathy, herbal therapy) in slowing the changes associated with aging.
- *Chapter 23: Body, Mind, and Soul* reminds us that aging is a spiritual adventure, as well as a physical and psychological one.

PART TWO

How to Die Young
... but as Late as Possible

CHAPTER FIVE

Making Changes That Last!

The Wright brothers flew right through the smoke screen of impossibility.   – Charles F. Kettering[1]

A Holistic View of Health and the Midlife Journey

We believe, as do all of the people we interviewed, that health is more than strong bones and low cholesterol levels. Feeling healthy is about mental, social, emotional, and spiritual well-being as well as physical health.

There are many factors that determine how healthy you will be. One of these is your personal lifestyle choices. This chapter and those that follow in the rest of this section provide solid information and advice on the key aspects of healthy living in midlife, and how you can make positive changes that will last into the next stage of your life. It also acknowledges that personal health practices are not the only determinants of health and well-being.

The good news is that healthy living is not about running marathons or denying ourselves pleasurable foods. It is about making realistic goals for change and then working toward those goals – one small step at a time.

The midlife journey is both an ending and a beginning. As we come to terms with the end of "youth," we open new doors that will help us establish our place in the next phase of our lives. Sometimes the changes will be dramatic: children leave home, parents die. Others will be more subtle: while we remain in the same job or intimate relationship, the nature of our involvement in those structures will change and evolve. Invariably, we will be faced with losses and new-found opportunities that touch our bodies, minds – and souls.

Whatever the changes that will be required of us in the coming years, we want to face them with grace and good humour. While some will be out of our control, there are many that we can take charge of. The first section of this book describes midlife as a journey. Here, we look at what will aid us in making the trip positive and life-affirming.

What Makes People Healthy? What Makes People Sick?

Since the early 1970s, North Americans have made enormous efforts to improve the way they live. On some fronts, we have made great strides. There are now more ex-smokers than smokers. We eat less fat and recycle more. On other fronts, in the gains we made in the early years, for example in fitness and weight management, we boomers are losing ground as we age. We have learned a great deal about the roles positive thinking and resiliency play in our health. Spiritual well-being has returned to the popular agenda: books about the soul have become best-sellers.

At the same time, we have become increasingly aware that factors in our socio-economic and physical environment have an extraordinary effect on our health. When we look at the overall health of Americans and Canadians, we find that poverty, unemployment, and disparities in income distribution damage health the most. Canadian men in the upper-income bracket can expect to live six years longer and to enjoy fourteen more years of living without a disability than men in the lowest income category. Women in the highest income bracket can expect to live five years longer and to have eight more disability-free years than women in the lowest income bracket.[2] In the United States, where disparities in income tend to be greater in some areas, these differences can be even more pronounced.

What can we learn from these kinds of statistics? Obviously, health is more than exercise and nutritious food. It is also more than medical care. Indeed, what makes a nation of people healthy has little to do with expensive, high-tech medicine. Yet, a comprehensive, accessible health-care system is an essential part of a civilized and compassionate society. More important are the ways that we organize and manage our wealth, our workplaces, our physical resources, our family lives, and our community supports. Ultimately, the values of peace, love, equity, and social justice that were so important to the boomers' experience of the sixties are the same values that create, maintain, and enhance the health of us all.

You Don't Need to Kill Yourself to Save Your Life

As we wrote this book, we were naturally anxious about fitting in everything we need to do to be healthy. At a workshop, one woman said, "I lie in bed at night and worry about the eight glasses of water I need for my skin, the three glasses of milk I need for my bones, my exercise plan, my plans for moving my office, the need to spend quality time with my daughter, and to have some time to listen to my husband . . . and, good grief, I forgot the anti-wrinkle cream for my face." We all laughed knowingly, sharing an important realization – healthy living should be a joy, not a chore. One of the downers in midlife is recognizing that we are no longer protected by the invincibility of youth. One of its joys is recognizing that we now have the wisdom and experience we need to take control of our health and make choices that matter.

The chapters that follow are filled with lots of sensible and practical suggestions based on the latest research. We would like to tell you that there is a new miracle drug to prevent cancer or reverse aging. That just isn't the case. We'd like to describe a hot new aphrodisiac that will improve your sex life. In reality, intimate relationships in midlife must struggle and evolve in the same way that the people involved adjust and change. We'd like to suggest that a multivitamin can replace a varied, healthy diet or that an exercise machine can do it for you. Alas, the road to good health in midlife remains largely dependent on three key ideas: a positive approach, moderation, and consistency.

At the same time, we believe that healthy living can be a lot more fun that it sounds. Humour, adventure, friendship, intimacy, optimism, good sex, challenge, relaxation, and pleasure are every bit as important to the quality of your life as eating well and staying active. When we view health-enhancing practices as pleasurable and allow ourselves to have fun we win twice: first in the immediate enjoyment and second in long-term health gains.[3]

Making Changes That Last

All of us have the ability to make changes in our lives. We can work to improve our economic situations, to become more nurturing people, to stop something that is hurting our health or to start something that will improve our health. When our goals for change are realistic and pleasurable, we stand a much better chance of succeeding.

Success is not always automatic or quick. How many of us have started an exercise program only to find that three weeks later we are back to old habits of working day and night? How many of us have lost and gained the same ten pounds a dozen times? How many of us have resolved to leave a painful relationship or an unsatisfying job only to find ourselves resigned to more of the same because we cannot move beyond contemplating the change we need?

When aikido master George Leonard teaches, he says that you must learn to "love the plateau," those long stretches of time and practice when nothing seems to be happening. It is in these periods that you consolidate your gains and ready yourself for the next growth spurt.[4]

After many years of studying the way that humans change, behavioural researcher James Prochaska and his colleagues have managed to explain the process of change through a model called the Stages of Change.[5] The model suggests that making changes involves a series of stages or steps through which we must progress. Whether you are trying to lose weight, quit smoking, or change the way you deal with stress, permanent change is best achieved in slow, steady stages that sometimes have to be repeated more than once or twice. Knowing which of the five stages you are in at any point can help you gauge your progress and choose strategies to help you move forward. Understanding that you are *not* a failure if you slip and that your efforts will help you succeed in the long run minimizes frustration and helps you believe in your own ability to change.

The Stages of Change Process

1. *Precontemplation*: In this stage you are not thinking seriously about change. This is a good time to seek information. What are the advantages and disadvantages of continuing the way things are?
2. *Contemplation*: You are thinking about making a change in the near future. You talk about wanting to change, but are not yet ready to actually do it. It is easy to get stuck in this stage. At this point you really need to understand your behaviour patterns. When do you react badly to stress? How much are you drinking or eating? When and where do you overeat? What will you gain by making a change?

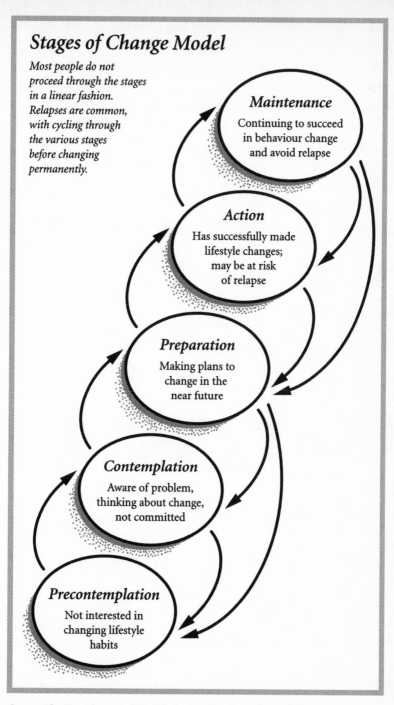

Stages of Change Model

Most people do not proceed through the stages in a linear fashion. Relapses are common, with cycling through the various stages before changing permanently.

Maintenance
Continuing to succeed in behaviour change and avoid relapse

Action
Has successfully made lifestyle changes; may be at risk of relapse

Preparation
Making plans to change in the near future

Contemplation
Aware of problem, thinking about change, not committed

Precontemplation
Not interested in changing lifestyle habits

Source: The Transtheoretical Model *developed by Prochaska and DiClemente*

3. *Preparation*: You are motivated to take action and you begin to take small steps – say you give up smoking after meals or start taking a walk at lunchtime. This is the time to make a firm decision to change and take steps to ensure that you will follow through. What has worked for you before? What strengths do you have when it comes to making a particular change? How can you build on these?

4. *Action*: You have overcome the major hurdles to getting started. You have cut down on your drinking or quit smoking. Give yourself a hand by substituting enjoyable activities – say going to a movie instead of a smoky hangout. Don't try to do too much too fast. Set yourself short-term goals and reward yourself.

5. *Maintenance*: You are starting to feel the benefits of your healthy change, even though you may still feel a sense of loss. Enjoy yourself and the knowledge that you have made a change that is good for you. Reinforce your commitment by telling others how you feel. Avoid temptation by making changes in your environment – get your family to agree to have fruit instead of sweet desserts for a few weeks, remove all ashtrays from the house, eliminate a weekly meeting that causes you stress.

Be prepared to relapse and repeat the cycle through several of these stages. This is a normal part of the process. Over time you will see that you do not go back to the starting point each time; gradually you gain ground. Each time, you learn from your previous experience. Ultimately you can succeed.

THE BOTTOM LINE

One of the joys of midlife is recognizing that we now have the wisdom and experience we need to take control of our health and make choices that matter. When our goals for change are realistic and pleasurable, we have a much better chance of succeeding. Making changes involves a series of stages or steps through which we must progress. Don't give up. Knowing where you are in this cycle and recognizing that you are *not* a failure if you slip will help you succeed in the long run.

Contacts and Further Information

Books

- *Changing for Good* by J. Prochaska, J. Norcross, and C. Diclemente. New York: Avon Books, 1995.
- *Healthy Pleasures* by R. Ornstein and D. Sobel. New York: Addison Wesley, 1989.
- *Life 101* by John-Roger McWilliams and Peter McWilliams. Los Angeles: Prelude Press, 1991.
- *Mastery: The Keys to Success and Long-Term Fulfillment* by George Leonard. New York: Plume Books, 1992.

Related Chapters in This Book

- The model of change described in this chapter can be applied to many of the personal health practices described in other chapters of this book.
- *Chapter 1: The Midlife Journey* will help you situate your plans for lifestyle changes within the broader context of the midlife journey.
- *Chapter 16: Partners in Health Care* provides additional information on how to seek out and use information on the Internet, and how to invest in preventive health care.
- *Chapter 23: Body, Mind, and Soul* reminds us that well-being is about more than physical health.

CHAPTER SIX

Wrinkles, Chin Hairs, and Baldness

Wrinkles should merely indicate where smiles have been.
— Mark Twain

Attached or unattached, male or female, fit or flabby, there comes a time when none of us can deny that our bodies are changing. We gain weight, we start to see "smile" lines on our faces that don't disappear. By age forty-five, many of us are wearing bifocals to correct problems in near vision. Midlife men bemoan hair loss, reduced muscle strength, and protruding bellies. Women are quietly dismayed over the mysterious appearance of chin hairs, skin tags, bunions, and woody toenails.

In this chapter, we'll look at some of the unrealistic media-driven standards of youth and beauty that we too often use to judge ourselves. With an eye to looking and feeling our best at any age, we'll examine two areas of particular interest to midlife women and men – aging skin and hair loss. Weight changes are discussed in Chapter 8. This chapter concludes with a key message about embracing change, learning to like the person we now see in the mirror, and looking outward to the riches of life around us.

Unrealistic Standards
The billions of dollars North American women and men spend on cosmetics, cosmetic surgery, diet books, and ab machines attest to the baby boomer's overwhelming desire to resist physical aging. "Forever Young" – singer Bob Dylan's anthem to a generation who believed they would never grow old – has become a common headline in newspaper and magazine articles that describe how midlife men and women can stop or reverse the passage of time.

Midlife men and women who find themselves in search of a new partner may be particularly vulnerable to worries about their appearance. One of the men we interviewed told us that he had been separated from his wife for eight months and was considering the idea of going out with a new woman. She was a colleague at work who was quite a bit younger than he was. "The truth is," he told us, "I'm worried about looking old. I'm starting to lose my hair and I've put on weight, even though I'm still pretty active. I'm afraid she won't think I'm attractive."

In many ways, boomers have succeeded in the quest to stay youthful. We are healthier and we live longer than the previous generation. Women in their forties and fifties are entering triathalons and having babies. Studies show that some men who stay lean and active into old age function as if they were twenty years younger.[1] Yet despite these real triumphs, many remain fixated on youth as the standard of beauty and virility for all of us.

Those standards have become increasingly unrealistic. In the 1990s, the average fashion model weighed twenty-five pounds less than a model in the 1950s.[2] Television, men's magazines, and movies portray male virility only as young, well-muscled men with full heads of hair who ski down glaciers and rock-climb in their spare time. Media images aimed at midlife women feature slim, taut bodies and wrinkle-free faces, with silver hair being the only concession to aging. Today, as never before, advertising compels us to shop for a new face, better hair, and a sculpted body. Aging has become a judgement we place on ourselves and others, rather than a biological reality."

The most visible signs of aging show up in our mirrors every day – frown and smile lines that don't disappear, sagging skin around the eyes. One woman laughed as she told us about bending over to touch her toes and having this strange sensation that something was pushing against her eyes. A glance in the mirror revealed that her cheeks, no longer youthfully elastic, were moving up and down with her!

Changes in body composition and in the skin and hair are a natural part of the aging process. However, as we experience these changes, we will be in serious trouble if we continue to look to media-driven, youth-centred standards for validation of our attractiveness – and, by extension, of our self-worth. Men who believe that their virility and attractiveness to women are dependent on looking like youthful idols Brad Pitt or Leonardo DiCaprio are sadly deluding themselves. They risk chasing a fantasy and missing out on the riches of this time in their lives. For most women, the overwhelming need to stay slim and youthful-looking is even greater.

Many midlife women describe themselves as feeling suddenly invisible to men. "I always got a reaction or at least a look from men when I walked into a room," said one woman. "Now they don't even know that I'm there." While some women may feel relieved by this new-found sense of freedom, those women who have defined themselves by the amount of attention men gave them may suffer a major loss of self-esteem when they feel male eyes pass over them.

This is not to say that we should let ourselves go to pot or refuse to consider cosmetic changes. While we cannot, and need not, stop the normal aging process, we can claim the beauty and richness of the age we are. Practising healthy living is one of the most important things we can do to keep our bodies both healthy and attractive. And with a grounded sense of self that celebrates our strengths in all areas, there is nothing wrong with wanting to look one's best. When Gloria Steinem turned fifty and people commented that she certainly didn't look her age, she replied, "This is what fifty looks like."

So, the challenge and opportunity of midlife become threefold:

- to reject the stereotypes that define us by inappropriate and distorted standards;
- to claim the beauty and virility of the age we are, both inwardly and outwardly; and
- to choose a healthy lifestyle and take care of our bodies as we grow older.

Healthy Skin for Life

As we age, our skin becomes drier, because of reduced oil production. To keep your skin moist, avoid the use of hot, soapy water and make use of moisturizing lotion.

Most women and men begin to show some signs of facial wrinkling by their mid-thirties. People with fair skin and blond or red hair tend to wrinkle earlier; in fact, the darker your complexion, the more wrinkle-resistant your skin is likely to be. What causes wrinkling? Smoking and drinking too much alcohol are both factors, but the number-one cause of premature wrinkling is the same risk factor as that for developing skin cancer – repeated exposure to the sun. Sun damage has a cumulative effect. In midlife, we begin to pay for all those times we fried ourselves on the beach as teenagers.

Ultraviolet skin damage, or "photo-aging," accounts for 90 to 95 per cent of all cosmetic skin blemishes and wrinkling.[3] Think of tanning as a dose of radiation – the UVB rays burn, tan, and damage the skin; the UVA rays (including those used in tanning salon lamps) exacerbate photo-aging as they penetrate deep into the skin's layers. The sun's rays also accelerate the degeneration of skin elastin and prematurely break down collagen, the protein that gives the skin its wrinkle-resistant elasticity.

Deadly Sunspots

In North America, the incidence of skin cancer, including malignant melanoma (its most serious form), has been steadily increasing since the late sixties. Obviously, protecting yourself from skin cancer is essential to your health. In so doing, you can also slow down the process of photo-aging.

In 1997 in Canada, new cases and deaths from melanoma among men were at an all-time high, and almost double the rates for women.[4] Cataracts – which can be a long-term outcome of excessive sun exposure – were reported by some 660,000 people.[5] In the United States, new cases of the often-fatal melanoma have also increased. For every 100,000 white women in the United States, 11.2 new cases of melanoma were diagnosed in 1992, compared to only 5.9 cases in 1973 – a 90-per-cent increase. White men were hit even harder: for every 100,000, there were 16.7 new cases in 1992, compared to 6.7 in 1973 – nearly a 150-per-cent increase. (African Americans rarely get melanoma.) This rise, however, shows signs of plateauing, perhaps because North Americans are starting to heed advice about staying out of the sun and using sunscreen.[6]

A national Canadian study has shown that there is little variation in sun exposure between men and women (except for outdoor workers, who often tend to be male). Men are far less likely than women to take routine sun-protection measures. For example, men were only half as likely as women to use sunblock.[7] Some key advice for preventing skin cancer is given in the box below. And to protect your eyes, wear good UV-resistant sunglasses.

SOME KEY ADVICE ON SUN PROTECTION

- Shun the sun between 11 a.m. and 3 p.m.
- Seek out shady spots at the beach and on outdoor patios.
- Be wary of reflected sunlight: 80 per cent of UV rays bounce off water, sand, cement, or snow.
- Wear long pants and long-sleeved shirts when you expect to be in the sun for a period of time; protect your face and head with a wide-brimmed hat (especially if you have hair loss).
- Beware of clouds: 80 per cent of UV rays can penetrate light clouds, mist, and fog.
- Cover exposed areas with sunscreen that has an SPF (sun protection factor) of 30. Apply sunscreen 30 to 60 minutes before you go out; it is not effective immediately. Re-apply it throughout the day, especially after swimming.
- Never use sun lamps or tanning salons.
- Ask your physician how to examine your skin for pre-cancerous spots.
- Be aware that certain prescription medicines and the use of Retin-A cream make the skin more vulnerable to sunlight.

Midlife Skin Indignities

Picture your aging mother or grandfather's hands. In all likelihood you remember that they were sprinkled with brown patches called age or liver spots. And now – God forbid – they have started to appear on *your* hands or forearms! Rest easy. These hyper-pigmented spots have nothing to do with your liver and little to do with your age. They are a reaction to years of overexposure to the sun – your skin's way of protecting itself from burning, by increasing its production of melanin, the substance that gives your skin colour.

Using a sunscreen with an SPF of 30 is the best way to avoid age spots or to keep them from darkening. If they really bother you, talk with a dermatologist about options for getting rid of the spots. She or he may suggest topical treatments that bleach spots, such as hydroquinone cream, creams containing Retin-A and/or alpha hydroxy acids, or liquid nitrogen.

Most liver spots are harmless, sun-induced patches. It is a good idea, however, to point out any new ones when you see your physician, since pre-cancerous spots can sometimes look like ordinary liver spots. If one appears suddenly, bleeds, or changes colour or shape, see a doctor immediately.

Three other skin indignities are:

- Cherry angiomas – These small, pinhead-size red dots are totally benign.
- Seborrheic keratosis – These soft, waxy, raised skin spots are benign; however, have them checked regularly.
- Skin tags – These small, benign pieces of skin can be embarrassing and annoying.

New Help for Wrinkles and Aging Skin

While creams and facials have traditionally been seen as a female concern, modern science and changing values have greatly increased men's interest in products and procedures that rejuvenate the skin. These techniques will not remove deep furrows, jowls, or bags under the eyes, but they can improve your skin's quality, texture, and glow. For good care of your skin, consider these three approaches:

1. Use sunscreen to prevent photo-aging. The best protection is prevention.
2. Use moisturizers in the morning and evening. The best remedy for dry skin is water. A good moisturizer works by restoring water to the outer layer of the skin. It does not penetrate the deeper layer of skin, so the effect is temporary.
3. Try medicated creams. Studies show that using creams containing tretinoin or AHA (alpha hydroxy acid derived from sugar cane, sour milk, or fruit) twice a day can lead to improvements in collagen, elastic fibres, pigmentation, and skin thickness. AHA is found in dozens of products in various strengths. Be aware that a concentration less than 8 per cent has not been shown to make a difference.[8] Tretinoin creams (a derivative of vitamin A) have been shown to reverse some of the milder signs of photo-aging. New variations of these creams such as Renova, Reversa, and Rejuva-A, designed especially for aging skin, are now on the market. Studies have shown a successful toning down of fine lines, age spots, and rough patches

after twenty-four weeks using these creams.[9] If you use vitamin A products, however, be aware that tretinoin increases the skin's sensitivity to sun, which can lead to sunburns if it is used during the day without a sunscreen. Tretinoin creams vary in cost, usually from $20 to $80 a tube or bottle.

Recently, scientists have also developed a liquid form of vitamin C, which appears to be effective in smoothing out wrinkles and could be used in the future to protect against skin cancer. Cosmetic companies have begun adding vitamins C, E, and beta-carotene to their skin-care products in the hope that these antioxidants can prevent skin damage.

4. Enjoy a healthy diet that includes yellow vegetables (vitamin A), nuts (vitamin E), and fruit (vitamin C), and drink six to eight glasses of water daily.
5. Exercise regularly.
6. Note that hormone replacement therapy (HRT) has been shown to thicken and moisturize the skin; however, it does not affect wrinkles.

Skin-Resurfacing Techniques

Skin-resurfacing techniques include chemical peels, dermabrasion, and laser therapy. They all take away the top layer of skin to expose and promote the growth of fresh, new skin.

Chemical peels vary in strength. The light "lunch-time peel" is quick and requires no recovery time. It is usually done in a series of four to six peels, and its benefits last about six months. Some dermatologists recommend a monthly regimen of the peels, which cost about $90 each time. Medium trichloroacetic acid (TCA) peels are used for more advanced skin damage; they usually require pain medication and seven to ten days to heal after each treatment. Heavy phenol peels effectively help reverse serious damage caused by the sun or acne; however, they are highly uncomfortable and it is recommended they be done by a dermatologist or cosmetic surgeon. Phenol peels cost about $2,000; TCA peels cost about $1,500 for a full face.

One woman told us that she felt a little embarrassed going for her first lunch-time peel. She said, "At first I felt I was buying into the cultural myth of trying to look younger than my years. But afterward, I realized that the benefit was not looking younger but feeling better."

Dermabrasion involves the use of a wire brush to remove deep wrinkles. Laser skin therapy uses a computerized laser to remove wrinkles that could previously be treated only with deep peels. Some dermatologists believe that this procedure will soon replace face-lifts as a preferred way to improve appearance and skin quality.

Laser therapy reduces superficial or moderately deep wrinkles and age spots, as well as removing spider veins and unwanted hair. Some of these procedures involve a general anesthetic and similar recovery time, and may cost up to $5,000. Cosmetic surgeons usually perform laser therapy and dermabrasion.

Other Procedures

There are now a great variety of plastic-surgery procedures performed under local anesthetic. The cost of these procedures can vary greatly. One of the most popular is blepharoplasty: surgically removing fat and excessive skin around the eyes. Goldie Hawn, in the made-for-boomers movie *The First Wives Club*, immortalized another common treatment called collagen injection, a low-risk procedure that helps to smooth out wrinkles (and, in Goldie's case, produce sexy, puffy lips). The effect lasts only three to six months, however, since collagen is biodegradable.

Liposuction is a surgical procedure used to remove fat from the chin and cheeks. Botulin injections may be used to relax frown lines; this will last for six months.

TREATMENT OPTIONS FOR AGING SKIN

Condition	Causes	Treatment(s)
Fine facial wrinkles	sun damage	➤ use sunscreen (SPF 30)
		➤ AHA and vitamin-A creams
	smoking	➤ quit smoking and drink water

Moderate wrinkles and age spots	sun damage	→ chemical peels with AHA (least aggressive), trichloroacetic acid or phenol (most aggressive)
Drooping eyelids	age and heredity	→ eyelid-lift
Deep wrinkles	sun damage	→ collagen injections → dermabrasion → botulin injections
Acne scarring	severe acne	→ laser therapy

If you are considering any of the surgical procedures, we suggest that you take some time to think about why you want to do it. These procedures are costly, temporary, often painful, and require substantial healing and recovery time. Will they help you look your best now, or are you on a futile search for your lost youth? For anything more severe than a "lunch-time peel," ask your family physician or dermatologist for a referral, or contact your state or provincial College of Physicians and Surgeons for names of reputable physicians who offer these treatments.

Hair Today, Gone Tomorrow?

Our hair turns grey as we age because the production of pigment at the root of the hair follicles gradually slows down. First, we find the odd grey hair around our temples; then, whole colonies of them seem to appear. By age fifty, half of the population (both men and women) has pronounced greying. While many people find grey hair attractive (especially on men), others vacillate between the decision to colour it or go "au natural."

Most of us can deal with grey hair. Losing your hair, on the other hand, can be very upsetting for midlife men. Conversely, midlife women are sometimes horrified to find that menopause triggers new hair growth, usually on the face or chin. The mention of chin hairs always brings a laugh of recognition in our seminars with midlife women. If you are faced with the occasional chin hair, it is easy enough to pluck it out. If you have excessive hair growth, contact your physician. Excessive growth of hair in women can have a number of causes, including the use of certain drugs and increased production of the male hormone testosterone. Your physician will advise you on appropriate treatment.

For most men, going bald can be painful. Take heart. The notion that bald men are unattractive or past their prime is passé in the 1990s. In fact, many athletes and younger men are shaving their heads in a bid to look more virile.

Balding is a common phenomenon: 12 per cent of men are balding at age 25, 37 per cent at age 35, and 45 per cent at age 45. By age 65, two-thirds of men are bald or balding.[10] Male-pattern baldness manifests itself in two ways: hair is lost over the temples (receding hairline) or from the crown of the head, forming a circular bald patch.

No one is quite sure why this occurs. Researchers suspect that male-pattern baldness – called androgenic alopecia in the medical literature – is related to testosterone action (although levels of testosterone remain normal in bald men). Severe stress, serious illness, and some medications can cause the hair to thin. Contrary to popular myth, though, male-pattern baldness is inherited from both parents.[11] Heredity also determines at what age thinning starts and the pattern of baldness that will follow.

If balding is in your family's history, it is probably best to come to terms with it. Keep your hair healthy by eating a diet that has adequate vitamins and minerals. Enrich your hair with conditioners that give the illusion of thicker hair. Wear it short, neat, and natural-looking. You might get a mild perm – it makes your hair look fuller.

If you are convinced that you cannot accept balding, however, there are several options available.

1. Propecia – a low-dose form of finasteride (a drug used to treat prostate problems) – has been shown to effectively combat male-pattern hair loss. In a controlled study, the drug promoted new hair growth in 66 per cent of men, compared to 7 per cent of men who used a placebo. Men with mild to moderate, but not complete, hair loss are most likely to benefit from the use of propecia. Taking one pill a day for three months is generally necessary to see if the medication

works for you. When you stop taking it, you start to lose your hair again within twelve months.[12]

2. The drug minoxidil was originally developed to treat high blood pressure. One of its side-effects was excessive hair growth. Now it is available under the brand name Rogaine as a hair-restoring treatment that you rub on your scalp twice a day. Tests have shown that it reduces hair loss in about 30 per cent of users. It works best on men who have just started to lose their hair; it will not grow hair back on a spot that is already bald.[13] Minoxidil does have some drawbacks. It takes four to six months to see if it works. If it does work, you have to continue treatment indefinitely at a cost of $45 to $85 a month.

3. Surgery is a more radical option that can be effective. Having administered a local anesthetic, doctors transplant hairs from the back of the head to the balding spot. The procedure is time-consuming and can cost anywhere from $5,000 to $15,000. A hair-lift, sometimes called a scalp reduction, is another option. The surgeon cuts away the bald spot from the top of the head, then stretches hair-bearing parts of your scalp over it. This procedure costs between $1,500 and $3,000.

4. Toupees have a bad reputation. There are probably more jokes about "rugs" than there are about baldness itself. But if you are willing to spend as much as $1,000, you can get an excellent artificial hairpiece that looks natural and stays in place.

DID YOU KNOW?

The normal scalp contains between 100,000 and 150,000 hairs. Normally, each hair grows two to four years, is dormant for two to four months and then falls out. At any time, 90 to 95 per cent of our hair is in a growing phase and we lose or shed approximately 100 hairs a day. When a man has androgen-induced hair loss, this cycle is disrupted, and he sheds more hair. Women lose less hair because they have higher estrogen levels and fewer androgens in their bodies.[14]

Male and Female Differences in Midlife

The following list of facts and fallacies highlights some of the differences and similarities between men and women in the areas discussed in this chapter:

Fallacy: Men in midlife tend to have rougher, older-looking skin than women do.

Fact: Despite the hours of skin care and the amount of money that women invest in skin products, men have a clear advantage. Men's skin is 10 to 15 per cent thicker, so it has more collagen to begin with; menopause accelerates collagen loss in women. Men also benefit from shaving, which helps keep the skin smooth by scraping off dead skin cells.

Fallacy: Midlife men are not interested in cosmetic-surgery techniques.

Fact: According to the American Society of Plastic and Reconstructive Surgeons, about 400,000 elective cosmetic surgeries are performed every year. A full 12 per cent of the people who undergo these procedures are men. Some individual cosmetic surgeons report that men make up about 20 per cent of their practices. Some of the most popular procedures are nose reshaping, eyelid surgery, scalp reduction, hair transplants, dermabrasion, and chemical peels.[15]

Fallacy: Men and women experience the same age-related changes in the body.

Fact: While men and women experience similar age-related changes in the body, some of these changes may occur earlier or be more severe in one particular sex (see chart below). Differences are usually mediated by the sex hormones.[16]

AGE-RELATED CHANGES IN WOMEN AND MEN

Change	*Who is most severely affected*
Dimming vision	women
Loss of brain cells	men

Loss of bone density	women
Grey hair	both
Excessive growth of eyebrows	both
Loss of facial hair	men
Growth of facial hair	women
Thinning, dry skin	women
Loss of height	both
Spreading feet	both
Decline in sex hormones	women

Liking the Person You See in Your Mirror

In her book *Mirror, Mirror: The Terror of Not Being Young*, Elissa Melamed writes, "Women are made to feel ashamed that they age and those that age less quickly are made to feel superior to those who don't. In this way, the double standard reinforces our denial of aging." She poses some tough questions worth considering by both women and men:

- Do you tell your real age? If not, when did you start concealing it?
- Does your real age match the age you feel inside?
- Can you imagine yourself older?
- How do you feel when you look in the mirror?[17]

Our feelings about how we look are dramatically intertwined with how we value ourselves and our potency in our relationships, communities, and cultures. The baby-boom generation has the opportunity to challenge the existing rigid definitions of youthful attractiveness and develop new, more appropriate expressions of mature beauty. When feminist writer Carolyn Heilbrun is complimented that she looks younger than her years, she replies, "No, I am not young. I am an older woman with pizazz, which is not the same thing."[18]

The journey through midlife is about looking inward to build upon the strengths, experience, and wisdom we have gained through these years. Focusing on trying to stay forever young cuts us off from the richness of who we have become and the beauty of life around us. As Germaine Greer puts it, "It is only when we stop the fretful struggle to be beautiful that we can look outward, find the beautiful, and feast on it."[19]

THE BOTTOM LINE
It's okay to take measures to help you look your best at any age. Ultimately, however, we will feel that inner glow when we are fulfilled, engaged with life, and affirming of our unique beauty and value.

Contacts and Further Information

Organizations
- American Academy of Dermatology, P.O. Box 4014, Schaumburg, IL. Tel.: (847) 330–0230; Fax: (847) 330–0050; Web: http://www.aad.org
- American Cancer Society, 1599 Clifton Rd. N.E., Atlanta, GA 30329. Tel.: (404) 320–3333; Fax: (512) 927–5791; Web: http://www.cancer.org
- American Society of Plastic and Reconstructive Surgeons, 444 East Algonquin Rd., Arlington Heights, IL 60005–4664. Tel.: (847) 228–9900; Fax: (847) 228–9131; Web: http://www.plasticsurgery.org
- Canadian Cancer Society, 10 Alcorn Ave., Toronto, ON M4V 3B1. Tel.: (416) 961–7223; Fax: (416) 961–4189; Web: http://www.cancer.ca
- Canadian Dermatology Association, 774 Echo Drive, Suite 521, Ottawa, ON K1S 5N8. Tel.: (613) 730–6262; Fax: (613) 730–1116
- Canadian Society of Plastic Surgeons, 30 St. Joseph Blvd. E., Suite 917, Montreal, QC H2T 1G9. Tel.: (514) 843–5415; Fax: (514) 843–7005; Web: http://www.plasticsurgery.ca

Websites
On Skin Care
- American Society of Aesthetic Plastic Surgery: http://surgery.org
- American Society of Dermatologists (sponsored by Pharmacia and Upjohn Inc.): http://www.asd.org
- University of British Columbia and the Vancouver Hospital and Health Sciences Centre: http://dermweb.com

On Melanoma
- American Cancer Society: http://www.cancer.org

- Canadian Cancer Society: http://cancer.ca
- Melanomanet (sponsored by the American Academy of Dermatologists): http://www.derm-infonet/melanomanet

On Hair Loss
- University of British Columbia Hair Research and Treatment Centre: http://dermweb.com/hairinfo/

Books
- *The Beauty Myth* by Naomi Wolf. Toronto: Vintage Books, 1991.
- *Mirror, Mirror: The Terror of Not Being Young* by Elissa Melamed. New York: Linden Press/Simon & Schuster, 1983.
- *Young as You Look: Medical and Natural Alternatives to Improve Your Appearance* by Dr. Don Groot and Patricia Johnston. Edmonton: InForum, 1993.
- *Young Skin for Life* by Julie Davis and the Editors of *Prevention* magazine. Emmaus, PA: Rodale Press, 1995.

Related Chapters in This Book
- *Chapter 1: The Midlife Journey* provides the larger context of the midlife journey.
- *Chapter 4: The Search for the Fountain of Youth* discusses theories of aging, the normal process of aging, and some emerging ideas on staying young.
- *Chapter 7: The Active Living Solution* and *Chapter 8: Food for Thought: Healthy Eating in Midlife* provide information on how regular exercise and healthy eating can influence how you age and how you look as you grow older.
- *Chapter 9: The Boomer's Drugs of Choice* provides information on quitting smoking and reducing alcohol intake – both of which can accelerate the aging of the skin.

The Active Living Solution

> Studies have shown that an eighty-year-old who leads an optimally active lifestyle can have the same functioning and energy capacity as a forty-year-old who is sedentary.
>
> – Dr. William Orban, exercise physiologist and creator of the Canadian 5BX exercise program for troops in the Second World War[1]

Denise's interest in active living began as a way to combat feelings of exhaustion and occasional insomnia. At fifty, she was beginning to experience menopausal symptoms. She found her job as a grade-three teacher increasingly stressful. When she told her best friend how she felt, her friend told her how much better she had felt since she started walking on a regular basis. After three weeks of procrastinating, Denise bought a hand-held cassette player and started going for long walks while listening to some of her favourite tapes. Her sleeping began to improve and she increased her walking time to forty-five minutes every other day.

At age forty-five, **Barry** decided to take up wind-surfing in order to spend more time with his teenaged sons. His first few attempts were frustrating. He was out of shape – he had given up running when he suffered a back injury and then got involved in a new project at work. He did not have the upper-body strength he needed to repeatedly haul the heavy sail out of the water each time he fell. His brother-in-law explained that technique was as important as strength and encouraged him to keep trying. After a few days, Barry was tacking across the lake with a happy, determined grin on his face. (Tacking back was another matter.)

"When we returned to the city, I was determined to keep it up," said Barry. "I joined the Y and started a fitness program that stressed strength, flexibility, and cardiovascular endurance. I bought a second-hand board and a book on wind-surfing. Now I keep in shape all year, partly because I feel better and partly so I can enjoy sailing with the boys in the summer."

The baby boomers made "fitness" not only acceptable but trendy in the 1970s and 1980s. Triathalons, aerobic dancing, cross-training, fitness testing, employee fitness, exercise videos, and a multi-billion-dollar sports-shoe industry are all products of the Big Generation's discovery that "working out" helps keep us energetic, youthful, and healthy. It is ironic, therefore, that many of us get out of the routine when we hit the middle years. Like Denise and Barry, we let work, family responsibilities, aging bodies, and excuses get in the way of doing something for ourselves that we know will make us feel and function better.

In this chapter, we give you the latest information on how to choose, start, and continue to enjoy an optimal active-living program in midlife. In doing so, we stress the importance of finding a routine that suits your needs, ability, and personal goals. We also deal with the role of physical activity in preventing and alleviating back pain – one of the most common musculoskeletal problems experienced in midlife – particularly by men.

The Real Fountain of Youth
There is solid evidence that moderate, regular physical activity can increase both the quantity and quality of the second forty or fifty years of your life. Regular exercise can help lower high blood pressure and improve blood cholesterol by increasing HDL levels (the good cholesterol). Active living protects you against heart disease, osteoporosis, diabetes, obesity, and some cancers.[2]

Barry's experience demonstrates how weight training and other activities can delay the decline in strength that usually accompanies aging. Some studies have shown improvements in strength and muscular endurance by 100 per cent in older adults.[3] This allows you to carry on with physical activities and sports that you enjoy. It also protects you from recurring back problems.

Physical activity is also good for your mental health. As Denise discovered, active people sleep better.[4] Regular physical activity can also help women deal with other menopausal discomforts, such as hot flashes, fatigue, and mood swings.[5] Aerobic exercise (the kind that makes your heart beat faster) reduces anxiety and improves a depressed mood and your ability to manage stress.[6] It provides a time for you to be free of the day's demands, to daydream, to be alone or with friends that you enjoy, to release pent-up emotions, and to feel strong. This is important for both men and women in midlife. Physical changes that accompany aging can lead to battered body images that are hard on self-esteem.

Studies have even reinforced the connection between regular exercise and a more vigorous sex life for both men and women. In a 1990 study by investigators at the University of California, a group of 500 middle-aged men who took part in a moderate aerobic exercise program reported more frequent sex and more satisfying orgasms than a control group who did not exercise. In addition to having more energy for sex, the men who exercised reduced their blood fat levels, encouraging better flow to the penile artery and thus stronger erections. Regular exercise may also keep you sexier longer. One study showed that master swimmers aged forty to seventy enjoyed making love about seven times a month, about the same frequency as twenty-six- to thirty-three-year-olds in the general population.[7]

Benefits of Various Activities

The following chart may help you choose the activities that will most benefit different aspects of your health.

ACTIVITY RATING CHART

\+ = some benefit

\++ = good benefit

\+++ = very good benefit

Activity	Weight control	Heart health	Bone strength	Muscle tone	Flexibility	Stress relief
aerobic dance	+++	+++	+++	++	++	++
basketball	++	++	+++	+	+	+++
bowling/curling	+	+	++	+	++	++
cycling						
5 mph (8.5 kmh)	+	+		+		+
10 mph (16 kmh)	++	+++		+		++

Activity	Weight control	Heart health	Bone strength	Muscle tone	Flexibility	Stress relief
calisthenics (incl. stretching)	+		+	+++	+++	
fast dancing	+	+	+	+	+	+++
golf (walking)	+	+	++	+	+	+++
hiking (some hills)	+++	+++	+++	+		+++
jogging	+++	+++	+++	+		+++
gardening & yard work	+	+	+	+	+	++
racquet sports (moderate)	+	+	++	+	+	++
rowing, canoeing	++	+++		+	+	+
skating & in-line skating	+++	+++	++	+	+	++
skiing downhill	+	+	+	+	+	++
cross-country	+++	+++	+++	++	++	+++
softball	+	+	+		+	+
stair climber	+++	+++	+++	+		++
swimming (continuous)	++	+++		+	+	+
volleyball	+	+	++	+	+	++
walking (4–5 mph/ 6–8 kmh)	++	++	+++			+++
weight training	++		+++	+++		
yoga, tai chi			++		+++	+++

Midlife Inaction

In light of the benefits of physical activity, you would think that the majority of boomers would be briskly walking and jogging their way to eternal youth. Unfortunately, this is not the case.

Approximately one-third of midlife women in the United States do not meet the basic requirements for moderate exercise; another one-third practise no leisure-time activity at all. In Canada, midlife women are only slightly more active (approximately 38 per cent) than their American sisters. Approximately 40 per cent of midlife men in the United States and Canada are active on a regular basis.[8, 9]

Why has the generation that created the fitness revolution and made marathon running a national pastime become a generation of couch potatoes? Surveys show that there are two main reasons: lack of time and lack of motivation. These are both legitimate reasons. Midlife is a busy time, when most men and women are at the height of career and family obligations. At the end of a long day, there is little appeal in the thought of jogging in the dark or climbing into a spandex outfit and feeling fat in a class full of hyped-up young exercisers. Humorist Erma Bombeck said, "The only reason I would take up jogging is so that I could hear heavy breathing again."[10]

But now there is a solution! Research has shown that you do not need to run marathons or spend two hours a day exercising to reap the benefits of active living. Active living is a kinder, gentler solution, and one that you can make part of your everyday routine. Even if you have never been active before or if you suffer from chronic health problems, you can reap the benefits of mild to moderate physical activity.

The Active Living Solution

Remember when your high-school coach used to say, "If it doesn't hurt, you aren't working hard enough," and the fitness gurus urged us to "go for the burn"? No more. Active living is a shift away from highly organized, high-intensity fitness approaches toward lifetime activities that place as much emphasis on enjoyment, sociability, quality of life, and personal growth as they do on aerobic capacity. So how much is enough? Will taking the stairs twice a day do it? How about housework or playing with the kids in the snow?

According to the recently released Surgeon General's *Report on Physical Activity and Health* and Canada's newly released *Physical Activity Guide to Healthy Active Living*, the basic recipe for disease prevention and healthy living is to be moderately active for a minimum of thirty minutes at least every other day (every day is preferred).[11] Moderate is defined as a bout of activity such as walking or raking leaves that burns about 150 calories (see the chart that follows). The key factor here seems to be fitting the thirty minutes, which does not have to be continuous, into your existing schedule. For example, get off the bus or subway a stop early and walk, take the stairs instead of the escalator, walk one or two flights before boarding the elevator. Every bit of exercise you do helps your heart, bones, and muscles as well as improving your mood and clearing your head.

If you like strenuous activity or are already active at least every other day for longer than thirty minutes, all the better. People who exercise more than the recommended guidelines will further improve their cardiovascular fitness, energy level, and overall well-being.

Ideally, in midlife you should also try to engage in some strengthening activities at least twice a week to improve the structure and functioning of your bones, joints, and muscles, and to rev up your calorie-burning capacity. This could be in the form of weight training, calisthenics, or activities that develop certain muscle groups (for example, canoeing and chopping wood develop upper-body strength; stair-climbing and skiing strengthen the legs). Everyday tasks such as pushing a stroller or carrying groceries are also good ways to develop your strength.

Midlife women should choose "weight-bearing" activities (in which you carry your weight) such as walking, dancing, skating, or skiing instead of "weight-supported" activities such as swimming or cycling, as well as working with small weights two to three times a week. These activities protect you from menopausal bone loss and strengthen your bone mass.[12]

THE ACTIVE LIVING SOLUTION IN MIDLIFE

1. Try to be active for 30 minutes every day (not necessarily continuous).
2. Every other day make your 30 minutes of activity continuous, moderate aerobic activity, such as brisk walking or cycling.
3. Stretch every day.
4. Add strength training two to three times per week.

Make physical activity a regular part of your schedule. Many of the beneficial effects of exercise training diminish within two weeks if physical activity is substantially reduced, and the effects disappear within two to eight months if physical activity is not resumed.

Sedentary people who are unused to exercise should start with short periods of moderate activity and gradually increase the duration or intensity until they reach their goal. People with chronic diseases such as heart problems or diabetes should consult with a physician before starting a new physical activity program and begin with small, gradual increases in everyday activities.

MODERATE ACTIVITIES THAT EXPEND 150 CALORIES

45 to 60 minutes of washing a car

45 to 60 minutes of washing floors or windows

45 minutes of recreational volleyball

30 to 45 minutes of touch football

30 to 40 minutes of wheeling self in wheelchair

35 minutes of walking (20-minute-mile pace)

30 minutes of golf (carrying clubs)

30 minutes of shooting baskets

30 minutes of cycling (5-miles-in-30-min. pace)

30 minutes of fast social dancing

30 minutes of pushing a stroller or wheelchair (1½ miles)

30 minutes of raking leaves

30 minutes of walking (15-minute-mile pace)

30 minutes of water aerobics

20 minutes of swimming laps

20 minutes of wheelchair basketball

15 to 20 minutes of basketball

15 minutes of cycling (4-miles-in-30-min. pace)

15 minutes of jumping rope

15 minutes of jogging (10-minute mile)

15 minutes of shovelling snow

15 minutes of stair climbing

The Time-and-Motivation Crunch

At forty-seven, **Carletta** understood that being active thirty minutes a day was good for her health, but other obligations always stood in the way. "I already put in eighteen-hour days," she said. "Where am I going to find thirty extra minutes?"

Then her family physician told her that her blood pressure was high. He urged her to get some exercise and lose a few pounds to avoid the necessity of going on medication. Carletta was frightened. Her mother had suffered chronic high blood pressure and had died of a stroke. She began to swim three mornings a week before work and she and her husband cycled on Sundays in preparation for a three-day bicycle trip. Her blood pressure dropped and she really enjoyed the activity.

Her resolve lasted three months. Her sisters were annoyed that Carletta had abandoned their traditional weekend brunch for cycling. After a month involving a lot of work-related travel, Carletta got out of the swimming habit. She still left home early, but she used the extra time to get caught up on extra office work. She took on a large commitment to run a local campaign for a voluntary agency. Six months later she was ragged and tired. Her blood pressure was higher than ever.

Carletta and her best friend talked about her inability to exercise regularly. "It's not that I dislike exercise," she said. "In fact I really like it when I am into it. It's just that other things seem more important, than, you know . . . me."

Carletta's realization that she valued work, other people's happiness, and charitable giving more than her own health was an eye-opener to her. She decided to take a practical approach, setting priorities, delegating more tasks, and letting some minor things go. This way she was able to build thirty minutes a day into her schedule in ways that would still allow her to do other things that were important to her. She told herself that time for herself was as important as time for others. "After all," she mused, "if I die, what use will I be to anyone?"

Carletta's experience is a common one. If active living is to become a way we live each day, we must learn to value our own needs and to enjoy the time we spend being active. For some, the initial motivation is health. For others it may be appearance or the desire to keep up with teenaged children. Tell yourself that you deserve it. If you persevere with activities that suit you, you will inevitably find the value of activity itself.

Tips for Starting and Sticking with It

People are at different stages of readiness when it comes to beginning an exercise program (see Chapter 5). The important thing is to start; any activity is better than none. Don't get discouraged if you stop after a time; just start again as soon as possible. Here are some ideas for increasing your motivation and commitment to active living.

Starting

- Join a club or group in an activity you enjoy or would like to learn (e.g., birding, nature hiking, tennis, curling). Take advantage of instruction and club activities that match you up for games and introduce you to others.
- Schedule time for exercise in your daybook, just as you do for meetings and other important tasks.
- Set realistic, short-term goals (e.g., to walk briskly for fifteen minutes at lunchtime, to exercise every second day). Keep track on the calendar and reward yourself for success. Tie your goals to physical accomplishments and feeling better, not to weight loss (which can diminish your enjoyment and commitment).
- Plan an active holiday with your partner, friends, or family members. Get in shape for a week of cycling, hiking, tennis, or camping. Studies show that people who exercise with others are more likely to stick with it.
- Commute the active way: cycle to work or walk partway. Think before you jump into the car. Can you walk or cycle on a particular errand or task?
- "Read" while you exercise. Books on tape are wonderful company on a long walk or when you are sitting on a stationary exercise bicycle. Some people keep themselves motivated by listening to music or a phone-in show.
- Consider investing in a few sessions with a personal trainer – he or she can provide you with a personalized plan, some company, and added motivation.

Sticking with It

- Train for and participate in active charity events (osteoporosis walk, runs for breast-cancer research, cycling for AIDS, walking for international development).

- Cross-training is a fancy word for variety. By combining activities you get a better work-out and you never get bored. Vary your pace, your space, and your fun.
- Take rest days when you need them.
- When you feel stressed is when you most need to exercise and are least inclined to do so. Even some stretching or a short walk can help you shift your energy.
- Concentrate on three-month stages. Research shows that exercisers who go past the first three months are more likely to stick with it.
- Use a birthday (turning forty, fifty, or sixty) as a an activity goal. Aim to run your first five-mile event, hike up a particular trail, or cycle to a predetermined spot by a particular date.
- Don't let travelling derail you. Use hotel fitness facilities and pools, walk to meetings or to explore a new city.
- If you stop working out, don't criticize yourself. Just start again.

From Fat to Fit

Yvonne had been trying to exercise regularly in order to lose a few pounds – with no success. Then she and two friends went on a holiday to London. They walked everywhere for twelve days. To Yvonne's surprise, she lost three pounds, despite her visits to British pubs.

Yvonne's experience is supported by Covert Bailey, exercise physiologist and author of *The New Fit or Fat*. Bailey makes the case that exercise (not dieting) is the only way to make the metabolic and chemical changes you need to lose weight and keep it off.[13] As we age, we inevitably lose muscle and gain fat, because we exercise less and often eat more. Even adults who weigh the same at age fifty-five as they did at age twenty-five have, in all likelihood, become fatter. They have replaced weight that once was muscle with weight in fat.

Two things happen as a result of this loss of musculature: changes in the chemistry within the muscle itself (which requires fewer calories) and a decrease in your overall body requirement for calories. Dieting may get rid of the fat under the skin, but only steady, aerobic exercise can change the body's chemistry from one that stores fat to one that burns fat. What kind of activity is best? Continuous (20 to 40 minutes) moderate aerobic activity that uses large muscle groups.

TOP TEN FAT BUSTERS

jogging*
cross-country skiing*
hiking
brisk walking (with or without a dog)*
skating, roller-blading
cycling*
aerobic dance
stair-climbing*
rowing,* paddling
swimming (least effective of the ten)

* outdoors or indoors on machines

Getting Strong

By age seventy, most people have lost 20 per cent of the muscle tissue they had at age thirty. Menopause may accelerate this decline. One study reported that menopausal women lost six times as much muscle tissue as women who were not menopausal.[14] Men start out with and continue to have a higher muscle-to-fat ratio than women; however, as men age, declines in testosterone levels and inactivity lead to a significant decline in their muscular strength and endurance. Muscle loss can dramatically affect how you look and function. Your strength declines (a major factor in sport performance and in everyday activities such as yard work and climbing stairs) and you put on fat because you have less active muscle tissue burning energy on a daily basis.

Benefits of Weight Training

Research has shown that moderate, regular strength training (or weight training) with free weights or machines can slow down and even reverse the muscle and strength loss that normally accompanies aging. Research at Tufts University has shown that men and women in their seventies who lifted weights (½ to 1 pound) strengthened the muscles in their legs, abdomens, and buttocks by 35 to 75 per cent. Participants in the weight-training program were also more likely than a control group to be active in recreational activities such as canoeing and cycling, and to have fewer falls and fewer difficulties performing tasks such as yard work and carrying groceries.[15]

What will weight training do for your appearance? Men will see some changes in the shape and size of their muscles over time. Women don't need to worry – weight training will not make you look like Arnold Schwarzenegger. To build muscle bulk (as opposed to muscle strength) you need to lift very heavy weights and have more testosterone in your system than women normally have. With a moderate resistance program, both men and women will see a loss of fat and a reduction in clothing sizes over time (as long as you do not overeat). Weight loss may not be dramatic since muscle weighs more than fat, but you will look more toned and fit. (Remember, if weight loss is your main goal, aerobic exercise is still the most important kind of activity, although adding strength training will accelerate the chemical changes in the muscle that increase fat burning.)

The benefits of weight training inside your body are just as important as the results you see outside. Strength training strengthens bones in both men and women. This is especially important for women at high risk for osteoporosis. Getting stronger is also a positive mood lifter. "Weight training made a tremendous difference in my downhill skiing," said one man we interviewed. "I could take the mountain without stopping, something I hadn't been able to do for the last four or five years. What a great feeling, to be able to keep up with my daughter and her boyfriend!" One fifty-year-old woman said, "Feeling strong makes me feel more in charge of my body and my life. I walk taller and I feel less tired at the end of the day."

How to Use Weights

How often should you train with weights? Research suggests that two to three times a week is enough – it is important to take a rest day in between. Most people do a combination of eight to ten exercises for all the major muscle groups: legs, trunk, shoulders, back, abdomen, and arms. If time is an issue, you can do the upper body one day, the lower body the next day, and then rest for a day. Lifting is done in "sets" of eight to twelve. Start with one set at a weight that allows you to do eight repetitions but challenges you at the same time; work your way up to two sets. Once you can comfortably perform two sets, it is time to bump up your weights.

Weight training can be done at home with free weights (dumbbells and ankle weights) or at a gym or club with machines. Technique (how you lift) is *very* important; it is easy to injure yourself if you lift the wrong way or start with too heavy a weight. As a result, the best way to begin weight training is to attend a course or one-on-one session with a qualified fitness instructor who will show you the proper way to lift or use the machines. If you are unused to exercise, or have joint problems or old athletic injuries, this is particularly important. You can also ask that a physiotherapist join the fitness instructor in helping design a routine that suits you. See Contacts and Further Information at the end of the chapter for help in finding a qualified fitness instructor.

Flat Abs and Back Pain

More than any other part of the body, "abs" have become an obsession in North America – owing largely to those muscled young models in television infomercials who demonstrate the latest ab trainer on television ten to twelve hours a day. In reality, most of these gadgets are no better than what you can do yourself with a form of sit-ups called abdominal crunches. Indeed, the improper use of ab machines can lead to back pain. And forget the guarantee of a "washboard stomach" in thirty days. Reducing a fat belly will take more than thirty days and you will need to do whole-body aerobic exercise, not just abdominal work. There is no such thing as spot reducing.

This does not mean you should abandon abdominal work. More than 80 per cent of North Americans experience back pain at some time, usually in mid- and later life. Back pain is a major cause of disability, particularly among men.

Most back problems are caused by weak abdominal muscles and underused back muscles, not by serious injury or disease. Fortunately, about 90 per cent of acute back problems spontaneously recover within one month. Persistent or chronic back pain, however, will likely require long-term treatment.

Exercise is essential in both preventing and treating back pain. Traditional guidelines suggesting bed rest for two weeks has been replaced by more positive advice to start gentle exercises and to move about every day when back pain strikes. Avoid activities that aggravate the pain (such as twisting or lifting), as well as prolonged sitting or driving. Gentle pelvic-tilt exercises (which flatten the lower back) are generally recommended, as well as a slow and gradual return to swimming, walking, or stationary bicycling.

Many people who have a tendency toward low back pain use a series of abdominal and back exercises to prevent recurrences of pain. One fifty-three-year-old man we interviewed explained that these exercises were as important to him as brushing his teeth every day. "It only takes five minutes in the morning," he said, "but if I don't do them, I pay the price."

Other advice on how to prevent back pain includes the following:

- wear low-heeled shoes;
- use a comfortable, ergonomically correct chair at work and at home;
- rest one foot on a low stool when standing or sitting;
- take breaks and walk around if you are sitting or standing for long periods of time;
- lose weight if you are overweight;
- sleep on your side in bed and put a pillow between your knees.

Flexibility and Aging

As we age, our flexibility (ability to stretch and move our joints through a full range of motion) naturally declines. You can prevent this decline with simple stretching exercises and staying active with gardening, dancing, and other activities that make you bend and stretch. Flexibility exercises can be done any time, anywhere, including the office. They will relieve tension and increase blood flow to the joints and muscles. This is especially important if you sit at a computer all day.

Get in the habit of warming up before activities with walking and stretching; stretch again at the end of your exercise session. This will prevent joint injuries and improve your flexibility. Yoga and tai chi (an ancient form of Chinese exercise) are also wonderful for flexibility, relaxation, and "calming" your thoughts and feelings. Why not visit a class in your community to see if these are activities you would like to try? One woman told us that she reluctantly went with a friend to her first yoga class and was amazed by the sense of well-being she had at the end of the class.

"It wasn't just the exercise," she said. "It was the feeling in the room that was so important. It has helped my depression and now I go regularly."

Are You Ready for an Active Lifestyle?

Most people can begin a moderate exercise program such as walking without worrying about getting hurt. The Physical Activity Readiness Questionnaire will help you decide if you should talk with your physician first.

PHYSICAL ACTIVITY READINESS QUESTIONNAIRE

If you answer "No" to the following 7 questions, you can be assured that it is safe for you to start on a gradual, sensible exercise program.

1. Has your doctor ever told you that you have a heart problem?
2. Do you frequently have pain in your chest or heart?
3. Do you often feel faint and weak or have spells of dizziness?
4. Has your doctor ever told you that you have high blood pressure?
5. Do you have a bone or joint problem that may get worse with exercise?
6. Is there a physical reason why you should not exercise?
7. Are you over 65 and unaccustomed to exercise?

If you answer "Yes" to one or more of these questions, talk with your physician about your intention to exercise. He or she may suggest an exercise stress test if you have several of the risk factors for heart disease or are experiencing any chest discomfort. One of the major advantages of this test (which is carried out on a treadmill in a laboratory) is the tailored exercise prescription and advice you will get from the exercise physiologist who administers the test. Make sure that this service is part of the procedure before you decide where to take it.

Fortunately, midlife is not too late to start to get active. Judy Flannery, a mother of five, started exercising at age thirty-eight. In 1997, at age forty-one, she was named Master Female Triathlete of the Year. Freelance writer

Denny Owen Harrigan began competitive rowing at age forty-five after a life on the sidelines. Psychotherapist Betty Larsen started practising yoga at age forty to help deal with chronic neck pain and stress. At age fifty-five she gave up counselling to teach yoga and run her own yoga studio.[16]

Whatever your age, be sensible about safety. Wear proper shoes and reflective tape if you walk at night. Wear a helmet when you cycle. Listen to your body and stop exercising if you feel pain. It is also important to pace yourself, both in terms of intensity and how often you participate in a particular activity. Runners are particularly prone to overuse injuries from constant pounding on the joints and muscles. "Weekend warriors," who do nothing all week then play full out in a weekend hockey or three-on-three basketball tournament, are asking for trouble. Train for sports and vary your activities. Be kind to your body . . . it's the only one you've got!

THE BOTTOM LINE

We all know that it's difficult to make the time commitment to an exercise routine. We also know that, when we do, we feel a lot better. Enjoy active living every day. Make exercise as enjoyable as you can, combining it with music you love, doing it with friends, or making it a relaxing time to be alone. Fit it into your existing routine whenever you can. Every little bit counts. If you stop being active, don't beat yourself up. Just start again.

Contacts and Further Information

Organizations

- Active Living Canada, 1600 James Naismith Dr., Suite 601, Gloucester, ON K1B 5N4. Tel.: (613) 748–5743; Fax: (613) 748–5734; E-mail: alc@rtm.activeliving.ca
- American Council of Exercise, 5820 Overland Dr., Suite 102, San Diego, CA 92121. Tel.: (800) 529–8227; Fax: (888) 348–3299.
- Melpomene Institute for Women's Health Research, 1010 University Ave., St. Paul, MN 55104. Tel.: (612) 642–1951.

- President's Council on Physical Fitness and Sports, 200 Independence Ave. S.W., Suite 738–H, Washington, DC 20201. Tel.: (202) 690–9000; Fax: (202) 690–5211.
- YMCA-USA, 101 N. Wacker Drive, Chicago, IL 60606. Tel.: (800) USA–YMCA; Fax: (312) 977–9063 or contact your local Y.
- YMCA of Canada, 42 Charles St. E., 6th Floor, Toronto, ON M4Y 1T4. Tel.: (416) 967–9622; Fax: (416) 967–9618, or contact your local Y.
- YWCA of/du Canada, 590 Jarvis St., 5th Floor, Toronto, ON M4Y 2J4. Tel.: (416) 962–8881; Fax: (416) 962–8084, or contact your local Y.

Websites
- Active Living Canada: http://www.activeliving.ca
- Active Trainer (sponsored by Laser Media): http://www.interactivefitness.com
- Fitness Link (sponsored by the American Council on Exercise): http://www.fitnesslink.com
- Fitness on the Net (sponsored by Balance Magazine): http://balance.net:80/
- Fitness Partner Connection Jumpsite (Fitness Partner): http://primusweb.com/fitnesspartner/
- Great Outdoor Recreation (various commercial sponsors): http://www.gorp.com/default.html
- Healthy Way (sponsored by Sympatico, trademark of Media Linx Interactive): http://www.sympatico.ca/healthyway
- Melpomene Institute: http://www.melpomene.org
- YMCA of Canada: http://www.ymca.ca

Books
- *Active Living: The Miracle Medicine for a Long and Healthy Life* by Gordon Stewart. Champaign, IL: Human Kinetics, 1995.
- *The Bodywise Woman* (2nd ed.) by Judy Mahle Lutter and Lynn Jaffee, Melpomene Institute for Women's Health Research. Champaign, IL: Human Kinetics, 1996.
- *Canada's Physical Activity Guide to Healthy Active Living*. To order (free) call 1–888–334–9769 (toll free) or fax 1–819–779–2833.

- *Fit over Forty* by James Rippe. New York: William Morrow, 1997.
- *LifeFit: An Effective Exercise Program for Optimal Health and a Longer Life* by Ralph Paffenbarger and Eric Olsen. Champaign, IL: Human Kinetics, 1996.
- *Smart Exercise* (1994) and *The New Fit or Fat* (1991) by Covert Bailey. Boston: Houghton Mifflin.
- *Stretching* by Bob Anderson. Bolinas, CA: Shelter Publications, 1977.
- *Strong Women Stay Young* by Miriam Nelson. New York: Bantam Books, 1997.

Related Chapters in This Book

- *Chapter 2: Understanding the Female Menopause* and *Chapter 3: Is There a Male Menopause?* show how physical activity can help you overcome both the short- and long-term concerns associated with the menopausal period.
- *Chapter 4: The Search for the Fountain of Youth* describes the use-it-or-lose-it theory of how active living prolongs life and prevents disease.
- *Chapter 5: Making Changes That Last!* walks you through the stages of making a permanent lifestyle change.
- *Chapter 8: Food for Thought: Healthy Eating in Midlife* provides more information on healthy eating and how to achieve and maintain a healthy weight.
- *Chapter 13: Stress-Proofing in Midlife* talks about how exercise and mind-body activities in particular can help you manage stress.
- *Chapter 17: Keep Your Bones Strong* helps you assess your risk for osteoporosis and provides information on preventing this disease.
- *Chapter 20: You Gotta Have Heart!* provides additional information on active living and heart health.
- *Chapter 23: Body, Mind, and Soul* touches on the links between physical activity, body-mind activities, and spirituality.

CHAPTER EIGHT

Food for Thought:
Healthy Eating in Midlife

There is no love sincerer than the love of food.
— George Bernard Shaw[1]

Nutrition in Midlife: What's New?

"Soy," "flaxseed," "cholesterol-free products," "tofu," "olestra." Hardly a day goes by that we do not hear of some nutrition breakthrough that may be the secret to preventing disease, stalling aging, and helping us keep our collective waists from expanding still further. But what is really important about eating in midlife? Why should it be any different than eating for good health at any age?

The answer is twofold. First, as we age our risk for chronic illness increases. Cardiovascular disease, cancer, osteoporosis, and diabetes are no longer vague health problems that apply to "older" people. As we approach ages forty-five or fifty, even those who have paid attention to nutrition throughout their lives become more aware of the need to understand how healthy eating can reduce our chances of developing a serious illness.

The second concern in midlife is the "creeping overweight syndrome." Every year that we age, our metabolism slows down. Unless we eat more carefully and exercise regularly, a few pounds creep on each year. Ten years later, an annual weight gain of two or three pounds has become a total of thirty pounds – an increase that could contribute to the development of a serious health problem. This change is compounded by an increase in fat tissue and a decrease in lean muscle tissue. As we will see later in this chapter, increased fat in the abdominal area is associated with a higher risk for cardiovascular disease.

Surveys suggest that most educated consumers recognize the link between what they eat and how they feel and perform. But often they are confused by the vast number of (sometimes conflicting) messages about nutrition. And while we recognize the importance of healthy eating, we need food options that are fast and flexible, that enable us to eat on the run and that are quick and easy to prepare.[2]

This chapter gives you the information you need to make informed decisions about healthy eating in midlife. It encourages you to make an investment in your health by paying attention to what and how you eat. It does not offer magic solutions, instant weight loss, or empty guarantees of a disease-free, long life. It does provide you with solid advice based on what science currently has to say about healthy eating and healthy weight in midlife. Our main conclusion is no surprise! Variety, balance, and moderation are still the best ways to stay healthy and add pleasure and good taste to your meals and snacks.

Back to Basics

Before we discuss the two main concerns about nutrition in midlife, let's review the basic guidelines that apply to all of us at all ages. Most people are familiar with the Canadian rainbow or the American pyramid, which illustrate the basic principles of healthy eating. But before you skip this section because (ho-hum) you've seen it all before, take a minute to review these common-sense guidelines, to think about what they mean in midlife, and to ask yourself how you put them into practice.

These guidelines fall within the context of what nutritionists call the "total diet concept." This theory contends that no single food is "good" or "bad." Your overall pattern of eating over a period of time is what matters. The nutritional characteristics of any one food or meal can be balanced by the choices you make at other meals and on other days to build a pattern of healthy eating.

Think about food in two categories:

- "Everyday" foods are nutrient-rich ones – fruits, vegetables, whole grains, protein foods, and low-fat milk products – which we need to eat every day to stay healthy.
- "Sometimes" foods are high in energy – pop, ice cream, potato

chips, cookies. Enjoy these foods in moderation, because they are lower in nutrients and higher in calories than everyday foods.

Guidelines to Healthy Eating

Enjoy a variety of foods. Did you know that most families have ten basic recipes that they recycle week after week? Try adding one new meal to that repertoire, perhaps one based on vegetables, beans, or a recipe from another culture. Eating foods with a variety of tastes, textures, and colours increases our enjoyment of eating, while ensuring that we get the nutrients and other food components we need.

Emphasize cereals, breads, other grain products, vegetables, and fruit. Build your meals and snacks around whole-grain products, vegetables, and fruit. While this guideline is important at any age, the link between these foods and the prevention of cancer and heart disease becomes especially important as we get older.

Choose lower-fat dairy products, leaner meats, and foods prepared with little or no fat. Most North Americans still consume too much fat; yet cutting down on fat does not mean cutting it out entirely. You can limit the portion size of meat, use cooking methods other than frying, choose reduced-fat milk products, and make other small changes in how you eat. For example, switching from cream to 2-per-cent milk in your two daily cups of coffee can eliminate some 100 calories' worth of fat each day – the equivalent of eating approximately two pats of butter. Since each gram of fat contains almost twice as many calories as a gram of protein or carbohydrate, this point is especially important if you are concerned about maintaining a healthy weight. Lowering the fat in your diet at the same time that you increase the amount of fruits, vegetables (including legumes), and fibre-rich grain products you eat may also reduce your risk of developing high blood pressure, heart disease, and certain cancers. (See the next section.)

Achieve and maintain a healthy body weight by enjoying regular physical activity and healthy eating. Some 45 per cent of Canadian men and 40 per cent of women aged forty-five to sixty-four are at high risk for health problems because they are overweight.[3] In the United States the proportion of Caucasian men and women in this age group is similar. Among African Americans, 45 per cent of women are overweight compared to 22 per cent of men.[4] There is as yet no biological explanation for this difference. As you will read later in this chapter, the secret to weight management is to concentrate on regular exercise and healthy eating rather than restrictive dieting.

Limit salt, alcohol, and caffeine. This guideline increases in importance with age since excessive amounts of sodium, caffeine, and alcohol can negatively affect your bone health. As bone loss is a consequence of aging in both women and men (and a factor in the development of osteoporosis), it is increasingly important in our midlife years to eat a calcium-rich diet that strengthens our bones and to limit our consumption of products that weaken them. Eliminating or limiting our intake of alcohol was a key recommendation in a recently released report from the World Cancer Research Fund and the American Institute for Cancer Research. Alcohol has been linked with an increased risk for certain cancers, especially breast cancer.[5] Limiting salt is also prudent, since salt can aggravate high blood pressure in people who are sensitive to sodium.

Eat to Beat Chronic Diseases That Appear after Age Forty

"Antioxidants," "isoflavones," "lyco . . . who?" A new language has emerged from our growing knowledge about the critical role that plant foods play in preventing heart disease, cancer, and other chronic illnesses.

Vegetables, fruits, legumes, and whole grains supply us with many of the nutrients our bodies require. They also are a rich source of fibre, which can provide protection against heart disease, stroke, and some cancers. However, the health benefits of these foods extend beyond these well-known factors. Plant foods also contain phytochemicals – the term used to define some health-enhancing, but non-nutrient, components in plant foods.

Phytoestrogens in plants can either block or enhance estrogen in the body. Research is currently under way to investigate their potential to alleviate menopausal symptoms such as hot flashes, as well as their potential in protecting against heart disease, bone loss, and cancer (more about this later in this chapter).

Other phytochemicals act as antioxidants – scavengers that protect against the harmful effects of oxidation in the cells. As mentioned in Chapter 4, when body cells use oxygen, they form "free radicals," which can damage cells and tissues, just as exposing metal to the air will cause it to rust. This cell damage may lead to health problems such as cancer, heart disease, arthritis, and other deterioration that accompanies aging. Antioxidants convert free radicals into harmless waste products that are eliminated before they do any damage; in addition, they may help undo damage that is already done.

GOOD FOOD SOURCES FOR PHYTOCHEMICALS

Food Sources	Phytochemical	Possible Benefits
Cruciferous vegetables (broccoli, cabbage, cauliflower, brussels sprouts)	Indoles: isothiocyanates such as carotenoids	May prevent cell damage that can lead to some forms of cancer.
Orange and yellow fruits and vegetables (carrots, sweet potatoes, winter squash, cantaloupe)	Carotenoids such as beta-carotene, lutein	May strengthen immune system, prevent retinal damage, help prevent cancer.
Tomatoes (especially cooked)	Lycopene	Antioxidant, may reduce risk for prostate cancer.
Soy foods (e.g., tofu, soy milk, etc.)	Isoflavonoids	Weak source of estrogen which acts in a selected way. May help reduce blood cholesterol, protect against breast cancer, and provide relief for menopausal symptoms.

Flax products	Lignans	Estrogenic effect may help reduce blood cholesterol, protect against breast cancer, and provide relief for symptoms associated with menopause.
Garlic, onions, chives, leeks	Allylic sulphides Phytosterols	May reduce risk for stomach and colon cancer.
Legumes (lima, kidney and navy beans, lentils)	Isoflavonoids Phytoserols	May help prevent cancer and heart disease.
Red grapes, red wine	Flavonols	May benefit the heart, prevent damage to cells, and curb tumour growth.
Citrus fruits	Flavanones Carotenoids	May fight cancer and act as an antioxidant.
Tea (green, black, oolong)	Flavonols Polyphenols	May reduce cancer risk and act as an antioxidant.

Source: "Beyond Vitamins: The New Nutrition Revolution," *University of California at Berkeley Wellness Letter*, April 1999.

Eating Fruits, Vegetables, and Whole Grains Does Make a Difference
More than 200 studies from around the world show that populations eating five or more servings of vegetables and fruit per day are less likely to develop heart disease and cancer.[6] This is the basis of the well-known

American campaign "Eat five a day," which urges people to eat at least five fruits and vegetables each day.

Canada's Food Guide to Healthy Eating recommends five to ten servings of vegetables and fruit a day, and the U.S. Food Pyramid recommends eating between three and five servings of vegetables and between two and four servings of fruits each day, depending on calorie needs. Only one in five adults meets these guidelines; the average person eats only three servings per day. In addition most adults eat only one serving per day of whole grains (versus the recommended three servings).[7]

Finding the time to plan ahead and make sure that you eat at least five fruits and vegetables and three servings of whole-grain products each day can be challenging. Here are some painless, non-time-consuming ways to make sure that you get the number of servings of vegetables, fruits, and whole grains that you require:

- Start your day with fruit and whole-grain cereal. Studies show that those who include fruit or juice in their breakfast are virtually the only people to reach the magic number of five a day or more.
- Rethink your meals. Make meat an accompaniment to your meal, not the main dish. Build your meals and snacks around grain products, vegetables, and fruit by filling three-quarters of your plate with these foods.
- Go for variety. Did you know that red peppers, mangoes, and kiwis have as much as or more vitamin C than oranges?
- Chase the food rainbow (a new, visual presentation of Canada's Food Guide to Healthy Eating). Aim to eat a fruit or vegetable of every fall colour each day: red, orange, yellow, and dark green. Try carrots, sweet potatoes, kale, broccoli, various squashes, and dark-coloured salad greens like spinach. Choose romaine lettuce over iceberg – the darker the colour, the richer the food is in nutrients.
- Add a meatless meal to your weekly repertoire. Plan it around whole grains, legumes, and other veggies. Red beans with rice or lentils with pasta are high-protein, low-fat, delicious alternatives to meat dishes. Bean salads and soups can be part of both hearty and light meals.
- Make canned tomatoes and beans (chickpeas, kidney beans, etc.) shopping staples. Add them to soups, chilies, and pastas for quick meals. Keep frozen beans, corn, and peas on hand.

- Whip up a delicious fruit smoothie, made with fresh or frozen fruit, skim or 1-per-cent milk or fortified soya beverage, and low-fat yogurt.
- No time to prepare vegetables? Use convenient bagged and ready-to-serve salads, baby carrots, and frozen vegetables. Get in the habit of washing and chopping your vegetables as soon as you bring them home from the grocery store. For example, wash, chop, and store carrots, celery, cauliflower, and broccoli for use any time you need them. Wash and dry lettuce, then wrap it in a tea-towel or put it in a crisper for easy use.
- Snack on cut vegetables and fruits. Low-fat cottage cheese or yogurt make great dips. Try roasted soy beans or chickpeas for crunchy snacks or as toppings on salads.
- Slip an apple or orange into your briefcase. Planning to work over lunch? Bring along some whole-wheat pitas or "wraps" filled with veggies and bean dips.

Wash fresh fruits and vegetables thoroughly with water to remove surface dirt and pesticides. Use a vegetable brush on produce like carrots, squash, apples, and pears. Remove the outer leaves on lettuce, cabbage, and other leafy greens. If you are still concerned about pesticides, consider purchasing organically grown fruits and vegetables. More and more are available at local supermarkets.

The Vitamin and Mineral Connection

Almost every week a new headline claims that certain vitamins and minerals can help ward off disease. Some of these claims have solid evidence to back them up; some show promise in preliminary results and are awaiting results from larger studies. Others, which are based on small studies with conflicting results, are exaggerated or misleading. As of the spring of 1999, here are some of the most promising findings for women and men in midlife to consider.

Folate (folic acid, folacin): Scientists now have proof positive that folic acid helps prevent birth disorders such as spina bifida. If you know a woman who is planning to conceive or is pregnant now (or if you are planning to have a baby yourself), suggest that she take a multivitamin containing 400 mcg of folic acid every day.[8] Even if you are beyond the thought of having a child, ensure that your diet is rich in folate by eating plenty of legumes, fruits, and vegetables. Studies have shown that people who eat a diet high in folic acid have a reduced risk for heart disease.[9, 10] A daily intake of 0.4 mg of folic acid appears to lower homocysteine levels in the blood (high levels of homocysteine are linked to increased risk for heart disease). Vitamin B6, found in non-citrus fruits, poultry, beef, beans, and certain vegetables, is thought to work along with folate to control homocysteine (see Chapter 20). Do not take higher doses of folic-acid supplements than are recommended: taking too much can mask the symptoms of B12 deficiency, which results in neurological damage.

SOME GOOD FOOD SOURCES OF FOLIC ACID

Fruits and vegetables	*Legumes*
• asparagus	• baked beans
• brussels sprouts	• chickpeas
• spinach	• kidney beans
• broccoli	• peanuts, peanut butter
• cauliflower	• sunflower seeds
• corn	
• beets	
• peas	
• bean sprouts	
• tomato juice	
• oranges, orange juice	
• cantaloupe	
• honeydew melon	

Vitamin E Several studies have shown a significant reduction in heart disease among men taking a high dose of supplemental vitamin E (400–800 international units (IU) per day).[11] Other large studies have shown a reduction in heart disease in men and women who took at least 100 IU a day.[12] A 1998 study of some 30,000 men showed that an even smaller dose (50 IU a day) appears to protect against prostate cancer.[13] In addition, many women find that vitamin E supplements relieve hot flashes associated with menopause. Vitamin E is found in vegetable oils, salad dressings, margarine, wheat germ, seeds, nuts, and peanut butter. While we await clinical trials to decide on both proof and recommended amounts, some dietitians suggest that it may be prudent to take a vitamin E supplement, since optimal levels (400 IU) are very difficult to obtain through diet alone.[14]

Beta-Carotene Beta-carotene is found in yellow-orange fruits and vegetables such as cantaloupes, peaches, carrots, apricots, and sweet potatoes, as well as dark-green leafy vegetables such as collard and spinach. Beta-carotene has consistently been shown to provide protection against cervical cancer and possible protection against breast cancer. However, the 1995 U.S. Physicians Health Study of 22,000 mostly non-smoking males showed that taking 50 mg of beta-carotene every other day for twelve years had no effect, positive or negative, on whether they developed cancer. Then another study of Finnish smokers and ex-smokers was halted when they found an increased risk of lung cancer by 18 per cent among smokers taking a beta-carotene supplement. What to do? Eat plenty of beta-carotene-rich foods but forget the supplements for now, especially if you are a smoker.[15]

Vitamin C Vitamin C is found in many fruits and vegetables, including grapefruit, oranges, strawberries, broccoli, kale, red peppers, and potatoes. Convincing studies have demonstrated a protective effect of vitamin C against cancers of the upper digestive tract and possibly for breast cancer. Most people can get the recommended intake of 250 to 500 mg of vitamin C per day. Since the body cannot absorb more than 500 mg per day, large doses above this amount are counterproductive and could be harmful.[16]

Selenium In the spring of 1997, a major study appeared in which 1,300 people who had been treated for skin cancer were given 22 mcg of selenium every day for four years. While the supplement did not prevent the recurrence of skin cancer, the selenium group did have a significantly lowered risk of developing prostate, colon, and lung cancer.[17] Since this evidence is preliminary, food, not supplements, is still your best source. You find selenium in a wide variety of foods, including meat, chicken, seafood, and grains, so eating a healthy diet should give you the amount you require.

Calcium This main builder of bones and teeth is found in dairy products, canned salmon, or sardines eaten with the bones, almonds, tofu (especially the kind made with calcium), kale, seaweed, and broccoli. Most plant foods contain small amounts of calcium compared to milk products, however, and it is not readily absorbed. Aging and menopause decrease the amount of calcium we absorb, which can increase your risk for osteoporosis. Women over age fifty and men over sixty-five require at least 1,200 mg of calcium each day. If you eat or drink three to four servings of milk products or fortified soya beverage per day and eat a varied, healthy diet, you are probably consuming enough calcium. Calcium-rich milk also contains other important nutrients such as vitamin D and magnesium, which help the body absorb and use calcium. If you cannot get enough calcium in your daily diet, consider taking a calcium supplement.

Iron In women, iron deficiency can be an outcome of heavy bleeding during the menopausal period. This can lead to anemia, which causes fatigue, weakness, and poor performance. Iron is found in animal sources such as red meat (heme iron) and plant sources such as legumes, soybeans, peanut butter, and enriched cereals (non-heme iron). Heme iron is absorbed more readily than non-heme iron. Vegetarians and others who prefer not to eat much meat can enhance the absorption of non-heme iron by eating a food that is rich in vitamin C at the same time.

Should I Take Vitamin and Mineral Supplements?

Contrary to the media hype suggesting that supplements are the answer to ensuring health and longevity, research suggests that supplements do not provide the same health benefits that food does. If you regularly eat a healthy diet of at least 1,800 calories that follows Canada's Food Guide to Healthy Eating or the U.S. Food Pyramid, you are probably getting the amount and variety of vitamins and minerals that your body needs. However, there are several exceptions:

- Vegans (who eat no animal products whatsoever) may require extra vitamin B12, vitamin D, and calcium.
- People who are ill or regularly take medications may require a vitamin supplement (for example, the long-term use of Aspirin for arthritis).

- Smoking increases the body's need for vitamin C. Drinking excessive amounts of alcohol can interfere with the body's use of some vitamins.
- Perimenopausal women who have very heavy periods may require an iron supplement.
- Women in midlife who do not drink milk or who have below-normal bone density will benefit from a calcium supplement.
- If you have a family history of heart disease or have several risk factors for heart disease, it may be wise to take vitamin E supplements, since it is difficult to get enough through foods alone. You may also want to take folic-acid supplements.
- Lastly, people who are unable (or unwilling) to consume a healthy diet may benefit from taking a multivitamin supplement as insurance.

If you are unsure about your nutritional status or your need to take supplements, consult a registered dietitian. To find one, call your local public health department or hospital, or ask your family physician. Just as a personal trainer can help you design a safe and effective exercise program, a registered dietitian can help you plan and manage a healthy diet that suits your needs. You can also contact one of the organizations listed at the end of this chapter.

If you do decide to take a supplement, remember that no supplement will replace a healthy diet. Choose a vitamin-mineral combination that addresses your midlife needs. Buy supplements from a reputable company. If you have further questions, ask a dietitian, pharmacist, or your health care provider for advice.

The Phytoestrogen Story
There are two main categories of phytoestrogens:
- **Lignans** are highly concentrated in flaxseed (also called linseed) and are also found in much smaller amounts in seaweed, whole grains, and some fruits and vegetables. Compared to hormone medications, the amount of estrogen in these foods is very small. However, when eaten in fairly large amounts, they can have an estrogen-like effect on the body.
- **Isoflavonoids** are mainly found in soy products, and to a lesser extent in chickpeas and other legumes. The level of isoflavonoids

found in a particular product can vary greatly according to how they are prepared.

The idea that foods containing phytoestrogens might relieve hot flashes was inspired by the finding that only 18 per cent of women in China and 14 per cent of women in Singapore – who typically eat many more soy foods than Western women do – have hot flashes, compared to 70 to 80 per cent of women in Western countries. Several studies have shown that this is the case: soy ingestion does appear to lessen the severity of hot flashes.[18] This is exciting news for women who are looking for alternatives to HRT as they go through menopause. One forty-eight-year-old woman told us, "My mother and sister had breast cancer, so the idea of using HRT scares me. I started to eat a lot of flaxseed and soy to control my hot flashes. Now I feel great!"

It has also been proposed that phytoestrogen consumption may protect against osteoporosis, since Asian women have much a much lower risk for hip fractures than Western women; at this point, this may relate to any number of factors, and cannot be attributed solely to diet.[19]

Studies suggest that populations with a higher intake of foods containing phytoestrogens have a lowered incidence of cancer of the breast, endometrium, and prostate.[20] In addition, a 1995 study published in the *New England Journal of Medicine*, which pooled data from several studies, concluded that eating soy products that are rich in phytoestrogens helped to lower levels of blood cholesterol and triglycerides.[21] So, while more research is needed, the potential benefits of food containing phytoestrogens seems very promising for both women and men.

Flaxseed breads are now available in most food stores. You can add your own seeds to hot cereal or granola or add ground seeds to muffins, pancakes, and loaves. The next section also gives you some practical ideas on how to include soy products in your diet.

Soy: More than Just a Hill of Beans

Dr. James Anderson, well-known for his research in fibre and soy protein, recommends at least seven servings of soy per week for healthy people, 14 servings a week for those aiming to prevent hot flashes and heart disease, and 21 servings per week for those who want to try to reverse osteoporosis or current heart disease.[22]

HOW MUCH SOY DO I NEED?

	Servings/day*	Isoflavones per day
Healthy person	1	16–20 mg
Prevent heart disease and hot flashes	2	32–40 mg
Reverse heart disease and osteoporosis	3	48–60 mg

* One serving = 4 oz. tofu or 8 oz. soy beverage or 2 soy muffins or 1 tbsp. isolated soy protein

Fine, but how do you eat it? One woman told us the answer was to be inventive: "My children joke about how, next time, there will probably be soy in their birthday cakes."

A growing number of soy products are now available in your grocery store or health-food store including:

- **Tofu** is white, odourless, and sold covered in water. Buy firm tofu with a cheese-like texture and marinate it in garlic, ginger, soy sauce, and sesame oil for use in stir fries, pizzas, pasta dishes, kabobs, tacos, stews, and salads. Use soft tofu in sauces, dips, and as a substitute for cottage cheese in lasagna. Look for tofu processed with calcium instead of magnesium if you want to add calcium to your diet, too.
- **Tempeh**, a fermented bean product, has a walnut-like taste and can replace meat in any dish.
- **Miso** is a salty fermented soybean paste that is often used in Asian soups.
- **Soy beverages** can substitute for milk in soups and puddings or as an additional beverage. Look for brands fortified with calcium.
- **Soy nuts**, roasted, are rich in isoflavones and make a delicious crunchy snack.
- **Soy flour** can substitute for a one-quarter cup of flour in most cases, except in bread recipes that require gluten to work.
- **Soy-powder isolate** is one of the most effective ways to eat soy. Be

sure to get powders that have not been washed in alcohol (this destroys the isoflavones) and do not buy powders mixed with other supplements. Try a soy smoothie: add two scoops of plain vanilla or chocolate soy-protein isolate to low-fat milk or juice. Add fruit and whip it up in the blender. Delicious!

- **Soy-protein low-fat bars** are now available in many stores.

Forget about soy sauce and soy cheeses – the isoflavones are washed away during processing. Many brands of soy hot dogs and burgers have the same problem. Nor are supplements the answer. There are not yet enough studies on the quality of soy supplements and whether or not they produce benefits similar to the real thing.

The Skinny on Fat

As we age, our potential for heart attacks and strokes increases. This makes it imperative to keep our dietary fat intake to 30 per cent or less of the total calories we take in each day. You also need to watch the kinds of fats you eat. Most dietitians recommend the following:

- Reduce your intake of saturated (hard) fatty acids found in meat, cheese, butter, and most pastries and cakes. High intakes of saturated fatty acid raise your risk for heart disease and possibly for colon and prostate cancer.
- Trans fatty acids (formed when oils are partially hydrogenated to make margarine and shortening) may raise blood cholesterol as much as saturated fats, so eat margarine, french fries, and dough-nuts sparingly.
- Unsaturated fatty acids (liquid oils) are preferred. Many foods with monounsaturated fats (found in olive oil, canola oil, peanut oil, avo-cadoes, nuts, and seeds) contain antioxidants. Polyunsaturated fatty acids (found in most vegetable oils, fish oil, and oily fishes) contain fatty acids, which may in fact help reduce heart-disease risks. So stir-fry in small amounts of canola oil and enjoy a small amount of olive oil on your salad. When it comes to fat, think small!

Are Low-Fat Products Worth It?

In some cases, the efforts of the food industry to introduce lower-fat products have been a boon to healthy eating. For example, the addition of

1-per-cent-fat milk has helped many middle-aged North Americans who did not enjoy skim milk lower their fat intake while continuing to get the calcium they need from dairy products. Using small amounts of lower-fat salad dressings also helps reduce the overall amount of fat in your diet.

On the other hand, eating a lot of the latest low-fat processed products (such as cakes, cookies, and snacks) can be a big mistake – especially if they replace more nutritious foods such as fruits, vegetables, and whole-grain products. Low-fat or no-fat products are usually expensive, and often they contain the same calories that the regular versions do! In addition, there is a temptation to ignore our internal cues and eat more of these products – because they are low fat.

What about olestra and other "fake fats," which taste like fat and pass right through the body undigested? A dieter's dream? Hardly. The problem with a compound that slips straight through the digestive tract is twofold: it may cause cramps and diarrhea, and it takes the fat-soluble vitamins and carotenoids in the stomach along with it.

The Creeping Overweight Syndrome

As we have already mentioned, in our forties and fifties, three dramatic changes that affect our weight and appearance take place:

- The first is that a change in body composition – reduced muscle mass and increased body fat – becomes increasingly obvious. To some extent, this is part of the natural aging process. Even people who maintain their weight at the same level will find an increase in their fat level and a loss of lean muscle tissue.
- Second, the body's metabolism (the rate at which you burn calories at rest), which begins to slow down in our early twenties, continues to decrease about 10 per cent for every decade that follows. This means that, if you want to maintain your weight (and your fat-free mass) as you get older, you need to choose your foods more carefully.
- Third, changes in the distribution of body fat are common as we age. Men and women tend to deposit more fat around their middles. Unfortunately, these changes are associated with a higher risk for cardiovascular disease. The theory is that fat cells in the abdomen metabolize more quickly than fat cells in other parts of the body

and, therefore, release more fatty acids into the blood. This can translate into elevated blood fat levels.

Does menopause or the use of HRT (hormone replacement therapy) cause weight gain? While weight gain is common at menopause, the contributing factors are not yet clearly understood. When Rena Wing and her colleagues studied weight change in 485 midlife women, they concluded that weight gain owed more to other factors than merely to menopause and hormone changes.[23] Another study of 875 women aged forty-five to sixty-five discovered that women taking HRT gained less weight than those taking a placebo. The investigation concluded that their weight gain had more to do with lifestyle changes such as a lack of exercise than the use of HRT.[24]

So what does make a difference? Henry Kahn and colleagues surveyed 80,000 healthy Caucasians, forty to fifty-four years old, in 1982 and again in 1992. The approximately 25,000 who did not gain weight were compared with the approximately 50,000 who did. They found that weight gain was less likely in people who reported eating more vegetables (at least 20 servings per week) and in those who exercised regularly (jogging at least one to three hours a week or walking, doing aerobics, gardening, or doing yard work at least four hours a week).[25]

Coming to Terms with a Middle-Aged Body

By the time we reach midlife, most of us understand that healthy bodies come in many different sizes and shapes. This intellectual understanding, however, almost never applies to ourselves.

Many of the men we interviewed talked about their concerns over weight gain and growing bellies. The women we talked with expressed even greater concerns. One woman described her experience: "After age forty, I started to gain weight, despite all my efforts to stay slim. I went back on the Pill to sort out my periods and my weight shot up another fifteen pounds. I paid more attention to how I dressed, and I got rid of the grey hair. But the weight really affected my self-esteem. I was embarrassed in a bathing suit. I was uncomfortable standing naked in front of my husband. I felt like an old woman in an unattractive body."

Negative body images and a preoccupation with weight are not new in midlife. Studies show that many young women (and increasingly young men) who have healthy weights or are underweight see themselves as overweight. This distorted perception is the result of social conditioning in a culture that worships thinness and perpetuates unrealistic weight standards, especially for women. Barbie and Ken recently turned fifty years of age. And neither has gained an ounce of fat or an inch around their middles!

There is nothing wrong with wanting to maintain a healthy weight. The problem comes when women and men measure their self-worth with the scales and see their maturing figures as personal failures. This can lead to a preoccupation with weight, excessive dieting, over-exercising, or despair – the very opposite of what we know creates and maintains a healthy weight.

What Should You Weigh?

When it comes right down to it, health – not unrealistic social standards – should be the way we determine our weight goal. Fortunately, there are two tools to help you predict health risk – the Body Mass Index and the Waist-Measurement Test (see the next section).[26]

The Body Mass Index

The Body Mass Index (BMI) can help you judge whether you are at risk for health problems associated with an unhealthy weight. It is designed for adult men and women aged twenty to sixty-five years (except for pregnant or lactating women). It may not apply to very muscular people and endurance athletes like marathon runners.

How to Find Your BMI

1. Mark an X at your height on line A.
2. Mark an X at your weight on line B.
3. Use a ruler to join the two Xs.
4. To find your BMI, extend the ruler to line C.
    Example:
*   If Tom is 5' 11" (1.80 m) and weighs 188 lbs (85 kg), his BMI is 26.
*   If Susan is 5' 4" (1.62 m) and weighs 132 lbs (60 kg), her BMI is 23.

What Your BMI Means

Under 20: A BMI under 20 may be associated with health problems for some people. Consult a dietitian or physician for advice.

20 to 25: This is the healthy weight–range zone. It is associated with the lowest

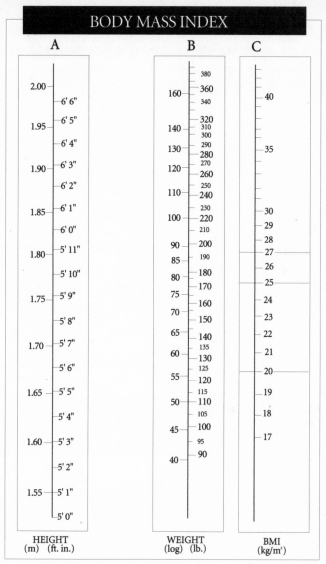

Adapted from a chart produced by Health and Welfare Canada

risk of illness and with living longer. This is the range you want to stay in.

25 to 27: A BMI over 25 is associated with health problems for some people. Caution is suggested if your BMI is in this zone.

Over 27: A BMI over 27 is associated with increased risk of health problems, such as heart disease, high blood pressure, and diabetes. Consult a dietitian or physician for advice.

Are You an Apple or a Pear?

When it comes to health, being shaped like an apple (with more fat deposited around your middle) can be riskier than being shaped like a pear (with extra fat deposited around the hips and thigh area). As mentioned earlier, studies show that extra fat in the abdominal area is more closely linked to heart disease than fat deposited elsewhere.[27]

An easy way to find out if you are a pear or an apple is to measure your waist circumference. Men whose waist measurements are more than 40 inches (102 cm) and women whose waists are more than 35 inches (90 cm) are at higher risk for illness and early mortality.[28]

What can you do if you turn out to be an apple? While fat distribution is partially influenced by genes, smoking and drinking too many alcoholic beverages also seem to increase the fat we carry in the stomach area. What about spot-reducing exercises? Unfortunately, expensive aerobic machines and multiple abdominal crunches will do little if nothing to reduce fat in the abdominal region (although the latter will strengthen and tone your muscles). Aerobic exercise and strength training will help you lose fat all over your body, not in one specific place. After all, if spot reduction really worked, gum-chewers would have thin faces!

Focus on Healthy Behaviours

Genetics, age, health, culture, eating patterns, and physical-activity habits all play a role in determining body weight. And people can be healthy at a number of weights. It is time to stop thinking about weight loss as an end in itself and to think about improving our eating and physical-activity habits as worth-while goals in their own right.

While the Body Mass Index gives you an idea of what science says is a healthy weight range for you, the real sign of success is lasting improvements in lifestyle habits and learning to feel comfortable with your body. A healthy weight is the weight that you can naturally maintain through healthy eating and regular physical activity, not a weight that you can maintain only by ignoring body cues, starving yourself, or over-exercising.

New fad diets hit the media almost weekly. They appeal to us because they promise fast, easy results. These diets do not work over the long term.

When they go "off" the diet and resume old eating habits, most people regain all of the weight they have lost. Some people actually gain *more* weight, because their bodies store energy as protection against future deprivation. The emotional and social costs of dieting are also high – dieting isolates us and leaves us feeling frustrated and irritable.

So what is the answer? Enjoy food in moderate quantities and refocus attention on regular physical activity and positive self-esteem. Lasting weight loss and improved health can only happen when we make permanent changes in all of these areas. When our expectations are realistic and we do not try to follow strict eating plans, we have a better chance of achieving lasting success.

Enjoy Healthy Eating, Not Dieting

If you are a constant dieter and rely on being told how much, what, and when to eat, you have probably lost touch with your sense of hunger and feeling full. Here are some tips to help re-acquaint yourself with your body's natural cues for regulating food intake.

Hunger rating. Learn the difference between body hunger ("I need to eat") and appetite ("It tastes good. I want to eat more"). Try to recognize your "just full" feeling on a scale from starved to stuffed. If you substituted a package of stale crackers for that second helping, would you still eat more? When we are truly hungry, we would eat even the stale crackers.

Meal spacing. Starving usually leads to stuffing. Don't skip breakfast and other meals. Eat when your body tells you it is running out of fuel. This may be every three to four hours. Eating a snack at four o'clock in the afternoon helps prevent gorging at dinner by taking the edge off your hunger.

Rate of eating. Your body will send you the message that you are full, but it takes about twenty minutes. If you slow down your intake, you will end up eating less by the time the "full" signal reaches your brain.

Physical activity. Activity increases the amount of energy you burn. This allows you to eat enough food to feel satisfied and to get the nutrients your body needs. Physical activity also helps you recognize true hunger, and helps control eating due to boredom and stress by alleviating those conditions. It promotes positive self-esteem and an improved body image. These feelings help you maintain positive changes in how you eat.

Enjoy food. Retrain your taste buds to enjoy the fresh flavours of food without a lot of added fat. Strike a balance between "everyday" foods and "sometimes" foods. Savour the flavour, especially for your "sometimes" choices. Pretend that each bite is worth $100, and you want to get your money's worth out of each mouthful. When it comes to sweet treats, one bite is often enough.

Be a Savvy Consumer

Every week some new nutrition claim hits the headlines. Often, the reports are contradictory and confusing. What can a savvy consumer do?

- Use common sense to make sense of it all. Be suspicious of miracle claims and absolutes. One study is not enough. True nutrition breakthroughs are the result of repeated findings from many studies.
- Take a critical look at the research. Who did the work? What do other experts say? Was the research with humans or animals? How many subjects were there? How old were they? Were women included? How do the results fit within the broader context of healthy eating?
- Don't jump to conclusions. The words "suggests," "linked to," and "associated with" do not mean proof or cause. Check with a qualified dietitian before you make a major change in your eating style. Even reliable research results may not apply to you.

THE BOTTOM LINE

Nutrition in midlife is not about forbidden foods, fad diets, or supplements that promise to slow the aging process. It is about moderation and enjoying a variety of foods. So, go ahead. Experiment with new tastes, try new foods and different cuisines. Make "nutritious" equal "delicious."

Contacts and Further Information

To find a dietitian in your area, check with a public health unit or a local hospital, or ask your family physician for a referral. "RD," or "registered dietitian," is a protected title. The websites of the American Dietetic Association and the Dietitians of Canada provide local listings of registered dietitians.

Organizations

- American Dietetic Association, National Center for Nutrition and Dietetics, 216 W. Jackson Blvd., Chicago, IL 60606–6995. Tel.: 1–800–877–1600; Consumer Hot Line: 1–800–366–1655.
- Centre for Science in the Public Interest, P.O. Box 70373, Toronto Station A, Toronto, ON M5W 2X5. Web: http://www.cspinet.org (Publishes a useful newsletter called *Nutrition Action* ten times a year.)
- Dietitians of Canada, 480 University Ave., Suite 604, Toronto, ON M5G 1V2. Tel.: (416) 596–0857; Fax: (416) 596–0603.
- Food and Nutrition Information Center, National Agricultural Library, U.S. Dept. of Agriculture, 10301 Baltimore Ave., Suite 304, Beltsville, MD 20705–251. Tel.: (301) 504–5719; E-mail: fnic@nalsvsda.gov
- North American Vegetarian Society, P.O. Box 72, Dolgeville, NY 13329. Tel.: (518) 568–7970.

Websites

- American Dietetic Association: http://www.eatright.org
- Arbor Nutrition Guide (complete set of nutrition-related links): http://www.arborcom.com
- Canadian Diabetes Association: http://www.diabetes.ca
- CyberKITCHEN (sponsored by the U.S. Government (Shape Up America! Campaign)): http://www2.shapeup.org/cyberkitchen
- Dietitians of Canada: http://www.dietitians.ca
- Food & Nutrition Information Center (sponsored by U.S. Department of Agriculture): http://www.nal.usda.gov/fnic
- Heart & Stroke Foundation of Canada: http://www.hsf.ca
- Jean Fremont's Food and Nutrition Page (sponsored by Simon Fraser University): http://www.sfu.ca/~jfremont

- Nutrition and Healthy Eating Unit (sponsored by Health Canada): http://www.hc-sc.gc.ca/nutrition
- Nutrition Navigator (sponsored by Tufts University, on-line rating and review guide for nutrition websites): http://navigator.tufts.edu
- Nutrition News Focus (free daily newsletter sponsored by Department of Nutrition and Food Science, Wayne State University, Detroit): http://www.nutritionnewsfocus.com
- Quackwatch: Your Guide to Health Fraud, Quackery and Intelligent Decisions. Operated by Stephen Barrett, MD (sponsored by Quackwatch Inc.): http://www.quackwatch.com
- Soy information (sponsored by United Soybean Board): http://www.talksoy.com

Books

- *The American Dietetic Association's Complete Food and Nutrition Guide* by Roberta Larson Duyff. Minneapolis: Chronimed Publishing, 1986. Call 1–800–877–1600, ext. 5000; catalogue #6032.
- *Becoming Vegetarian: The Complete Guide to Adopting a Healthy Vegetarian Diet* by Vesanto Melina, Brenda Davis, and Victoria Harrison. Toronto: Macmillan Canada, 1994.
- *Eat Well for a Healthy Menopause* by Elaine Moquette-Mague. New York: John Wiley, 1996.
- *Estrogen the Natural Way: Over 250 Easy and Delicious Recipes for Menopause* by Nina Shandler. New York: Villard Books/Random House, 1998.
- *Intuitive Eating: A Recovery Book for the Chronic Dieter/Rediscover the Pleasures of Eating and Rebuilding Your Body Image* by Evelyn Tribole and Elyse Resch. New York: St. Martin's Press, 1995.
- *Get Fresh!: How to Cook a Kumquat and Other Useful Tips for More than 100 Fruits and Vegetables* by Madeleine Greey. Toronto: Macmillan Canada, 1999.
- *Real Food for a Change* by Wayne Roberts, Rod MacRae, and Lori Stahlbrand. Toronto: Random House, 1999.
- *When in Doubt, Eat Broccoli* by Liz Pearson. Toronto: Penguin Books, 1998.

- *You Count, Calories Don't* by Linda Omichinski. Winnipeg: Tamros Books, 1993.
- The Heart and Stroke Foundation publishes and sells a number of excellent cookbooks, including *Simply HeartSmart Cooking* and *More Simply HeartSmart Cooking* by Bonnie Stern, *HeartSmart Chinese Cooking* by Stephen Wong, *Light Hearted Everyday Cooking* by Anne Lindsay, and *The HeartSmart Shopper: Nutrition on the Run* by Ramona Josephson.

Related Chapters in This Book

- *Chapter 4: The Search for the Fountain of Youth* gives you more information on the role of antioxidants in aging.
- *Chapter 5: Making Changes That Last!* describes a cycle of personal change that can help you take up and maintain new eating behaviours.
- *Chapter 6: Wrinkles, Chin Hairs, and Baldness* explores some of the unrealistic standards for appearance that we set for ourselves as we grow older.
- *Chapter 7: The Active Living Solution* is the companion chapter to this one. Physical activity and healthy eating are partners in good health.
- *Chapter 9: The Boomer's Drugs of Choice* gives you more information on alcohol use and how much is too much.
- *Chapter 17: Keep Your Bones Strong* provides detailed information on dietary sources of calcium and how our calcium needs change as we get older.
- *Chapter 20: You Gotta Have Heart!* provides more information on nutrition and heart health plus a self-test of your risk factors.
- *Chapter 21: Complementary and Alternative Medicine Is Coming on Strong* gives you more information on herbal therapies that may complement a healthy eating approach.

CHAPTER NINE

The Boomer's Drugs of Choice

First you take a drink, then the drink takes a drink, then the
drink takes you.   – F. Scott Fitzgerald[1]

More than any previous generation, the boomers liked to experiment with
illegal drugs. Most of us probably know some middle-aged boomers who
still enjoy the occasional joint (even if they don't inhale!). But the reality
of most drug use in midlife is largely the same as it was for our parents.
Alcohol and tobacco are the drugs of choice. And while both are legal and
readily available, they are not without their own dangers.

Despite what we know about the effect of tobacco on our health, about
one-third of North Americans in the age group forty-five to sixty-five still
smoke. Middle-aged men are slightly more likely than middle-aged women
to smoke; however, women are quickly catching up. This is because more
men in this age category are likely to have quit (43 per cent) than women
(30 per cent).[2]

Alcohol use is associated with more than 100,000 deaths from diseases
and injuries in the United States each year.[3] The majority of middle-aged
North Americans drink alcohol. Men are twice as likely to drink daily than
women. They are also more likely to drink heavily. In 1995, one in five male
drinkers in Canada reported consuming more than five drinks at a time at
least once a month.[4]

There is an important difference, however, between drinking and
smoking. As we will see in this chapter, moderate drinking may sometimes
be good for some people's health. Smoking, on the other hand, is hurtful to
everyone in any amount.

This chapter looks at smoking, the pros and cons of moderate drinking, and a fairly new idea called "risky drinking." For those who smoke and would like to quit, there is hope. You can give up tobacco and maintain your sanity at the same time. It all depends on readiness.

The French Paradox
By now you have probably heard of the French Paradox. It goes like this. People in France, who pride themselves on cream sauces and duck paté, and have far fewer restrictions on smoking, must have more heart disease than North Americans. Right? Wrong – that's the paradox.

How can this be? A number of researchers claim that the French are protected from heart disease because of a moderate intake of alcohol, especially red wine, which they traditionally enjoy with their meals. Indeed, research over the last ten years has shown that some people who drink moderately (two drinks per day or less) have a 40-per-cent lower risk of heart disease than others who abstain. Despite these impressive statistics, of course, drinking for health reasons is not as straightforward as it sounds.

The Pros and Cons of Moderate Drinking
The theory is that moderate amounts of alcohol protect against heart disease by interfering with the formation of blood clots and the build-up of plaque in the arteries. Remember, moderation is the key word. Studies of drinking and total mortality show a J-shaped curve with a shallow dip in mortality when small amounts are consumed (no more than two drinks per day) and significant increases in total mortality with higher levels of drinking.[5]

Scientists and health professionals are quick to point out that, beyond a small reduction in coronary heart disease, there are no other important reasons to drink alcohol. Heavy drinking can lead to accidents, injuries, and the development of some cancers, cirrhosis (liver disease), and stroke. It can also be a precipitating factor in situations of domestic and work-related conflict and violence.

So, is it advisable to drink moderately or not? It depends on you, your medical history, your current drinking habits, and your current state of health.[6]

- For women and men who are middle-aged and older and are in good health, moderate drinking (defined as two or fewer drinks per day) may be beneficial to heart health.

- Two drinks may be too many if you are not accustomed to drinking or if you have a history of substance abuse.
- Men in midlife who are concerned about their sex lives should be cautious about their use of alcohol. While evidence about the effects of alcohol on impotence is not as clear as that for nicotine, it makes sense to avoid over-indulging (especially if you are having problems getting and maintaining an erection). Most men can relate to Shakespeare's suggestion in *Macbeth* that alcohol "provokes the desire but takes away the performance." Heavy drinking over a long period of time may result in chronic liver damage, which may lower testosterone levels and increase estrogen levels, causing a man's breasts to enlarge and his testicles to shrink.
- Because alcohol impedes the absorption of calcium, women and men at high risk for osteoporosis should restrict their intake of alcohol (see Chapter 17).
- Some fifty studies have shown an increase in breast-cancer risk among women who drink daily. Alcohol raises estrogen levels, so women who are at risk for breast cancer or who are using hormone replacement therapy should be cautious about their use of alcohol (see Chapter 19).
- Abstain from drinking if you are pregnant, breast-feeding, or taking certain medications (as indicated by your pharmacist).
- Do not drink if you have uncontrolled hypertension, liver disease, peptic ulcers, and certain other disorders (your physician can advise you).
- If you currently do not drink, or drink very occasionally, do not begin to drink as a way to reduce your risk for heart disease. Taking up regular exercise and reducing the amount of fat in your diet are far healthier ways to improve your heart health.

Risky Drinking: How Much Is Too Much?

Most North American adults who drink alcohol do not drink every day. When they do drink, they consume moderate amounts. However, anyone who drinks can develop alcohol problems – either by binging (drinking too much at one time) or by developing a pattern of ongoing, daily drinking that creeps into the "risky" category.

The Risky-Drinking Checklist
Answer the following questions honestly. If you check Yes to any question, your drinking may be having a negative effect on your health.

YES	NO	
_____	_____	Do you regularly drink more than 2 standard* drinks a day?
_____	_____	Do you drink every day?
_____	_____	Do you drink and drive?
_____	_____	Do you drink when swimming, boating, hunting, or using power tools?
_____	_____	Do you drink and are you pregnant?
_____	_____	Do you drink and take medication?
_____	_____	Do you drink to excess or binge-drink on occasion?
_____	_____	Do you feel guilty or defensive about the amount you drink?
_____	_____	Has drinking caused problems for you?
_____	_____	Is drinking alcohol your primary way of dealing with stress?
_____	_____	Has your partner or co-worker expressed concern about your drinking?

* Standard drink = 1 bottle of regular beer
= 5 oz. glass of wine
= 1.5 oz. liquor

Source: Adapted with permission from the Toronto Public Health Department's *DrinkThink* campaign and published in the *CrownLife ParticipACTION Quality of Life* newsletter, fall 1997.

How to Cut Down on Your Drinking
If you are concerned about your drinking or the drinking of someone close to you, here are some practical ideas for drinking less.

- Remember, it is always okay to not drink. You can have a good time without alcohol.
- Plan some alcohol-free days each week (e.g., don't drink from Monday to Thursday).
- Limit yourself to two drinks if you are a man and one drink if you are a woman.
- Do not drink more than twelve drinks in a week.
- Plan ahead. Decide when, where, and how much you will drink.
- Volunteer to be the designated driver.
- Try alternatives to drinking when you are under stress – talking with a friend, enjoying some music, taking a walk.
- Always measure your drinks. Cut down on the amount of alcohol and add more mix.
- Pace your drinking. Have a glass of water or juice before each drink. Don't have more than one drink in one hour.
- Choose beer and wine with a lower alcohol content or try alcohol-free beer (it tastes great!).
- Always have something to eat when you drink.
- Don't drink alcohol to satisfy your thirst. Drink a large glass of water first.

DID YOU KNOW?[7]

- Beer contains about 5-per-cent alcohol, wine contains between 8-per-cent and 19-per-cent, and liquor about 40-per-cent.
- Alcohol affects women more powerfully than men. Women reach a higher blood-alcohol level than men do after drinking the same amount of alcohol in relation to their body weight. Women's reactions also vary at different stages of the menstrual cycle because of their changing hormone levels.
- One gin-and-tonic has as many calories as a large ice cream cone; a pint of beer has as many calories as two large ice cream cones.
- Your driving can be impaired well below the legal blood-alcohol level of .08. Taking a shower, drinking coffee, or eating will not sober you up any faster.

When Drinking Becomes a Problem[8]

The CAGE Questionnaire is one of the most widely used screening tools for the detection of alcohol abuse and addiction.

If you or a family member answers Yes to even one of the CAGE questions that follow, it is time to consult with a physician, employee-assistance (EAP) counsellor, or addictions counsellor.

1. Do you feel you ought to **C**ut down on your drinking?
2. Do people **A**nnoy you by criticizing your drinking?
3. Do you ever feel **G**uilty about your drinking?
4. Have you ever had a drink first thing in the morning to steady your nerves or get over a hangover (an **E**ye-opener).

If you or a family member has a problem with alcohol, it is important to get help right away. Your physician or an EAP counsellor at work can assist you. Several of the men we interviewed talked about their own experiences with Alcoholics Anonymous (AA) or of the experiences of friends who belonged. One man told us he attended an AA meeting with some old high-school buddies while on a ski vacation. "In high school, they were party animals," he said. "Now they are responsible guys who took a major step in getting control of their problem."

Alcoholics Anonymous is a self-help group of alcoholics. AA is the grandparent of numerous other self-help groups that help people deal with various addictions. (See the end of this chapter for how to reach both AA and AlAnon, which is for families and friends of alcoholics.)

One More Reason to Butt Out[9]

Smoking is the most important cause of preventable illness, disability, and premature death in North America. In fact, the use of tobacco products kills more North Americans than alcohol, AIDS, illicit drugs, car accidents, suicides, and murders combined. While there is no need to repeat the long list of well-known effects of tobacco on health, here are some lesser-known facts that may be of particular interest to men and women in midlife.

- Nicotine belongs to the same family of drugs as morphine and cocaine. Experiments rank it ahead of alcohol, heroin, and cocaine in terms of severity of dependence resulting from use.
- There is now strong evidence that smoking causes cervical cancer in

women. Components of tobacco smoke have been found in the cervical secretions of smokers.

- Smokers are more likely than non-smokers to lose their teeth, to have tooth decay, and to have gum disease.
- Smoking decreases blood flow in the small vessels of the skin, causing wrinkling and the appearance of premature aging in both women and men.
- Smoking and using oral contraceptives at the same time greatly increases a woman's risk for heart disease and stroke.
- Smoking makes natural menopause occur earlier.
- The Environmental Protection Agency in the United States has declared environmental tobacco smoke a human carcinogen that causes lung cancer and heart disease in non-smokers.
- Cigarette smoking, which impedes arterial blood flow, has been clearly linked to impotence. The more cigarettes smoked per day, the greater the problem. One recent study at the University of Boston showed that men who smoke a pack a day for twenty years run a 60-per-cent risk of becoming impotent.[10] A group of Israeli doctors believes that fear of impotence may be a stronger incentive to men to give up smoking than fear of death! In a study of 886 smokers suffering from impotence, 80 per cent quit after they were encouraged to do so in the hope of improving their sex lives.[11]
- Long-term smokers are four times more likely to get grey hair prematurely and men who smoke are twice as likely to be bald or balding.[12]
- Smoking is linked to a reduction in bone density.[13] A recent study of female twins suggests that a woman who smokes one pack of cigarettes daily may experience a 5-per-cent to 10-per-cent reduction in bone density by the time of menopause.[14]

Why Bother to Quit Now?[15]

No matter how long you have smoked or how much you smoke, the message is clear. Anyone who quits can enjoy health benefits, even those who already have a smoking-related disease.

- Smokers who quit before age fifty cut in half their risk of dying in the next fifteen years compared to those who continue to smoke.

- A smoker's increased risk of dying from heart disease is reduced by half after only one year of abstinence.
- A smoker's increased risk of dying from lung cancer is reduced by half after ten years of abstinence.
- For a smoker who has had a heart attack, quitting reduces the risk of a second attack or premature death by 50 per cent, compared to someone who continues to smoke.

How to Quit for Good

It takes the average smoker five or more attempts to quit before he or she quits completely. While it is not easy to do so, you can beat an addiction to nicotine. In Canada, more than seven million men and women have quit smoking; indeed, ex-smokers now outnumber smokers.

The Stages-of-Change theory described in Chapter 5 suggests that successful quitters go through a process involving five stages:

- precontemplation: denial, no interest in quitting;
- contemplation: thinking about it but not yet ready to quit;
- preparation: getting ready to quit;
- action: quitting; and
- maintenance: remaining a non-smoker.

The trick is to understand which stage you are in and to choose activities that support where you are and help you move on to the next stage. The story that follows demonstrates how awareness of the stages of change can affect your ability to succeed.[16]

Mary and Jack are a newly married midlife couple. Mary was anxious that Jack quit smoking and she reminded him often of the danger of his habit to his health and hers. Jack was at the contemplation stage, thinking that this might be a good time to take action. He was open to information on quitting and to the idea of cutting down. But after six weeks of encouragement, Mary put her foot down and insisted that he join a smoking-cessation program. Jack made it to quit day, then resumed smoking one week later when he was faced with a crisis at work. He felt like a failure and blamed Mary for forcing him into something he did not want to do.

To some extent, Jack was right. He had allowed himself to be threatened into action, a rationale for change that invariably fails. His efforts to quit were based on someone else's readiness, not his own.

Does this mean that we must sit quietly by and watch the people we love destroy their health? Does this mean that Jack is doomed to smoke the rest of his life? The answer is no on both counts.

Jack's attempt at quitting, half-hearted as it was, was still a positive step. Indeed, as mentioned earlier, the average smoker makes five or more attempts to quit before he or she actually becomes smoke-free for good. With this failed attempt, Jack will not fall back into the first phase of pre-contemplation. With time (and support from those around him) he will identify what he did right in this first attempt and what the barriers were in his environment that stopped him from making it to the maintenance stage. Next time, he will make plans in the preparatory stage to overcome those barriers, such as finding other ways to cope with stress at work, and making it his decision, not Mary's, to quit. In the action stage, he may decide to ask his doctor for a prescription for a nicotine patch or Zyban to help him through the initial withdrawal symptoms. Jack may quit, enter the maintenance stage, then relapse three more times. But with persistence and the knowledge that he can eventually succeed, he will do it. In maintenance, he will anticipate the situations that lead to relapse – stressful situations, poker nights with friends who smoke – and gain confidence as he learns to deal with these situations without smoking. Eventually, Jack will see himself as a non-smoker. This shift in his self-perception will help him refrain from starting again.

How can Mary help Jack through this process? In the early stages, she can encourage Jack to talk about what he sees as the advantages and disadvantages of smoking. It is only when he decides for himself that the cons of smoking outweigh the pros that he will successfully move on. As he prepares to take action, she can reinforce his strengths and provide information on various programs or self-help guides that might assist him. With Jack's agreement, she can create a supportive environment for change, for example, by asking visitors not to smoke in the house, by having friends to the house for a drink rather than going to the pub where smoking is heavy, and by cleaning out the car ashtray and filling it with peppermints. If Jack relapses, she can express confidence in his ability to succeed next time.

Similarly, a good relationship with a family physician who continues to be supportive at each visit can help a person eventually quit. A forty-five-year-old man was very pleased to announce at his annual check-up that, after many failed attempts, he had quit smoking. He thanked his physician for always bringing up the smoking issue. He said, "You never gave up on me. Your encouragement really helped."

DID YOU KNOW?

- Teenage smoking has recently increased, and adolescent girls are now smoking more than boys.[18]
- Lung cancer has already replaced breast cancer as the number-one cause of cancer death among women. If increased rates of smoking among young women continue, there will be a virtual epidemic of lung cancer among women twenty years from now.

Helping You Quit

While the majority of smokers eventually quit "on their own," most make use of a variety of tools and aids for quitting at various times. Here are some options that have varying degrees of success:

- Self-help guides to quitting are available from a variety of sources. These are particularly useful for people in the preparation stage. (See the Contacts section at the end of this chapter.)
- Group programs offered by the Lung Association and others are especially effective for people who find it helpful to share the process with others in the same struggle.
- The use of nicotine gum or the nicotine patch may be especially helpful for heavy smokers who experience physical withdrawal symptoms when they quit. But be sure that you don't end up with a double dose of nicotine by smoking at the same time!
- Marketed under the name Zyban, the antidepressant bupropion (Wellbutrin) also serves as an aid to smoking cessation. Zyban reduces the withdrawal symptoms of tobacco addiction by controlling the anxiety, depressed mood, or irritability many people experience while trying to quit. Smokers who begin the use of Zyban set a quit date two to three weeks into therapy. If the smoker does not

successfully quit, he or she may use Zyban in conjunction with the nicotine patch. People at risk of having seizures or who are taking other antidepressants should not take this drug.

- Some people find acupuncture or hypnosis helps them focus their efforts in the action stage and lessens their cravings for cigarettes.
- Others find it helpful to start an exercise program in the preparatory phase, and to continue with it as they proceed through quitting and maintenance. Physical activity provides stress release and weight management, as well as reminding you daily that you are taking positive steps to improve your health.

Do Women Have a Harder Time Quitting than Men?[17]

While it has long been suggested that women have greater difficulty quitting than men, recent reviews suggest that few gender differences actually exist. What may differ are the strategies each requires. High rates of smoking among women are associated with stressful experiences, especially for women in high-demand, low-control jobs, such as nursing or hospitality services. It has also been shown that women find support for quitting from a partner and from friends especially important.

Women (and many men) in midlife are particularly concerned about gaining weight after they quit, the average increase being five to ten pounds. However distressing this may be, the risks of smoking far exceed the risks associated with this temporary weight gain. Once you have securely established the non-smoking routine, then you can address the matter of losing weight.

THE BOTTOM LINE

If you are a smoker, quitting is the most important thing you can do to improve both the quality and quantity of your life. Do not give up; the process takes time. Many people do not succeed on their first, second, or even third try, but, with perseverance and support, you can eventually reach your goal. Drink moderately (or not at all) and seek help if you drink too much.

Contacts and Further Information

Organizations and Websites

A number of organizations provide information and help to quit smoking. Use your telephone book to find local offices of the following associations or visit their websites on the Internet.

- American Cancer Society: http://www.cancer.org/
- American Heart and Stroke Foundation: http://www.amhrt.org
- American Lung Association: http://www.lungusa.org
- Canadian Cancer Society: http://www.cancer.ca (Tel. (toll-free): 1–888–939–3333).
- Canadian Lung Association: http://www.lung.ca (Tel. (toll-free): 1–888–972–2636).
- Heart and Stroke Foundation of Canada: http://www.hsf.ca

For help with alcohol problems, contact your employee-assistance (EAP) counsellor at work, your physician or spiritual leader, or use your local telephone book to find help from addiction agencies or self-help groups in your area, such as Alcoholics Anonymous (for the drinker) and AlAnon (for family members and friends).

Other Websites

- Alcoholics Anonymous Home Page: http://www.solar.rtd.utk.edu/~al-anon
- Canadian Centre for Substance Abuse: http://www.ccsa.ca
- A Guide to AA-Related Literature (Alcoholics Anonymous): http://www.moscow.com/resources/selfhelp/AA
- Information on smoking cessation from Health Canada: http://www.hc-sc.gc.ca/hppb/tobaccoreduction/public.html
- National Clearinghouse on Tobacco and Health (Canada): http://www.cctc.ca/ncth
- Nicotine Anonymous: http://www.slip.net/~billh/nicahome.html
- QuitNet (sponsored by Massachusetts Tobacco Control Program): http://www.quitnet.org
- Smoking Cessation Guidelines and Tips for Clinicians and Smokers (sponsored by Center for Cardiovascular Education (U.S.)): http://www.heartinfo.org

Related Chapters in This Book

- *Chapter 5: Making Changes That Last!* describes in more detail the Stages-of-Change theory that is used in this chapter to describe the process of quitting smoking.
- *Chapter 7: The Active Living Solution* and *Chapter 8: Food for Thought: Healthy Eating in Midlife* will help you develop healthy lifestyle practices that support your efforts to reduce drinking or quit smoking.
- *Chapter 12: Dealing with Impotence* discusses the relationship between smoking, excessive drinking, and erection problems. Read this chapter for good incentive to quit or cut down.
- *Chapter 13: Stress-Proofing in Midlife* provides tips on ways to deal with stress without drinking or smoking.
- *Chapter 15: When Times Are Tough: Depression, Anxiety, and Insomnia* helps you recognize depression and anxiety, which some people try to cover up with alcohol use. It explains that alcohol will disrupt your sleep and suggests other ways to get a good night's rest.
- *Chapter 17: Keep Your Bones Strong* will help you identify your risk for osteoporosis, which both drinking and smoking accelerate.
- *Chapter 19: Breast Health* points out that smoking and drinking can increase your risk for breast cancer.
- *Chapter 20: You Gotta Have Heart!* explains more about your risks for heart disease and its relation to tobacco use.
- *Chapter 23: Body, Mind, and Soul* explores spiritual well-being, which AA and other groups believe is central to beating addiction.

CHAPTER TEN

Growing Apart and Together: Relationships in Midlife

Stand together yet not too near together. For the pillars of the temple stand apart, and the oak tree and the cyprus grow not in each other's shadow   – Kahlil Gibran[1]

Midlife relationships take many different forms. They include relationships with intimate partners, family members, and friends. Intimate partnerships may be heterosexual relationships inside and outside conventional marriage and same-sex relationships. Many people in midlife are in new partnerships, often with children from previous relationships. Others are newly separated, divorced, or widowed and find themselves seeking intimacy again after ten or twenty years out of the dating scene. Some find satisfaction in same-sex relationships after ending traditional marriages. Others are without intimate partners and are questioning what this means for them at this stage of their lives.

However an intimate relationship is structured, it is invariably rich, complex, demanding, and confusing. The stresses and changes in midlife tend to amplify both the positive and the troubling aspects of a relationship.

In this chapter, we focus on partnerships between men and women who are in midlife. We look at some of the common difficulties that arise, provide a framework for understanding why they arise, and offer some direction for improving communications. We also discuss other key relationships in midlife – with friends, parents, and our children.

We can hardly do justice to the importance of intimate relationships in one short chapter. We do hope that reading it will stimulate you to talk further with your partner or a friend and to search out other sources of information on this important topic.

Nurturing Intimate Relationships

Recent research tells us that marriages tend to be less happy, fulfilling, and affectionate in midlife than in their earlier and later stages, even though the number of manifested problems (mortgage payments, child-rearing) gradually decline over the life cycle.[2] Early reports from a ten-year study of eight thousand midlife Americans suggest that, while overall satisfaction with marriage is fairly high, finances and sexual difficulties provide the greatest stress.[3] This finding is in keeping with what our interviewees told us. The hopeful news is that there seems to be greater satisfaction and contentment in later years.[4]

What are the factors that lead to the sense of unhappiness or restless uneasiness so common in midlife relationships? The stresses seem to be both external and internal. Unlike our parents' generation, many boomers begin second marriages and second families in midlife. Children now often require longer periods of financial and family support at the same time that aging parents require assistance. Changes in the workplace have greatly eroded our sense of job and economic security. What used to be a time of life when things eased up now seems fraught with increased worry and strain. These pressures make it extremely difficult for a midlife couple to set aside significant time for their own relationship. After a period of time, many people wake up one day feeling that they really do not know the people they are living with.

The internal pressures of midlife add to the strain. The process of re-evaluating your life, questioning what you are doing and what you want to do in the finite numbers of years ahead can be hard on intimate relationships. A fifty-two-year-old woman said, "My partner can barely support himself as a result of his own prolonged midlife crisis. He is in no way able to support me." A forty-eight-year-old man, married for twenty years, said, "I would like my partner to attempt to see things from my perspective more often. She clearly resents the time my job requires, but I feel so pressured to maintain our standard of living."

Very often, both partners feel they are carrying a top-heavy load of responsibility with only a fragile base of support. This makes both partners more vulnerable to a self-defeating cycle in which they seek support that the other is unable to give at that time, and then withdraw in disappointment. Consider the fifty-year-old self-employed businesswoman who is experiencing sleepless nights, hot flashes, and irritability owing to menopause, and is dealing with adolescents and increasingly dependent parents, while her forty-eight-year-old partner of fifteen years is worried about his company's downsizing, his best friend who just had triple-bypass surgery, and his growing inability to relate to his children. At the least, the relationship between the two is going to be strained.

The internal and external stresses of this time test the foundation of the relationship at the very time that each partner's personal resources are also strained. Yet a midlife breakdown of support and communication does not have to lead to an irreparable meltdown. Indeed, it can be the beginning of a healthier, sturdier, and more satisfying restructuring of an intimate relationship.

The Legacy of the Past

The most significant relationships any of us ever have are with our mothers and fathers. What we experience growing up in a family shapes our later view and understanding of intimacy. Those who are fortunate enough to have parents who were strong individuals and who forged a loving and stable bond with each other and with their children are likely to carry this legacy into adulthood. Those whose parents were unable to resolve conflict or were angry, depressed, distant, smothering, invasive, or manipulative are more likely to experience difficulties related to trust and vulnerability in their own adult relationships.

Poet Robert Bly once described the "secret ceremony" that takes place in the basement of the church or synagogue, while the traditional marriage service occurs above. In this metaphor, the father of the bride is seen to address the groom, saying that all the ideals, dreams, and disappointments that the bride has projected onto her father over the years will now be directed toward the groom. Similarly the mother of the groom addresses the bride, telling her that all of the unmet needs and dissatisfactions that her son has projected onto his mother will now be directed toward his bride.[5] In this way, our mates become (by virtue of the closeness and commitment that we share) the repositories of all the unmet needs, unresolved conflicts, and unfulfilled wishes of our childhoods.

Those parts of ourselves that still function in the realm of childhood bring considerable pain to our intimate relationships. The accusations

"You're just like my father!" or "You sound just like my mother!" are deeply disturbing. Most people who found growing up with Mom or Dad less than ideal have made a conscious effort to be different and to choose a partner who is different. How can our partners now seem just like them? Were we so blind? Has our partner changed so much from the amazing, too-good-to-be-true person we fell in love with? Probably not.

While we consciously try to find someone different, many of us unconsciously choose someone with characteristics similar to a parent with whom we have unresolved conflicts. Freud saw this "compulsion to repeat" certain patterns in our relationships arising from a deep desire to resolve these early difficulties.[6] This need can wreck havoc with a relationship unless you and your partner can recognize that certain areas of conflict may be rooted in a much earlier time in your lives.

It is unlikely that the perfect partner with whom we fell in love has changed so radically. It is just that he or she is much more human than we first realized. As we spend time together, the illusory cloak of perfection begins to slip off the shoulders and to wear thin along the hem and collar. We face the complexity of being with another human being who brings his or her own conflicts and confusions to the mix. When both partners bear wounds from the past, they are vulnerable to mistrusting or blaming each other, feeling blamed themselves, or setting up unrealistic expectations of each other.

Bly's story tells us that we must come to terms with our parents as real human beings who had their own unmet dreams, needs, and shortcomings. They could not possibly have been the perfect beings that we as young children expected them to be. In all likelihood, they did the best they could with the resources available to them. Now, we must take responsibility for our own choices and decisions in life. Otherwise we risk filling the living space of our current relationship with so much baggage from the past that we cannot see who our partner really is. We risk losing our ability to adapt to the inevitable changes in a shared intimate relationship.

An Opportunity for Growth

The difficulties faced by midlife couples can be a catalyst for personal development and an impetus to help the parts of ourselves that still respond in childlike ways – such as making unrealistic demands or behaving like a judgemental parent – to grow up. Just as the individual journey of midlife begins with a sense of loss and moves into a period of turmoil, so must the couple in midlife come to terms with past disappointments and hurts in order to move on (see Chapter 1).

In her book *Intimate Partners*, Maggie Scarf suggests that we have a choice at midlife. Because of the soul-searching nature of this time, we can choose to comfort each other and be true companions or to withdraw, distance ourselves emotionally, and rail at each other about the disappointments and resentments of a lifetime. Scarf says we must abandon the desperate, hopeless effort to remake the past in the context of current relationships if we are going to have a satisfying partnership for the next few decades of our lives.[7]

Confronting the difficulties together can lead to what is sometimes called the midlife "remarriage." **Phil and Marion**, a couple in their early fifties who fell passionately in love in their late thirties, provide a concrete example. Phil and Marion told us of their efforts to create the perfect relationship and family, each bringing two children from previous marriages. Four years later they separated, because of the enormous difficulties and power struggles that a blended family encounters; despite this, they continued to be lovers and friends. Marion developed a successful business of her own and each became a single parent to their own children. Five years later when the children had all left home, they chose to live together again as equals in a much more satisfying relationship. When they moved back in together, Marion remembers saying, "Thank heavens the honeymoon is over and the real love can begin." While most people do not have such a dramatic story, it is the willingness to confront the difference between our dreams of each other and the reality of each other that leads to true partnership.

If you find yourself and your partner bogged down in old resentments and disappointments and unable to constructively make changes, it may be very helpful to consider marital therapy. Too often, people wait until they are in a serious crisis before seeking help – and then it may be too late. A relationship and family therapist can help you build understanding and compassion for each other, so that difficulties don't become insurmountable.

Ingredients of a Healthy Relationship

While there is no one recipe for nurturing a healthy relationship, five key ingredients seem to form the basis of success. These are:

- adaptability to change;
- tolerance of ambivalent feelings;
- acceptance of differences and similarities;
- open, effective communication; and
- friendship.

Adaptability to Change

If you are in a long-term relationship, you need to recognize that the relationship you signed on for X number of years ago is not the one you have now, nor is it the one that you will have as older partners. One man told us "our relationship is very different now, but the essence of how we relate is still the same." The "happily ever after" myth is from the fairy tales, and is not the reality of our lives. While long-term relationships rely on a foundation of liking, loving, and trust, there must also be flexibility in allowing ourselves and our partners to evolve and be different.

Researcher Carolyn Maltas points out that, when midlife women feel freer of child-rearing responsibilities, they are more able to assert their own needs and move out into public life.[8] At the same time, men have the opportunity to become more nurturing and attentive to their children. While these shifts may look like another case of men and women growing apart, the result may in fact be greater ease and understanding between the two partners.

People who find themselves alone in midlife, as a result of divorce or death or an earlier life choice, also confront the need to be adaptable as they consider whether they want to enter into a new relationship or to take a solo journey.

Tolerance of Ambivalent Feelings

We won't always like our partner or what he or she does, and that person won't always like us. It is a difficult but important development in a relationship to be able to hold onto our love for each other even when we feel angry (and sometimes hateful) toward our partner. One man talked about the need to be aware of his partner's strengths and limitations at the same time and to make accommodations for his ambivalent feelings. "She's not perfect," he said, "but she is rather good enough!" In this way, we more realistically see each other as we really are, and not as some exaggerated all-good or all-bad Other.

Acceptance of Differences and Similarities

It helps to remember your similarities – the attitudes and values you share which foster mutual respect. But clearly, there are differences. Such recent best-sellers as John Gray's *Men Are from Mars, Women Are from Venus* and Deborah Tannen's *You Just Don't Understand* continually make the point of how differently men and women approach problems and express both needs and feelings. When these disparities are viewed as differences between men and women rather than personal slights and antagonisms, we are more likely to find peaceful solutions to interpersonal difficulties.

One forty-five-year-old lawyer who has been married for twenty years said that the ideas in these books helped her deal with her anger with her husband when his responses were different from what she wants. "It's not that he doesn't care about me," she said, "it's just that he's from a different planet!" Understanding these differences allowed this couple to find humour where only tension existed before. Paradoxically, the acknowledgement of differences has created more closeness. A man we talked with described how he understood the different ways that he and his partner approached a problem. "I immediately pick up the tool box of ways to fix the problem; she just wants to talk it out."

Deborah Tannen writes that, when things go awry, we most often want to send our partner in for repairs, rather than consider changing our own style. "Believing that 'you don't care about me as much as I care about you' is a dead end," she says, "while believing 'you have a different way of showing you care' leaves room for negotiation without the casting or taking on of blame or shame."[9]

Open, Effective Communication

Most of us know that the ultimate requirement for effective communication in a relationship is making time to listen, really listen. But knowing and doing are two different things. Finding time together can be difficult when you have two careers, children to care for, ailing parents to visit, and households to maintain. Listening is also difficult: studies repeatedly show that most people are poor listeners and that we tend to interrupt to get our own point across more often than we truly listen.

All of us have experienced the disappointed feeling of having someone's half-hearted or distracted attention. We also know that the feeling of really being listened to helps us feel more secure and worth-while. What does it mean to really listen to someone you love? What does it mean to really be listened to?

- It means putting aside our own agenda: what we want to say the moment someone else has finished speaking, or what we think they should be saying to make us feel better.
- It means listening as we might to someone who speaks a language different from ours or how we might listen to a child learning to talk.

Listening also requires private time together when partners can show curiosity, interest, and caring. The way we live today makes this seemingly simple requirement extremely difficult. One woman we talked with pointed out that travelling together in the car had been a good time to talk with her partner before the advent of beepers and cell phones. Another said there is no time for spontaneous intimacy with her teenaged children constantly in and out of the house.

One midlife man explained how he and his partner had learned to make time for real listening. After psychotherapy helped them through some rocky times, they decided to make it a daily practice to listen to each other for five minutes without fail. While one speaks, the other pays close attention and does not comment; then they switch. This simple commitment has helped them stay connected during busy and strained times.

Friendship
One couple we know said that the strength of their relationship lies in the fact that they were good buddies for a number of years before they became intimately involved. One of them said, "When things are really stressful or when we're not getting along, we know that deep down we are friends, and that pulls us through." Current research about what makes a good marriage verifies this. John Gottman and Nan Silver, co-authors of the recent book *The Seven Principles for Making Marriage Work*, describe friendship in terms of partners having mutual respect, enjoying each other's company, and

intimately knowing each other's likes, dislikes, quirks, foibles, and dreams.

They go on to say that friendship provides the best protection against adversarial feelings between partners. Friendship engenders a surfeit of positive feelings, which tend to outweigh the negative feelings that get stirred up in arguments. Positive regard and trust cushion the stress of disagreements and prevent them from becoming major disruptions. It also facilitates the creation of shared meaning and a sense of purpose.[10]

DID YOU KNOW?

Couples who agree on what is funny are more likely to like and love each other than couples who don't laugh at the same things. Couples with a common sense of humour also tend to stay together longer. "A shared sense of what is funny," said the researchers, "is indicative of many other things: values, interests, preoccupations, intelligence, imagination, and needs."[11]

Families in Midlife

Many North American boomers will remember the Cleavers – June, Ward, Wally, and the Beaver – the perfect all-American family, with Mom at home, Dad the wise breadwinner, and two innocent kids, living in suburbia. Today, it is rare to see this classic nuclear family. Most women work outside the home. Some midlife couples are new parents, some are raising adolescents, and some are grandparents. Some middle-aged men and women have chosen to live on their own, yet play important roles in extended families of relatives and friends. Gay and lesbian couples are adopting children. Remarriage and blended families are common, as is single-parenting, especially by women. Most of us welcome an understanding of "family" that is defined more by the ties of love and commitment than strictly by blood affiliation. At the same time, we recognize that this expanded definition of the traditional family adds a great deal of complexity to our lives.

As we were writing this book, the wide variety of family-life experiences in midlife was constantly on our minds. While the three of us span only a four-year age difference, our family situations span the entire continuum.

One of us is recently remarried. She and her husband have adopted a newborn. While initially unsure of their ability to be first-time parents in their late forties and to alter their lifestyle so dramatically, both of them now believe that their new family is the best thing that could ever have happened to them. The second author is the mother of two teenagers and the daughter of an aging parent who is ill. She and her partner joke about residing in a house where the "raging hormones" of menopause and adolescence live together. The third author had her own two children in her early twenties and welcomed two stepdaughters into her life in her late thirties. Now, at age fifty-one, she is the delighted grandmother of five young boys. She believes that she is more relaxed and has more fun with her grandchildren than she did with her own children when they were young. At that time she was preoccupied with paying the bills and being a mother, when she did not feel fully grown-up herself.

The boomer generation's new experience of family has been driven by three overriding changes in demographics: delayed child-raising, the entry of women into the workforce en masse, and the aging of the population. By 2050, more than 5 per cent of the population will be over age eighty. And while older people are staying healthier longer, those over eighty are the most likely to have chronic health problems that require help from family members. For midlife families who find themselves caring for children and the needs of aging parents at the same time, the nest is far from empty.

The consequences for the so-called sandwich generation can be feelings of exhaustion, frustration, and guilt. You want to spend time with children who are still living at home, you need to give time to your career and your partner, and you know that your recently widowed mother needs both physical and psychological support. Faced with these competing demands and the limitations on your time, it is no wonder you feel like the middle of a grilled cheese sandwich!

Studies show that two of five Canadians aged thirty or older are providing some form of care for aging parents. Suddenly, we find that the pros and cons of retirement homes, estate planning, homecare, and how to handle a parent with Alzheimer disease have become common topics of conversation at dinner parties with friends.

It's not easy to admit that the people who nurtured you are now vulnerable and in need of nurturing themselves. When one or both of your parents die, it is hard to accept that you have moved to the head of the generational train, and that the people who gave you unconditional love are gone.

Several men told us how they regretted the distance between themselves and their fathers and that they were unable to build an emotional attachment with their fathers before they died. Some spoke of trying to break the cycle by becoming closer to their own children.

Most often when a parent becomes ill, it is the daughter or daughter-in-law who assumes the bulk of the caregiving responsibilities. Too often, boomer women who were raised to believe that denying themselves is the ideal end up exhausted, depressed, irritable, or vulnerable to substance abuse. Alcohol, nicotine, caffeine, and prescription drugs may help a woman maintain an exhausting schedule while denying the truth for a while – but not for long.

If you or a friend are caught in the sandwich-generation caregiving squeeze, it is essential that you do some things to avoid burnout:

- Consider attending a support group. Talk with friends, family members, and co-workers. Their support is important.
- Involve other family members in caregiving; don't assume total responsibility yourself.
- Make use of community services such as homecare, Meals on Wheels, seniors' clubs, church visitation, etc.
- Take time for yourself. Get away once in a while alone or with someone special.

Friends Are Good Medicine

There has been a lot of research in the past few decades on the positive links between a strong social support network and well-being. It is particularly important to have a good friend you can confide in, numerous acquaintances, and involvement in at least one community network (such as a church, club, or voluntary association). People who nurture these relationships live longer, healthier lives and have a reduced need for medical care. People who become isolated from friends due to illness, dislocation, divorce, or the death of a partner are particularly vulnerable to heart disease and other fatal illnesses.[12] Many of us have heard stories of widowers and widows who died soon after their partners, despite being physically healthy at the time their partners died.

Mobility and the time crunch of multiple responsibilities in midlife sometimes make it difficult to develop and nurture friendships. On the other hand, by midlife we have learned to be more tolerant and accommodating of others. As one woman said, "I now accept my friends as they are, even when some things they do are irritating." We have had the time and the experiences necessary to develop a social network that promotes health. This includes friends and acquaintances of all ages with whom we enjoy reciprocal give-and-take relationships. Work friends may be best able to help us with work stressors, friends who have been through a crisis (such as a divorce or the death of a parent) may best be able to help us deal with difficult midlife events of our own. An old school chum may be the person we need to confirm who we are and what is really important in life. A new friend who shares a passion for music, a love of tennis, or a challenging new work responsibility can help us sort through and take advantage of the growth opportunities at this stage in our lives.

Generally, women are more likely than men to have close friends that they confide in. If you are a man and your partner or one family member is your only confidant, it is important to make a friend, both for the pleasure friendship can bring and to ease the burden on your primary relationship. Close friendships can be with both women and men. One man told me that he was more comfortable sharing his feelings with women friends. He said, "They listen. They don't tell me to snap out of it."

The best way to make friends is to be one. However, many of the people we talked with said that they were concerned about the lack of time they have to spend with friends in light of their heavy career and family responsibilities. Happily, the quality of the time you spend with a friend is more important than the quantity. For example, some women described how they maintained supportive relationships with old friends who lived in different cities through telephone calls and occasional treasured visits. "It's like we were never apart when we get together," said one woman. "I see her once a year but I know I can call on her – and she on me – at any time."

Helping You Helps Me

In the last twenty years, self-help or mutual-aid groups have become increasingly popular. In a self-help group, people with a similar problem get together (or chat via the Internet) to share their experiences and solutions and support each other. Groups deal with all kinds of issues – from addictions to single-parenting to coping with a chronic illness or overeating.

Several of the women we talked with spoke about getting support from informal or formal groups of women in midlife. We also had the pleasure of spending a morning with a men's group that had been together (with some changes) for fifteen years. The members, who are now in midlife, shared an easy camaraderie and an unusual ability to express their feelings about a range of issues from relationships to careers and spirituality. All of them spoke about how the group had helped them and how they felt good about helping each other.

Why not consider joining or starting a midlife support group? All you need is one or two others who share your interest. Listed below are some books and organizations that can help you find or start a group.

THE BOTTOM LINE

Don't take your relationships for granted. Relationships need regular nurturing to survive and flourish over time. Make time for yourself and your partner away from the rest of the family. Do something you both love. Don't be afraid to go to marriage counselling, and *go* before you are in a crisis. Look after yourself as you look after others and welcome the joy and comfort that friends and self-help groups can bring.

Contacts and Further Information

Organizations
- American Association of Homes and Services for the Aging, Dept. 5119, Washington, DC 20061–5119. Tel.: (800) 508–9442; Fax: (301) 206–9789. (Information on continuing-care options for aging parents)
- American Self-Help Clearinghouse, North West Covenant Medical Center, 25 Pocono Rd., Denville, NJ 07834. Tel.: (201) 625–7101; Fax: (201) 625–8848; E-mail: ashc@bc.cybernex.net

- Children of Aging Parents, 1609 Woodbourne Rd., Suite 302A, Levittown, PA 19057. Tel.: (800) 227–7294.
- Self-Help Resource Centre (Canada), 40 Orchard View Blvd., Suite 219, Toronto, ON M4R 1B9. Tel.: (416) 487–4355; Fax: (416) 487–0344; E-mail: shrc@sympatico.ca

Websites
- American Self-Help Clearinghouse (sponsored by Mental Health Net): http://www.cmhc.com/selfhelp
- National Association for Home Care (U.S.): http://www.nahc.org
- Self-Help Resource Centre (Canada) (sponsored by Health Canada and others): http://www3.sympatico.ca/fcsn

Books
- *Don't Blame Mother: Mending the Mother-Daughter Relationship* by Paula Caplan. New York: Harper and Row, 1989.
- *Getting the Love You Want: A Guide for Couples* by Harville Hendrix. New York: HarperPerennial, 1992.
- *How Did I Become My Parents' Parent?* by Harriet Sarnoff Schiff. New York: Penguin Books, 1996.
- *Lesbians at Midlife: The Creative Transition* by B. Sang, J. Warshaw, and A. A. Smith (eds.). San Francisco: Spinsters Book Company, 1991.
- *Love and Survival: The Scientific Basis for the Healing Power of Intimacy* by Dean Ornish. New York: HarperCollins, 1998.
- *Men Are from Mars, Women Are from Venus* by John Gray. New York: HarperCollins, 1992.
- *The Self-Help Way: Mutual Aid and Health* by Jean-Marie Romeder. Ottawa: Canadian Council on Social Development, 1989.
- *The Seven Principles for Making Marriage Work* by John Gottman and Nan Silver. New York: Crown Publishers, 1999.
- *You Just Don't Understand: Women and Men in Conversation* by Deborah Tannen. New York: Ballantine Books, 1990.

Related Chapters in This Book
- *Chapter 1: The Midlife Journey* will help you think about the issues of midlife that affect all of us, including our partners and friends.

- If you are a man, reading *Chapter 2: Understanding the Female Menopause* will help you understand what your partner is going through. Women should read *Chapter 3: Is There a Male Menopause?*
- *Chapter 11: Enjoying Sex in Midlife* provides some good advice on keeping the sexual spark alive.
- *Chapter 13: Stress-Proofing in Midlife* will remind you how stress in midlife can affect relationships and suggest some ways you can deal with those stresses.
- *Chapter 15: When Times Are Tough: Depression, Anxiety, and Insomnia* will help you determine if you or your partner may be suffering from burnout, anxiety, or depression – all factors that strain relationships.

CHAPTER ELEVEN

Enjoying Sex in Midlife

> I still get turned on. It just takes me longer to get plugged in.
> — George Burns, age ninety-one

When Voltaire asked a famous courtesan who was eighty years old when women cease to feel sexual desire, she replied: "I do not know. I have not lived long enough."

Despite the jokes and stereotypes about sexless old age, sexuality is one of our last faculties to deteriorate (thank goodness!). But sex in midlife is rarely a straightforward matter. The physical aspects of aging, the emotional changes in relationships, and the stresses of midlife inevitably affect sex in the middle years. Work pressures, adolescents in the home, aging parents, and feelings of lost youth can all dramatically affect your sex life. Sometimes, health problems become an issue: a woman who undergoes a hysterectomy or surgery for breast cancer may feel less attractive; a man recuperating from a heart attack may be fearful of the stress associated with lovemaking.

Happily, most women and men we interviewed said that sex was a positive, fulfilling experience in midlife. They expressed a sense of comfort in their sexual relationships and a belief that sex and love had become more balanced and complementary in their lives. As one woman said, "Sex is important. Without sex and love, you lose both physical and emotional health." This chapter draws on their experiences in addition to information gathered from the contemporary literature on sexuality in order to:

- describe some of the common feelings and problems that are associated with sex in midlife;
- provide you with the factual information you need on birth control, sexually transmitted diseases, and how sexual functioning changes

with age, so that you and your partner(s) can enjoy the pleasures that healthy sexuality brings; and

- suggest some ways to enjoy and celebrate sexuality in midlife.

While we recognize and celebrate the equal importance of enjoying sex in gay and lesbian relationships, the scope of this chapter is limited to heterosexual relationships. We use the term "married" to also describe common-law and long-term relationships outside marriage.

Sexual Relationships in Midlife

An orgasm a day keeps the doctor away. – Mae West

Remember when you were growing up? The thought of "old folks" like your parents making love seemed incomprehensible. Now, the boomer generation is looking for ways to ensure that sex remains a rich part of their own experience of aging.

In a culture that worships youth, this is not an easy task. Popular magazines, television, and other media perpetuate the myths associated with sex and aging: that older women are not sexually attractive or active, and that all middle-aged men are looking for sex with young women. In her book *The Fountain of Age*, Betty Friedan reflects on these beliefs when she says, "Our denial of the personhood of age and its definition as a problem ensures the virtual blackout of people over fifty as sexual beings, especially women."[1]

The truth is just the opposite. Studies show that sexually active married men are happier with their sex lives at age sixty than twenty-year-old single men who have many sexual partners.[2] One man said, "Sex is still important and a lot more comfortable. Though less frequent, sex has become more of an expression of love. It plays an important role in keeping alive the romance in my relationship." Many women experience an increased interest in sex once children have moved out and the fear of pregnancy is eliminated. One woman said, "We have time for intimacy now that the children are gone." Another said, "I never realized how great sex could be again, until our kids went off to camp. Suddenly, we had privacy, more time to talk, and more time to make love."

Our interviews with both men and women confirm the subtle shift in midlife sexuality away from "raw sex" to enhanced feelings of intimacy and love. One man said, "I'm not as preoccupied with it as I was when I was twenty. I don't masturbate as much as I used to. . . . I acted more on sexual attraction then, now more maturity is involved. It's better in many ways. I can have female friends now; before it was harder because there was always an underlying sexual attraction."

The women in our seminars always breathe a sigh of relief when they hear that men's attitudes toward sex and love tend to shift in midlife. Many women find that their sexual confidence is threatened by physical changes of aging such as weight gain or wrinkles. It helps to know that your partner is also looking for less pressure on performance and more emphasis on intimacy. Indeed, despite the media hype about sex as a prerogative of the young, Tobi Klein, a sex therapist from Montreal, Canada, asserts that "in real life the plain, unglamorous couples are often the ones to have great sex, while the perfectly sculptured young couples struggle with ongoing sex problems."[3]

On the other hand, the middle years do not always accommodate a robust sex life. For women, in particular, the greatest problem is likely to be the lack of a partner. Since women who are divorced or widowed are far less likely than men to remarry, the man shortage can become critical in midlife and later. The other problem for older women is North American culture's tendency to equate sexuality in women with youth and reproduction. Until recently, the sexual lives of older women were rarely discussed. Now, a number of studies have shown that most women, as well as men, remain sexually active into very old age. In one study of 202 women between 80 and 102 years of age:

- 50 per cent fantasized or dreamed about sex often or very often;
- 63 per cent reported touching and caressing with sexual intercourse;
- 40 per cent continued self-pleasuring;
- 30 per cent continued to have intercourse.[4]

Interestingly, in tribal cultures where women gain status and freedom as they grow older, they report continuing sexual activity despite the loss of a partner, frequently with younger men.[5] One fifty-one-year-old woman told us about the restorative power of a new partner to both her sexuality and her self-confidence: "I am surprised by the level of my sex drive; it has never been like this before. Maybe it has something to do with my new partner!"

Effects of Aging on Your Sex Life

The aging process does not include a general sexual decline. Aging does, however, have an effect on each of the three phases of sexual response: desire, excitement, and orgasm.

EFFECTS OF AGING ON SEX: MEN AND WOMEN

Desire

Men

- Sexual passion or desire is controlled by testosterone. If levels drop too low (this is rare), a man loses his interest in sex. Hormone replacement therapy (HRT) can help.

Women

- Testosterone levels also affect sex drive in women. Hormone treatment must be used with caution because of side-effects.

Excitement

Men

- Increased blood flow to the genitals results in an erect penis. Erection is delayed and the penis becomes less rigid with age.
- In young men, either physical or psychological stimulation (fantasy) can produce an erection; older men require both to attain and maintain erection.

Women

- Increased blood flow to the genitals lubricates the vagina. At menopause when the ovaries stop producing estrogen, the walls of the vagina are less lubricated and elastic. They become thinner and more vulnerable to physical trauma. As with older men, arousal is delayed.
- HRT, regular intercourse, use of water-soluble lubricants, and estrogen cream or an estrogen ring can slow this process.

Orgasm

Men	Women
• Most men ejaculate normally until a very advanced age. While the interval between a first and second ejaculation is a few minutes at age 17, it can take 48 hours by age 80.	• Women may find the intensity of their contractions at orgasm decrease with age.
• Men have more control over the timing of their ejaculations as they get older.	• Women can experience multiple, rapid, repeated orgasms throughout life.

The changes that come with aging can actually lead to better sex. Because it takes men longer to get an erection and to ejaculate, and because they need both direct and indirect stimulation, foreplay is longer and more enjoyable for both partners. This is a particular bonus for women who take longer to reach orgasm than men at any age.

DID YOU KNOW?

The fact that men require longer to get an erection and to reach orgasm as they age can be a great relief for women. Here's why "quickies" don't work for women:

There are 6 physical stages in the sex act:

1. partial erection (man) / clitoral swelling (woman)
2. full erection (man) / vaginal lubrication (woman)
3. sustained erection (man) / sustained arousal (woman)
4. point of ejaculation inevitability (man) / point of orgasm inevitability (woman)
5. reflex ejaculation (man) / reflex orgasmic release (woman)
6. return to pre-excitement stage (man and woman)

Men between the ages of twenty-five and fifty go through all 6 stages in an average of 2.8 minutes, whereas women require about 13 minutes to complete this cycle![6]

When Sexual Desire Wanes

Low sexual desire is a common issue for both men and women in midlife. The causes of reduced sexual drive may be physical, psychological, or related to changes in the relationship over time:

- Common physical causes include the use of certain medications (for blood pressure, depression, and ulcers), problems associated with menopause (heavy bleeding, frequent periods, dry vagina), chronic pain (back pain, arthritis), and androgen (testosterone) deficiency.

- Common psychological problems include depression, the stress and distractions of work and financial concerns, repressed anger toward one's partner, and inhibitions about sexuality that were learned as a young person. Fatigue, negative beliefs about the attractiveness of middle-aged bodies, and a lack of privacy can all detract from sexual willingness in midlife.

- After many years together, couples who do not make an effort to keep novelty, excitement, and romance in their relationship may experience a loss of sexual desire or boredom. The lack of sexual desire in itself does not necessarily cause a problem if both partners feel the same way. "It does become an issue," one man told us, "when partners have different levels of sexual drive and expectations for sex." When one partner loses interest, the other may feel rejected and believe that his or her partner finds him or her unattractive or uninteresting.

When sexual desire wanes, it is important to determine whether the reason is physical, psychological, or due to a change in the relationship. Often it is a combination of these factors. Physical issues are the easiest to deal with. Menopausal women who experience pain with intercourse should contact their physicians immediately. A dry vagina is easily treated with vaginal creams or a hormonal ring that helps with lubrication. Men with erection problems should also see their physicians as a first step: the arrival of Viagra and other non-invasive treatments for impotence means that most men can successfully overcome sustained bouts of impotence (see the next chapter).

Such treatments, however, will not change a relationship already in trouble. For example, a woman recently came into our office whose husband had had surgery for prostate cancer two months earlier. It had left him impotent. She said, "I'm so afraid. I don't know what to do. He's coming home today with his prescription [for Viagra] and I haven't even dealt with his cancer yet." As with all relationship difficulties, good communication and sensitivity to our partners' feelings are essential.

How can you avoid sexual ennui? Make sex a priority in your life. Plan dates with your partner that focus on mutual interests and romance. A rich sexual life flourishes when you give it the time it deserves. Build love-making into your schedule, and take advantage of those unexpected moments. A lunch-time tryst or a leisurely Sunday morning of lovemaking can be a definite turn-on. Take holidays together, even if only for a weekend. Most of us can attest to having better sex during time away from work and children.

Once sufficiently aroused, the majority of women are orgasmic. However, orgasm can be inhibited by emotional difficulties. For some women, inhibitions about sex, based on upbringing or an earlier experience of sexual abuse, can seriously affect their ability to enjoy sex (about 15 per cent of women reported an inability to have an orgasm).[7] Psychotherapy (for you and your partner) can help.

It is not too late at age forty-five or fifty to discover the joys of pleasuring yourself and how your body responds to sexual touching. Sexual fantasies also become more important in midlife, since men now require both physical and psychological stimulation. Some couples find that talking about their fantasies (and sometimes acting them out) can be part of the fun.

Researchers now believe that the underlying mechanisms of male impotence and female inorgasmic response may be similar. Viagra trials with women are under way in Europe and in the United States, but present research suggests that it offers little help for women with sexual dysfunction (with the possible exception of women whose problems are related to the use of antidepressants).

When desire wanes for either sex, many therapists counsel taking the emphasis off intercourse itself and stressing necking, petting, caressing, passionate kissing, and laughing together. When couples realize that they do not need to have "the earth move" every time, they can relax and enjoy themselves more. There appear to be good physiological reasons for this advice. Touching releases oxytocin, a chemical that stimulates the desire for sex and creates an enveloping sense of contentment.

At the same time, you and your partner need to talk about your expectations of snuggling. Some women believe that being held close by their mates signals nothing more than "upper persuasion for a lower invasion." One woman told us, "My husband comes to the bathroom every morning and watches me shower. Then he wants to make love. All I want him to do is hold me and tell me that he loves me. Sex doesn't have to follow each time." Similarly some men may withdraw from hugging because they think it is a prelude to intercourse they don't want. This is not to say that orgasms are suddenly unimportant. When Ann Landers asked men readers if they "would settle for being held tenderly and be willing to forget about the act," she received more than 67,000 replies. Of that number, only 5,600 men were willing to settle for cuddling and forget the act. In the words of one man, "The older I get, the longer it takes, but I won't settle for cuddling until that is ALL I can do." Said another wise reader, "Don't those fools know that being held tenderly can lead to the act? It always does in our house!"[8]

In *The Seasons of a Woman's Life*,[9] Daniel Levinson describes how changes in a relationship affect women in the midlife transition who chose to make homemaking their careers earlier in their lives. Virtually all of the women he studied felt that their marriages were stagnant and that their husbands had no apparent interest in making love or even in having genuine personal contact. Because these women had devoted the previous stage of their lives to their husbands and children at the expense of their own development, they found themselves struggling in midlife to assert themselves. All of the women wanted more from their love relationships now that the homemaking project of their youth was coming to an end. They had more time and energy to invest in the relationships and they were looking for more frequent sex and more fun in these relationships.

Unfortunately, their husbands had largely lost interest in sex and become increasingly distant. Despite this, there was little talk of divorce. Both partners believed that their marriage was essential to their existence and worthy of the great sacrifices they had made. Unless these couples can reconnect as separate individuals with a shared mission that goes beyond the partnership they have known to date, it is unlikely that their sex life will flourish. In cases like this, couple counselling may be required.

In contrast to the homemakers, career women in Levinson's book talked about their workloads interfering with sexual intimacy, about "living on a treadmill, endlessly running to meet the requirements of a demanding career and needy family." Career women were anxious to establish equal partnerships with their mates in terms of love, passion, intimacy, play, and household management. When this equality was missing, sex became just one more tiring chore.

Keeping the Spark Alive

"Midlife is a time to make love, not just sex," said one man. "One of the differences in my relationship with my partner is the strong heart connection. I'm more connected emotionally, not just interested in a roll in the hay." Another forty-eight-year-old man told us, "Sexuality continues to be important. I feel more relaxed about it than I used to. It's like a move from a good Scotch to warm bread ... although I still like the Scotch sometimes!"

Like most good things in life, there is no one pattern or secret for successful lovemaking. What works for one couple may not work for another, so be open to experimenting and finding out what works for you. Many sex therapists agree on the following common-sense advice for keeping the spark alive:

1. *Express yourself.* Like most aspects of intimate relationships, communication is the key to good sex. Talk with each other about your love and attraction, about what turns you on and what feels good. Similarly, find a way to discuss things that bother you and get in the way of your pleasure. One sex therapist suggests that "oral sex" should mean talking to each other.[10] Talking about sex is sometimes difficult, but couples who learn to openly discuss sex and to solve problems in their relationships have better sex. Expressing yourself physically is also important. Couples who enjoy sex tend to be playful in their lovemaking.

2. *Make a commitment.* Most people experience sexual fulfilment in a relationship that is based on compatibility, familiarity, intimacy, and a joint commitment to sustain the relationship. Numerous surveys show that people in committed relationships have more and better sex than people who are not in committed relationships. One study showed that both men and women have less variety and experimentation in affairs than in marriage, and that women were more orgasmic with their husbands than with their lovers.[11]

3. *Break out of routine.* Bedtime, when androgen and energy levels are low, is not the best time for sex. Make a point of making love at unusual times in unusual places, so that it doesn't become routine.

4. *Rediscover the things that turned you on when you first met* (and find some new ones) – skinny-dipping, massages, romantic get-aways, kissing in public places. One couple told us how they love a series of travel guides titled "Best Places to Kiss In."

Love Potion Number Nine[12]

Since the beginning of recorded history, every culture claims to have discovered a love potion that stimulates sexual desire and stamina. While the efficacy of aphrodisiacs is far from proven, people all over the world enjoy experimenting with them. Before you imbibe, however, be aware that herbal preparations can be powerful medicines. Purchase them from an established health-food store and be sure that the bottle includes instructions, side-effects, and contraindications. Stop taking them if you experience problems.

Here are some of the best-known aphrodisiacs:

- *Yohimbine* from the African tree of the same name is said to strengthen sexual powers by increasing blood flow to the genitals. However, it can cause low blood pressure when taken in large amounts.
- *Ginseng,* used in China, India, and by North American native peoples is one of the most popular aphrodisiacs. Ginseng is a mild irritant and dilates blood vessels, which may contribute to sexual arousal.
- *Fenugreek* is renowned in Turkey as an aphrodisiac. Fenugreek contains vitamins A and D, which may strengthen sexual desire, as well as steroidal saponins, which are used to produce sex hormones.
- *Royal jelly* from bee pollen has been used to treat impotence since ancient times in Egypt, Persia, and China. Tests have demonstrated that pollen contains a form of the male hormone testosterone. *Bee pollen* and royal jelly can cause severe allergic reactions and should be avoided by anyone with allergies to pollen and other substances.
- *Sarsaparilla* and *saw palmetto* are used by North American native peoples for increasing sexual desire. *Saw palmetto* is also used to treat prostate inflammation in men and to stimulate milk production in women.

- *Oysters* may be regarded as an aphrodisiac because of the likeness of an oyster on a half shell to the female outer genitalia. More likely it is based on the fact that oysters are an excellent source of zinc, a mineral important for reproductive health. The Japanese eat clams to increase sexual potency, which are also high in zinc.

Fertility and Birth Control in Midlife

Birth-control needs in midlife differ today from what they were in our parents' time. Some couples delay having children until well into their forties. Women with heavy bleeding during the perimenopause are looking for reliable contraception that will also address the bleeding problem. Men and women who are entering new relationships are looking for both reliable contraception and protection from sexually transmitted diseases (STDs) and AIDS.

During the menopausal period, menstruation becomes less regular. This is a double-edged sword – while middle-aged women are less likely to become pregnant, missed or delayed periods can cause pregnancy scares. Fertility is reduced during the perimenopausal period, but as long as you are still menstruating you can become pregnant. The pregnancy rate for women who are not using contraception at age forty-five is 10 to 20 per cent; by age fifty, this risk drops to 5 per cent. Even though these are low rates, if you are not prepared for a pregnancy you must use birth control until you reach menopause (confirmed when you have not had a period for twelve consecutive months).

Unlike women, men are capable of conceiving children well into old age, although sperm production does decline with age. In theory, a man is fertile as long as he produces sufficient quantities of healthy sperm – at least 20 to 100 million sperm in a millilitre of ejaculate.

Most men and women in midlife decide that reliable birth control is in order. Today, they have more options than ever before, including oral contraceptives, which were previously thought to be dangerous in later life. Here is a short description of some of the most common and reliable methods of birth control to consider:

The Low-Dose Birth-Control Pill: A Positive Option for Many Midlife Women
Historically, physicians have advised against the use of oral contraceptives

after age thirty-five because studies done in the 1960s and 1970s linked use of the Pill in later life with an increased likelihood of suffering a stroke or blood clot. A re-evaluation of these studies, however, has shown that smoking, not oral-contraceptive use itself, caused the greater incidence of strokes among women after age thirty-five. This has paved the way for new guidelines on the use of the Pill among women in their later reproductive years.

For healthy, non-smoking women without any direct contraindications (such as breast cancer, thrombosis, high lipids, and liver dysfunction), oral contraceptives provide a safe method of contraception up to the point that your periods cease. The use of oral contraceptives (OCs) have a number of other impressive benefits, including:[13]

- relief from menopausal complaints such as hot flashes, irregular bleeding, and bloating;
- fewer ovarian cysts, which are common in perimenopause;
- a reduction in the incidence of endometrial cancer by 50 per cent and of ovarian cancer by 40 per cent. The protective effect of OCs may last for ten to fifteen years once a woman has discontinued use;
- a reduction in the number of women having fibroids and profuse bleeding, from 20 per cent to 5 per cent. The use of OCs minimizes the embarrassment of flooding and reduces the incidence of iron deficiency anemia (caused by excess flow) by 50 per cent;
- the prevention of bone loss and a possible increase in bone density when combined with exercise and a calcium-rich diet;
- a decrease in the incidence of benign breast disease (lumpy breasts);
- the prevention of thinning, drying, and loss of elasticity in the vagina and urinary tract, which can lead to stress incontinence (losing urine when you sneeze or jump) and painful intercourse.

While there is no clear link between OC use and breast cancer in older women, women at high risk should weigh the benefits of OCs against the risk of being exposed to additional estrogen (see Chapter 17).

Sterilization: Vasectomy and Tubal Ligation

Permanent sterilization is the second most popular method of birth control after the use of oral contraceptives. Of the two operations, vasectomy is easier, because general anesthesia is not required and there are fewer complications and side-effects. Conventional vasectomies are done on an out-patient basis under local anesthesia, although a new no-scalpel procedure is now available. The procedure has no effect on a man's sex drive or his ability to ejaculate. Pre-vasectomy counselling is important, however, to discuss short-term discomforts such as bruising or swelling and longer-term side-effects in a small number of men (0.3 per cent) who experience some psychosexual problems after the procedure.[14] It takes two to three months after a vasectomy before a man's ejaculate is free of sperm. Vasectomies can be reversed: the longer the time between the operation and the reversal, the lower the chance of an ensuing pregnancy (76 per cent chance of pregnancy after three years; 30 per cent chance after fifteen years).[15]

Some people worry about long-term adverse consequences with vasectomies, including an increased risk of prostate and testicular cancer. However, studies have shown no significant relationship between them. Studies showing an increase in heart disease among monkeys who have had vasectomies have not been replicated with humans.[16]

Tubal ligation is a surgical procedure carried out under general anesthesia, using an instrument called a laparoscope to make a small incision above the pubic hair and clamp off the woman's fallopian tubes. The operation is normally done in hospital as a one-day procedure.

Barrier Methods
Latex condoms and spermicidal gel or foam offer reliable protection against pregnancy, as well as protecting against sexually transmitted diseases (STDs). Condoms have the advantage of being easily purchased over the counter and slipping easily into your pocket or purse. This is the preferred method in new relationships. The cervical cap, diaphragm, and Lea's Shield are reliable if used regularly and properly; the cervical sponge has a 60- to 90-per-cent effectiveness rate when used alone. Spermicidal gels, creams, and foams have a high failure rate if they are not used in combination with condoms.

IUDs (Intrauterine Devices)
While they are well tolerated in some women, IUDs may present a major disadvantage in midlife by increasing a woman's tendency to heavy bleeding and spotting, symptoms already associated with menopause. However,

Progestasert, an IUD containing progesterone, may be beneficial for heavy bleeding.

The Morning-After Pill
When accidents happen, the morning-after pill (OCs, combined with Gravol, given in two doses) has a 98-per-cent success rate in preventing pregnancy if given within seventy-two hours after unprotected intercourse.

Injectables and Implants
These include Depo-Provera (an injection) or Norplant (hormone-containing rods inserted under the skin). These are not an ideal form of birth control in midlife because they can mask changes associated with menopause.

Oh No! I Can't Possibly Have an STD!
Ironically, the legacy of the 1960s era of free love may be having a devastating effect on aging boomers. Unlike our children, who have been raised in the era of AIDS, many boomers are unused to and uncomfortable with safe-sex practices. One middle-aged mother requested that her physician have a long talk about sexually transmitted diseases (STDs) and AIDS with her fifteen-year-old daughter, who had her first steady boyfriend. Six months later, the same woman, who was separated from her partner, was horrified to learn that she herself was infected with genital warts. To her chagrin, she realized that she had denied her own risk and showed greater concern for her daughter's sexual health than her own.

When the 1960s generation became sexually active, pregnancy was the greatest concern. Most of us were vaguely aware of gonorrhea and syphilis – horrible-sounding STDs that we were sure would never affect us. Today, the STD situation is vastly different. There are some twenty diseases that are sexually transmitted (including HIV, the virus that leads to AIDS), and some of them occur in North America in almost epidemic proportions. Sometimes, the symptoms are mild or unnoticeable until too late (for example, chlamydia may go unnoticed and eventually cause infertility).

Women in midlife are more susceptible to STDs than they were in their younger years, because declining estrogen levels cause the vaginal wall to become thinner and thus more prone to small cuts, which increase the risk of infection. Women are also more vulnerable than men to the long-term effects of STDs, such as sterility. Middle-aged men are also at risk for STDs, particularly because of increased travel and mobility and an increased acceptance of a variety of sexual practices.

In this short section we will concentrate on providing you with the basic information you need to practise safe sex and protect yourself from STDs, including HIV infection. Safe sex is any sexual practice that reduces the risk of passing STDs from one person to another. We urge you to contact your physician or public health clinic if you have further questions or concerns.

Most Common STDs

Genital warts (human papillomavirus) It is estimated that as much as 30 per cent of the North American population is infected with genital warts, although some people may show no outward symptoms. These highly infectious warts may appear on the cervix and the penis or in the vaginal or rectal areas. Most infections are transient (they come and go) and benign.

There are many types of papilloma viruses. Some are persistent and associated with increased risk for cervical and vulvar cancer in women and cancer of the penis and anus in men. Because of their association with cancer, genital warts should be treated promptly, and women who have had warts should have regular Pap smears.

Herpes simplex virus While some herpes lesions or blisters in the genital area are caused by oral-genital exposure to the typical cold-sore virus (herpes simplex Type 1), the majority of genital herpes cases are caused by the herpes simplex virus Type 2. The first outbreak is often accompanied by fever, genital pain, itchiness, discharge, and painful lesions that blister and crust over. There is no permanent cure for herpes caused by the Type 2 virus, although the frequency of subsequent outbreaks can be minimized with an oral antiviral medication. This medication can shorten the duration of outbreaks, reduce the number of them, speed up healing, and possibly prevent recurrence.

Gonorrhea Almost 400,000 cases of gonorrhea are reported in the United States each year.[17] Men with gonorrhea most often notice a discharge from the urethra and burning as they urinate. Women may have an abnormal vaginal discharge, burning with urination, abdominal pain, and fever; however, about half of the women infected do not present any noticeable symptoms. Untreated gonorrhea often leads to pelvic inflammatory disease, with accompanying scarring and infertility.

Chlamydia The symptoms of chlamydia are similar to those for gonorrhea. Many women experience no symptoms at all. Left untreated, chlamydia, which is three times more common than gonorrhea, can lead to pelvic inflammatory disease in women and infertility in both women and men.

Hepatitis B In acute cases, this virus causes fever, nausea, jaundice, headaches, dark urine, and an enlarged, painful liver. In its chronic form, it may go undetected for years, eventually leading to cirrhosis of the liver, liver cancer, and liver failure. Hepatitis B can be prevented by vaccination. Some jurisdictions now offer this vaccination to young people in school. If you have multiple sex partners, talk with your physician about getting the Hepatitis B vaccine.

Human immunodeficiency virus (HIV) While people infected with HIV are now living longer, thanks to better drug treatments, there is still no cure for HIV, which eventually leads to AIDS. HIV, which was first recognized in 1981, destroys the body's immune system, leaving it vulnerable to a host of diseases. HIV is a major cause of disability and AIDS is a major cause of death for people in midlife. The rate of AIDS infection in the United States is significantly higher than that in other industrialized countries (2,392 cases per million people).[18]

In Canada, the proportion of annual AIDS cases among women increased from 4 per cent in 1982 to 14 per cent in 1997, largely as a result of intercourse with infected male partners or injection drug use.[19] In the United States, 30 per cent of AIDS cases in women originated with heterosexual intercourse; the majority of cases arise from injection drug use.[20]

While the gay community has done an impressive job of reducing the transmission of HIV among older gay men, HIV and AIDS remain a major concern among bisexual men and younger gay men. Currently in the United States and some parts of Canada, the majority of new AIDS cases are among injection drug-users and their partners. The *only* way to protect yourself from HIV is to avoid intravenous drug use (sharing needles) and to use a condom every time you have sex when you do not know whether or not your partner has HIV.

How to Protect Yourself from STDs

- Follow safe-sex guidelines. If you are unsure or believe that your partner may have been exposed to STDs, choose activities that do not allow semen, vaginal secretions, or blood to enter the mouth, anus, vagina, or any open sores. Avoid sex when you or your partner has sores or an infection. Use a condom and spermicide every time, even if you are using other methods for birth control. Do not use petroleum jelly or other creams as they can damage the condom. Be aware that the risk of transmission is twice as high with anal inter-course as with vaginal intercourse.
- Make sure your partner has no apparent signs of infection, does not use intravenous drugs, and is not involved with multiple lovers. Refrain from casual sex. The more partners you have, the more you are exposed to infection.
- Talk about safe sex. Find out about your partner's sexual history and overall health. Discuss the need for safe sex *before* the passion heats up. Ask for and volunteer to have an AIDS/STD test before embark-ing on a sexual relationship.
- Be responsible. If you think you have been exposed to an STD, seek medical help, testing, and treatment. Urge your partner to do the same. Refrain from sex until you and your partner have finished treatment.

THE BOTTOM LINE

Be well informed about birth control, STDs, and safe sex so that you can relax and enjoy the benefits of mature sexuality. Remember, communication is the best aphrodisiac. Keep novelty and fun in your long-term sexual relationship. Practise safe sex in new rela-tionships. Midlife is a time to enjoy your sexuality and make love, not just have sex.

Contacts and Further Information

Organizations

- (In U.S.) American Academy of Family Physicians, 8880 Ward Parkway, Kansas City, KS. Tel.: (800) 274–2237; Fax: (816) 822–0907.
- The American Association of Sex Educators, Counsellors and Therapists, P.O. Box 238, Mount Vernon, IA 52314. Tel.: (319) 895–8407; Fax: (319) 895–6203. Provides names of qualified therapists in your area.
- American College of Obstetricians and Gynecologists, 409 12th St., S.W., Washington, DC 20024. Tel.: (800) 673–8444.
- (In Canada) No-Scalpel Vasectomy Inc., 29 Clemow Ave., Ottawa, ON K1S 2B1. Tel.: (613) 236–6772; Fax: (613) 237–8193.
- The North American Menopause Society (NAMS), P.O. Box 94527, Cleveland, OH 44101–4527. Tel.: (216) 844–8748.
- The Sex Information and Education Council of Canada, 850 Coxwell Ave., East York, ON M4C 5R1. Tel.: (416) 466–5304; Fax: (416) 778–0785; E-mail: sieccan@web.net.
- Sexuality Information and Education Council of the United States, 130 West 42nd St., Suite 350, New York, NY 10036. Tel.: (212) 819–9770. Call to request a list of publications or a list of certified sex therapists in your area.
- The Society of Obstetricians and Gynaecologists of Canada, 774 Promenade Echo Dr., Ottawa, ON K1S 5N8. Tel.: (613) 730–4192.

Websites

- AIDS Clearinghouse (Canada) (sponsored by Canadian Public Health Association): http://www.cpha.ca
- Best Years (columnist Mike Bellah, PhD): http://www.bestyears.com
- Centers for Disease Control and Prevention (U.S.) (for information on STDs, HIV, birth control, and AIDS): http://www.cdc.gov/nchwww/default.htm
- Health Canada (for information on STDs, HIV, and AIDS): http://www.hwc.ca

- Sexual Health Infocenter (sponsored by Renaissance Discovery): http://www.sexhealth.org/infocenter/infomain.htm

Newsletter
- *Sex over 40*, P.O. Box 1600, Chapel Hill, NC 27515. $36 U.S. annually.

Books
- *For Each Other: Sharing Sexual Intimacy* by Lonnie Barbach. Garden City, NY: Anchor Press/Doubleday, 1982.
- *For Yourself: The Fulfilment of Female Sexuality* by Lonnie Barbach. New York: Signet, 1975. It's old but still one of the best.
- *In Touch* by Dr. Beryl Chernick and Dr. Avinoam Chernick. Toronto: Macmillan, 1977.
- *The New Joy of Sex* by Alex Comfort. Westminster, MD: Random House, 1995.
- *The New Male Sexuality* by Bernie Zilbergeld. New York: Bantam Books, 1992.
- *Sex May Be Wasted on the Young* by Lee Stones and Michael Stones. York University (Toronto): Captus Press, 1996.

Related Chapters in This Book
- *Chapter 2: Understanding the Female Menopause* and *Chapter 3: Is There a Male Menopause?* discuss the effects of menopause on sexuality.
- *Chapter 6: Wrinkles, Chin Hairs, and Baldness* suggests that a positive, realistic body image, not an obsession with youth, is what keeps you vibrant, sexy, and feeling good.
- *Chapter 7: The Active Living Solution* reminds you that fit people make better lovers and suggests ways that you can get active now.
- *Chapter 9: The Boomer's Drugs of Choice* provides advice on moderate drinking and butting out for good. Alcohol and tobacco use can both have a negative effect on your sex life.
- *Chapter 10: Growing Apart and Together: Relationships in Midlife* suggests ways to nurture intimate relationships.
- *Chapter 12: Dealing with Impotence* gives you more details on the causes of impotence and how to deal with it.

- *Chapter 16: Partners in Health Care* gives you information on talking with your physician and how to find more information on the Internet.
- *Chapter 21: Hormone Replacement Therapy (HRT): The Big Decision* provides more information on the use of hormone therapy as a way to prevent vaginal dryness and other sexual discomforts that sometimes are part of the menopausal period.
- *Chapter 22: Complementary and Alternative Medicine Is Coming on Strong* provides additional information on the use of herbal remedies that increase vitality.

CHAPTER TWELVE

Dealing with Impotence

Viagra could give new meaning to the phrase "Don't worry, dear, I'm on the pill." — Sue Johansen, sex counsellor[1]

The Age of Viagra

Since man first walked on earth, his power (and often his sense of self-worth) has been directly related to his ability to have and maintain an erect penis. Indeed, in our interviews with middle-aged men, many stated that losing the ability to have an erection was one of their primary concerns about getting older. Researchers confirm what men say. At the 1994 annual meeting of the American Urologists Association, Dr. Irving Goldstein of Boston University reported that the most striking finding of his research on impotence was "its impact on men's ability to work, maintain social and family roles and sustain self-esteem.[2] Is it any wonder that when Viagra — the first effective oral medication for impotence — was released in the spring of 1998, 36,000 prescriptions were filled during its first two weeks on the market?

Our chapter on impotence had already been drafted when Viagra was released (we had predicted its coming, but the test results were not yet in). We knew immediately that this major breakthrough would affect not only this chapter but others as well. Finally, men had a convenient, painless option for dealing with an emotionally charged issue that affects more than 50 per cent of men between forty and seventy years of age at some time.

A review of our draft confirmed that considerable rewriting was necessary, especially around the investigation and treatment of impotence (what the medical community calls erectile dysfunction, or ED). Yet a lot of what we believed important was still pertinent. It is still important to understand how aging affects potency, how intimacy is involved, and how difficult it is to separate the physical and the psychological causes of erection problems. This chapter gives you this information, as well as what we could find out about Viagra and other new impotence drugs on the horizon.

Impotence and Aging

Virtually all men are occasionally unable to have an erection. For many, the first agonizing experience occurs at a relatively young age, when having sex after an evening of heavy drinking. The likelihood of impotence, however, increases with age.

The 1994 Massachusetts Male Aging Study of 1,290 men aged forty to seventy showed that more than 50 per cent experienced some degree of erectile dysfunction: the largest group (25 per cent) had moderate impotence (a problem attaining and keeping an erection half the time); 17 per cent experienced minimal impotence, and 10 per cent were completely impotent.[3]

After age fifty, some normal physiological changes occur. It takes longer to get an erection, and it is softer. There is a longer refractory period (after ejaculation it takes longer to get it up again), and the force of the ejaculation decreases. Men in midlife are more likely to experience emotional feelings of overload, pressure, and turmoil, which can all play a major role in impotence. Understanding and accepting this is important, since denying the changes associated with aging and stress can result in a vicious circle: a hint of performance problems leads to increased denial and anxiety – which in turn lead to increased erection difficulties. Fear of failure can also cause physical changes such as an increase in the secretion of the hormone epinephrine. This increase affects the muscles of the penis and can prevent an erection or mean the loss of erection sooner than desired.

A note of encouragement: If you keep yourself healthy and learn to accept some inevitable fluctuations in libido, *impotence is not an inevitable consequence of aging.* According to the 1993 James Report, some 40 per cent of men over age sixty-five enjoy sex several times a week.[4] One doctor we interviewed told us about an eighty-four-year-old who came to emergency late one night because he couldn't get an erection. The tired physician suggested that the gentleman's problem, while distressing at any age, was not really an emergency. The older man replied, "It may not be an emergency for you, Doc, but it sure is for me!"

Does the appearance of Viagra make the normal changes associated with aging irrelevant today? No, it does not. Viagra corrects erection problems when accompanied by sexual arousal and stimulation. It is not an aphrodisiac or a fountain of sexual youth. It does not affect libido or fix troubled relationships.

Viagra offers many men who are experiencing moderate or total erection problems a positive, easy-to-use treatment option to vacuums and penile injections. Later in this chapter we describe another new medication called Medicated Urethral System for Erection (MUSE), which may be even more effective for men with medical conditions. The appearance of these drugs on the market may also mean that many more men experiencing ED will visit their doctors, knowing that a non-invasive, more spontaneous form of treatment is now available. This benefit is important. Surveys indicate that, before Viagra, 80 per cent of men with impotence problems never sought treatment[5] and that most men waited three years before they sought help.[6] The longer a man waits to seek treatment, the more complex and difficult an impotence problem is likely to be. This is because a vicious circle of denial and lowered self-esteem is often the result of impotence. As one man told us, "I just don't talk about it. That way, nobody will know."

How Does an Erection Occur?
The hormone testosterone is responsible for male sex characteristics and libido; erections are controlled by the nervous system. The spinal nerves cause men to have an erection in response to genital touching; the nerves in the brain generate the response to sexual fantasies or to hugging and kissing.

Once a man is aroused, electrical activity in the brain sets off a series of reactions in the penis. Inside the shaft of the penis are two erectile cylinders, surrounded by a tight coat of fibre. Signals from the brain stimulate the release of a chemical in the penis called cyclic GMP (guanosine monophosphate). GMP causes the muscle layer in the cylinders to relax and the arteries to expand. This increases blood flow, which pours into the space, expanding it and squeezing shut the veins that normally carry the blood out of the penis. The cylinders become rigid, making the penis harden. Finally, a set of muscles at the base of the penis contracts, enlarging the penis and making it more rigid.

In men with erectile dysfunction, the veins that allow the blood to leave the penis do not get squeezed off, due to a shortage of cyclic GMP. Viagra works by increasing the cyclic GMP that is present, allowing for a full erection. Interestingly, Viagra (sildenafil) was first tested as a heart drug designed to increase blood flow to the heart. While it did not open coronary arteries, the fact that it did increase blood flow to the penis came to the attention of the researchers when the happy test subjects were reluctant to return their pills!

Determining the Causes of Impotence: Is It My Hormones or My Head?
At least half of North American men over age forty have experienced midlife impotence to varying degrees. When problems persist, it is time to see your physician and look for underlying causes. As we will see, the causes are varied and include both physical and psychological issues.

One of the concerns about Viagra is the North American tendency to jump to the magic-pill solution without considering the underlying causes of the problem. While Viagra may "fix the plumbing," you may compromise your health, well-being, and relationship if you fail to investigate the root cause. In her recent book *Male Passages*, Gail Sheehy sums it up this way: "The potency pill is a mixed blessing. If [a man] can walk into certain doctors' offices or fly-by-night clinics and ask for a potency pill, it may never be discovered that his impotence is a result of depression, or high cholesterol, diabetes, high blood pressure, or that he has evidence of prostate cancer, which is quite curable if detected early."[7]

Physical Causes of Erectile Dysfunction
Physicians used to believe that impotence was almost exclusively a psychological problem. They now know that more than half of impotence cases – some researchers report as many as 80 per cent – are caused primarily by physical problems.[8] Essentially, anything that disrupts blood flow to the penis or interferes with the nerve or gland functions of erection can impair sexual function.

There are numerous physical conditions that can affect erectile dysfunction:
- chronic illnesses, including hardening of the arteries, heart disease, high blood pressure, diabetes, and chronic peptic ulcers;

- insufficient testosterone production (which causes a less-firm erection and less-intense orgasm) or problems with other glandular and hormonal functions in the body;
- use of tobacco products (smoking reduces blood flow);
- complications resulting from prostate surgery (although new studies described in Chapter 18 suggest that impotence does not have to be a common consequence of surgery) or from other abdominal surgery;
- neurological diseases such as stroke, multiple sclerosis, and Parkinson disease;
- damage to the spinal cord overall or to the fine nerve tissues (such as diabetes);
- disease or deformity of the penis.

In addition, certain lifestyle practices and the use of certain drugs may also affect a man's ability to get and maintain an erection (usually on a temporary basis). These include:

- the use of certain prescription drugs, including those used to treat high blood pressure, elevated blood cholesterol, heart disease, and depression, and some over-the-counter drugs, such as some sinus and allergy medications and appetite suppressants;[9]
- excessive consumption of alcohol or the use of illicit drugs (cannabis, cocaine, or LSD).

Psychological Causes of Erectile Dysfunction

Psychological factors play an important role in impotence, both as a primary cause and because emotional concerns tend to aggravate physical causes. What are the key psychological factors?

- Depression (which is often accompanied by lethargy and lowered self-esteem) can interfere with your sex drive and cause physical changes that interfere with erection. Ironically, some antidepressant medications can cause erection failure as a side-effect.
- Anger is another important predictor of problems. Men who score high on tests of anger are more likely to have potency problems than men with lower scores.[10]
- Studies suggest that men with dominating personalities are less likely to be impotent than those who are less controlling.[11] Power and potency have always been linked. Indeed, the word impotence

comes from the Latin word *impotentia* meaning "lack of power." Henry Kissinger is often quoted as saying that power is the great aphrodisiac. This may explain why men who feel they are unsuccessful at work sometimes have erection problems. In North American culture, high incomes and success at work are still equated with personal power and status.

- Performance anxiety and fear of failure can lead to a vicious circle of anxiety —➤ failure to get an erection —➤ increased anxiety, and so on.
- Other psychological factors relate to one's response to stress, preoccupation with other issues such as work, and feelings of guilt.
- Relationship issues, such as discontent, a partner's emotional unavailability, and discrepancies in sexual drive and preferences, can also contribute to impotence.

IMPOTENCE: IS THE CAUSE PSYCHOLOGICAL?

The following set of questions helps determine whether or not impotence can be attributed largely to psychological reasons. "Adequate" is defined as sufficient for penetration.

1. Do you experience adequate spontaneous erections or erections upon waking two or more times each week?
2. Do you experience adequate erections during foreplay and/or masturbation?
3. Do you experience adequate erections with someone other than your partner or erections induced by fantasy?
4. Have you experienced an abrupt onset of impotence associated with psychosocial stress, such as a divorce, an illness in the family, the loss of a job, or some other trauma?
5. Have you experienced an abrupt onset of impotence that is *not* associated with a change in your medical status or use of medication?
6. Do you get an erection but have trouble maintaining it until penetration?

Answering Yes to the first 3 questions is clear evidence that the dysfunction is mainly psychological; answering Yes to questions 4 through 6 suggests the same conclusion (but not as strongly as questions 1 through 3).

Adapted from K. Blindt-Segraves and R. T. Segraves, "Psychogenic Impotence," in A. Bennett, ed., *Impotence: Diagnosis and Management of Erectile Dysfunction* (Philadelphia: W. B. Saunders, 1994), p. 94.

Impotence and Intimacy

The following three stories show how complex and interrelated the causes of impotence can be.

Impotence can be an outcome of an unhealthy lifestyle that leads to an unhappy relationship. **Margaret**, age forty, and **Colin**, age forty-five, were both upset about Colin's inability to get an erection. They had been living together for three years. Their sex life had been great until Colin's daily nightcap had turned into two beers and a bottle of wine. Colin's first failure to get an erection had been devastating for his self-image. He claimed that it was one of the reasons he was drinking more. He believed that alcohol would help him relax and get turned on. Colin loved Margaret and he could not understand what was wrong. Margaret was equally baffled. Colin seemed healthy and she knew there was no one else. But impotence was one of the ways her previous husband had expressed his anger with her. Was Colin losing interest in her, or was alcohol the problem?

Margaret became increasingly hurt and frustrated, not only with Colin's sexual performance, but also because she felt unloved. After six months of fighting, Colin agreed alcohol was probably a large part of the problem. With the help of a close friend, Colin joined Alcoholics Anonymous and managed to stop drinking. Three months later, Colin was able to get and maintain an erection; however, his intimate relationship with Margaret remained a problem.

After a thorough physical, Colin's doctor gave him a clean bill of health and applauded his abstinence. He explained that it would take time for Colin and Margaret to rebuild their relationship and for Margaret to trust that Colin would remain sober. Colin and Margaret agreed to see a psychotherapist for marital therapy. They both hoped that it was not too late.

Sometimes, the frustration of impotence can be the turning point that leads to personal re-assessment in midlife and more open communication between couples. **Robert**, a fifty-year-old lawyer in a large firm, was devastated when he was unable to get an erection on several occasions. His wife, **Susan**, was encouraging and suggested that the problem was related to stress at work. When Robert talked about going to his doctor, she supported the idea. After a thorough physical, Robert's physician asked him some questions about his marriage and his sex life. It became clear that there was no physical reason for Robert's problem, but that his emotional life was in turmoil. Robert was agonizing over whether or not he should stay in his marriage. The sexual spark with his wife was gone and another woman had become important to him. Robert's physician suggested that his problem was emotional, not physical, and that he go home to have a long, honest conversation with his wife. Since Robert was still unsure about what he wanted to do, his doctor suggested psychotherapy.

Frank, a fifty-eight-year-old businessman, had suffered partial impotence since prostate surgery five years earlier. He had tried numerous things, but both he and his wife were uncomfortable with the lack of spontaneity (and discomfort for Frank) of treatments such as penile injections. Frank's doctor prescribed MUSE. Frank went home apprehensive and excited and wondered how to approach his wife, **Chloe**. Then he remembered how a romantic dinner used to be a part of their lovemaking rituals. So Frank surprised Chloe with a candle-lit dinner he cooked himself. After dinner, Frank and Chloe inserted the small pellet into his penis and both of them enjoyed a long period of gentle physical and mental stimulation before penetration. Frank and Chloe lay in bed together for an hour afterward, laughing, touching, and reliving old times.

Investigating Impotence

What do you do when she says yes and your penis says no? Occasional failure to get an erection is not true impotence. You and your partner need to treat it as something that happens from time to time, especially in midlife when you have a lot of responsibilities and stress. Don't abandon your lovemaking when it happens. Instead, enjoy the opportunity to touch, cuddle, and experiment with each other.

Whatever the cause, persistent impotence is not just "his" problem. It is best treated as a couple's concern. Inevitably, impotence that remains a silent problem affects the woman partner as well as the man. Indeed, women whose partners are impotent may become withdrawn or hostile if both parties don't learn how to communicate with each other.[12]

Talking about your feelings and the situation with your partner is the first step. Of course, this is not easy. You might use this book to start a conversation. This worked for one of our patients, who told us that her husband had refused to discuss the issue. She left the draft chapter by his side of the bed. He read it and then began to talk with her about the problem. Understanding what was happening, and knowing that impotence is a common occurrence that, in most cases, can be treated without invasive side-effects, enabled one troubled man to break the silence with his partner.

Women can help by treating the problem as temporary, and by encouraging their partners to seek help. A loving partner who does not feel shut out and is able to remain sensitive can be an essential source of support during this stressful time. Men need to work hard to overcome the tendency to withdraw when feeling anxious or embarrassed – this will only make your partner feel rejected and confused. Stay connected and make time for your relationship. Some therapists suggest avoiding intercourse and concentrating on caressing, kissing, and other forms of sexual pleasuring the next few times you are together.

If problems persist, of course, it is time to see your physician. He will take a complete history, ask you questions about smoking, alcohol intake, and your use of prescription medicines, over-the-counter drugs, and herbal remedies. He will also ask about current frustrations and stresses in your life. He may recommend some lifestyle changes: quitting smoking, cutting back on drinking, and getting more exercise.

After a complete physical examination, including the prostate, penis, and testicles, your physician will likely order blood and urine tests. If there are no contraindications to the use of Viagra, he will likely suggest that you try it. If Viagra does not work, your physician will probably prescribe MUSE. If MUSE fails, further investigation is necessary. You may be referred to a urologist, or to an andrology clinic if there is one in your area. These clinics have a urologist, endocrinologist, and psychologist on staff and can assess the problem completely. More specific tests may be ordered, such as the nocturnal penile tumescence test, which is carried out in a sleep laboratory. This test measures the rigidity and number of erections a man has during sleep. If the penis becomes erect the normal number of times during sleep, he may be facing psychological issues that are causing the problem. Another test involves injection of an erection-producing drug into the side of the penis. If the injection does not produce an erection, the physician will proceed to investigate further physical causes.

DID YOU KNOW?

On average, men get an erection every 70 to 100 minutes while sleeping. The intervals between erections grows longer as they get older.

Treatment Options for Persistent Impotence

Treatment for erectile failure depends on the cause. If impotence is caused by a particular drug you are taking, a simple change in prescription should help. Because of the strong links between the physical and emotional causes of impotence, however, the treatment commonly involves both medical and psychological interventions.

1. *Lifestyle Changes.* Since excessive drinking and smoking and the use of certain medications or illicit drugs can cause impotence, lifestyle changes are the first treatment option. Living drug-free, eating healthy food, and exercising regularly will benefit your whole body and mind, not just your ability to perform sexually.

2. *Couples Counselling.* Couples counselling can be helpful, because impotence affects how a man feels about himself and how a couple interrelate.

3. *Viagra (sildenafil).* While Viagra is not a panacea, it is an effective drug for men who are experiencing persistent impotence. In carefully controlled studies, improvements in erection were reported by 63 per cent of men taking 25 mg, 74 per cent taking 50 mg, and 82 per cent taking 100 mg of the drug, compared to 24 per cent taking a placebo. About 10 per cent of men in the drug trial experienced mild headaches, nausea, indigestion, and facial flushing. On high doses, about 3 per cent of the participants were unable to distinguish

between green and blue. Viagra does not cause persistent erection (priapism), a major problem with penile drug injections.[13]

A man using Viagra takes a single pill about one hour before lovemaking; then he and his partner engage in sexual stimulation in order to achieve and sustain an erection. Viagra may also hold out some promise for women; while more research is needed, early studies suggest that it may also help women who have difficulties achieving orgasms.

Viagra should never be taken with nitrates such as nitroglycerin; together they may lower the blood pressure to dangerous levels. Some physicians are also concerned about possible interactions with medications for high blood pressure. As with any new drug, there are still many unanswered questions about Viagra. Will it work over an extended period of time? Will it cause negative interactions with other drugs? What are the long-term effects?

Paradoxically, using Viagra and other new impotence drugs, which is so much easier than earlier treatment options, is the reason behind some sex therapists' warnings to couples about using these drugs too quickly. Many couples have learned to deal with impotence over the years by enjoying forms of sexual intimacy other than penetration. Others have agreed to share their lives without sexual intercourse. Suddenly, there is a pill that may reverse the problem mechanically. Therapists fear that, without planning and good communication, this abrupt change may send a relationship into chaos. Women unaccustomed to intercourse may find it physically uncomfortable or fear that they will lose their now-potent partners to younger women. Men who have regained the ability to engage in intercourse may forget how important foreplay, cuddling, and other forms of sexual intimacy are to their partners.

4. *Medicated Urethral System for Erection or* MUSE *(alprostadil).* Sildenafil (Viagra) will not work for everyone; for example, it may be not be effective with some men who have medical conditions such as diabetes, vascular disease (plugged arteries), or impotence following prostate or abdominal surgery. MUSE may be the treatment of choice for these men. MUSE comes in the form of very small pellets or suppositories, which can be inserted painlessly into the tip

of the penis to widen the blood vessels and increase the flow of blood to the penis. Studies show that two-thirds of men who tried this system found it effective. Lowered blood pressure is one possible side-effect; some men may experience mild pain or burning in the penis while using the medication.[14] When using MUSE, it is important to work it into lovemaking, just as putting on a condom is best done as part of intimate foreplay. Because MUSE causes an erection independent of stimulation, it may minimize the loving interaction between a couple, unless both parties make a conscious effort to include caressing and stimulation before penetration.

MUSE differs considerably from Viagra. Unlike oral medications, it works locally on the penile tissue and does not have to be absorbed into the body. An additional advantage is that there are no known drug interactions.

5. *Other Treatment Options*:

- Self-administered penile drug injections before intercourse produce an erection that lasts for three hours. Ironically, the most worrisome side-effect is possible priapism, or persistent erection. After six hours, this condition must be treated in a hospital emergency department, before permanent damage is done to the spongy tissue of the penis.

- Hormone (testosterone) replacement therapy in the form of injections, tablets, or skin patches may be used if hormone levels are low (after a check to rule out prostate cancer). Men with low levels of testosterone report significant increases in sexual arousal and sexual activity with testosterone supplements.[15]

- Yohimbine, one of the oldest aphrodisiacs known to man, is a chemical extracted from the bark of an African tree. It has been shown to improve erections in 30 to 40 per cent of subjects (the same percentage who improved with a placebo).[16]

- Trazodone is an antidepressant that causes a prolonged erection as a side-effect. This drug is sometimes used to treat men who suffer from depression and performance anxiety at the same time.

- Creams containing nitroglycerin and minoxidil rubbed on the penis before intercourse increase the blood flow to the penis and produce a stiffer erection. These creams, however, can cause your partner to get headaches if the nitroglycerin enters her blood through the vagina and goes to the brain.

- Surgical implants are prosthetic, mechanical devices that supplement or replace the function of the penis. There are two types of implants – semi-rigid rods that provide half an erection all the time and inflatable implants that are activated by squeezing a pump implanted in the scrotum. While these devices can malfunction, a 1991 study in the *American Family Physician* showed that 80 to 90 per cent of men who have implants said they were satisfied.[17]
- Vascular surgery can sometimes correct a narrowing in the artery that supplies blood to the penis.
- External vacuum devices, which have been around in various forms since 1917, usually consist of a vacuum chamber, a pump, connector tubing, and penile-constriction bands. Men using these devices (and their partners) report improved sexual functioning, despite some minor side-effects.[18]

THE BOTTOM LINE

Most midlife men will experience impotence once in a while or for a short period of time. You and your partner should not let an occasional occurrence of impotence become a major upset. Keep talking and spend more time on affectionate touching. If the problem persists, see your doctor about it. In the vast majority of cases, impotence can be helped in an unobtrusive way. Treatment is most successful when both partners support one another and are involved in treatment.

Contacts and Further Information

Organizations

- The American Association of Sex Educators, Counsellors and Therapists, P.O. Box 238, Mount Vernon, IA 52314. Tel.: (319) 895–8407; Fax: (319) 895–6203. Provides names of qualified therapists in your area.

- Canadian Diabetic Association, 78 Bond St., Toronto, ON M5B 2J8. Tel.: (416) 363–3373.
- Impotence Institute of America, 10400 Little Patuxent Parkway, Suite 485, Columbia, MD 21044–3502. Helpline: (800) 669–1603; Tel.: (410) 715–9605; Fax: (410) 715–9609. Provides information and referrals to local support groups.
- The Sex Information and Education Council of Canada, 850 Coxwell Ave., East York, ON M4C 5R1. Tel.: (416) 466–5304; Fax: (416) 778–0785; E-mail: sieccan@web.net

Please see Chapter 11 for other helpful organizations.

Websites and Toll-Free Telephone Numbers
- Impotence Site (sponsored by Pharmacia and Upjohn Pharmaceuticals): http://www.impotent.com/
- Urology Information (sponsored by American Urological Society): http://www.auanet.org
- Urology Nurses of Canada: http://www.unc.org
- Vivus (sponsored by Vivus Corporate, a pharmaceutical company): http://www.vivus.com
- Toll-free Erectile Dysfunction Information Centre: 1–888–678–2820.

Please see Chapters 3 and 11 for additional websites.

Books
- *BioPotency: Your Guide to Problem-Free Sexual Fulfilment* by Richard Berger and Deborah Berger. New York: Avon Books, 1990.
- *Male Sexual Health: A Couple's Guide* by Richard Spark. New York: Consumer Reports Books, 1991.
- *Midlife Man* by Art Hister. Vancouver: Greystone Books, 1998.
- *The New Male Sexuality* by Bernie Zilbergeld. New York: Bantam Books, 1992.
- *Understanding Male Sexual Health* by Dorothy Baldwin and Richard Berger. New York: Hippocrene Books, 1995.

Please see Chapter 11 for additional related books.

Related Chapters in This Book

- *Chapter 3: Is There a Male Menopause?* provides more information on the male midlife passage.

- *Chapter 9: The Boomer's Drugs of Choice* gives some practical suggestions on how to cut down on drinking and quit smoking.

- *Chapter 10: Growing Apart and Together: Relationships in Midlife* discusses ways to nurture intimate relationships in midlife.

- *Chapter 11: Enjoying Sex in Midlife* explains the changes in sexuality we can expect as we grow older.

- *Chapter 13: Stress-Proofing in Midlife* provides tips on de-stressing your life and improving your emotional well-being.

- *Chapter 15: When Times Are Tough: Depression, Anxiety, and Insomnia* will help you determine whether you should seek help for depression or anxiety; these are common causes of impotence.

- *Chapter 18: Prostate Health* describes how the prostate gland changes with age. Prostate problems or treatments may be linked to impotence.

CHAPTER THIRTEEN

Stress-Proofing in Midlife

Stress is the spice of life – Hans Selye[1]

The experience of stress is a given in our lives, and it is, as Hans Selye suggests, "the spice of life." Stress can save us from complacency and boredom. But most of us have trouble seeing stress as adding spice, zest, and flavour to our lives. More often, it gives us heartburn, headaches, and back problems. We complain to each other that we are "stressed to the max," and that "we can't handle the stress any more." Too often, we find ourselves in a stressful situation, too exhausted to see that we might be able to do something to change it.

This chapter is designed to help you take better charge of your relationship to stress, become more resilient in the face of stressful situations, and be more "stress-hardy."[2] Just as some plants learn to thrive in harsh climates through adaptation, so too do we need to learn to be hardy in the face of the challenging and ever-changing circumstances of our lives.

This chapter begins by identifying some of the major midlife stressors, then discusses what stress is and what it isn't. It takes a look at how stress has an impact on our work life and how to avoid burnout. These two issues are of particular concern to people in midlife. Then the chapter shifts focus, by presenting a useful and engaging exercise for assessing your stress level, followed by a practical approach to improve your stress-proofing quotient.

Midlife Stressors
While the experience of stress is not unique to any particular age group, there are certain issues that seem to come into sharp focus in midlife. Here are some of them:

- *Being in the sandwich generation.* Women in particular often find themselves squeezed between providing care for elderly parents while still looking after young children. This squeeze is often accompanied by a gap in support, due to geographical distance from other siblings and less involvement in community and religious centres, which traditionally have provided support to families.
- *The changing face of the midlife family.* Many boomers divorce, remarry, and start second families and/or live in blended families with children from previous marriages. Some find themselves "empty nesters," with children leaving home, or "boomerangers," with adult children returning.
- *Hormonal fluxes.* For women especially, the shifting hormonal tides that influence mood, sexual desire, and sleep can erode the calm and confidence needed to cope with external changes. Many women try to be "superwomen," thinking that they should be able to handle the demands of career, children, parents, spouse, and hot flashes, without blinking an eye. They are dismayed when they collapse or become depressed or seriously ill.
- *Work-related stress.* Corporate restructuring, downsizing, rapid technological advances, and early retirement have all contributed to dramatic changes in our work lives, as we will see later in this chapter.
- *Financial insecurity.* Our interviewees repeatedly named financial insecurity as one of the major stressors in midlife. Dwindling government resources, people living longer, and children requiring lengthier periods of support have all contributed to this growing concern.
- *Awareness of mortality.* The death of a parent, good friend, or colleague, a life-threatening illness, or turning fifty are some of the events that get us thinking about the time we have left in our lives. Not only can we not "have it all," we will not be "forever young," either. This awareness can become either a major stressor or a useful wake-up call.
- *Worrying.* Finding time and energy to do everything we need to do to stay well can be stressful in itself, according to some women. We become stressed about being stressed! That's the point at which we need to laugh and learn to take ourselves a little more lightly.

What Stress Is and Isn't

Human beings – like most animals – want to be safe, comfortable, and well-fed. By nature, we seek homeostasis, an inner stability and balance. Once we achieve a sense of well-being, we want things to stay like that ... forever. We quickly try to negate or overlook the one irrefutable constant in our lives: change. In the face of constant flux, we are required to adapt. Our difficulties with adaptation and flexibility are what lead to stress.

In the mid-1950s, Canadian researcher Hans Selye popularized the term "stress." He called it "the nonspecific response of the organism to any pressure or demand on it."[3] In other words, stress is not the cause of our upsets; rather it is our total response – physical, mental, emotional, and behavioural – to anything that disrupts our sense of equilibrium. Stress is a normal part of life, and can't be avoided. There can be good stress (called eustress) that results from a happy occurrence, such as getting married, being promoted, or winning the lottery. Bad stress (more familiar to us as distress) occurs in the face of events we construe negatively, such as being fired from a job, getting divorced, or missing that green light. The stressor, according to Selye, is "that which produces stress."[4]

Jon Kabat-Zinn, author of *Full Catastrophe Living* and founder of the Stress Reduction Clinic at the University of Massachusetts Medical Center, further clarifies Selye's definition. He points out that "a stressor can be (and often is) an internal occurrence as well as an external one."[5] For example, on a roller-coaster ride, one person may be up in the front car, squealing with glee, while another sits white-knuckled in the back seat, praying for the ride to end. They are having the same external experience, yet a completely different inner experience. In this case, the perception of your degree of choice or control determines your level of stress. What constitutes stress for each of us is unique; we each have our own version of it, which is always changing, yet generally maintains some basic pattern.

The basic stress reaction is as old as humankind. When we experience something as a danger to our well-being, the famous "fight or flight" response kicks in and we once again become the hapless cave-dweller face to face with the sabre-toothed tiger. Our automatic physiological response remains the same as it was thousands of years ago, although the nature of our stressors has changed enormously.

When we move into the "fight or flight" position, a chain reaction of physiological responses occurs. The mind sounds the alarm to the body. The pituitary gland releases adrenalin and other stress hormones to sharpen our perceptions. Heart rate and blood pressure increase to maximize blood flow. The liver releases sugars, cholesterol, and fatty acids into the bloodstream for energy, and we move into high gear. This chain reaction (called the "General Adaptation Syndrome" by Selye) has helped us survive for thousands of years by getting us ready to either flee the situation or fight to survive when we sense danger.

The problem is that "the fight or flight response is a physiologically neurotic response for twentieth-century living," according to Dr. Robert Eliot, former director of Preventive and Rehabilitative Cardiology at St. Luke's Hospital in Phoenix, Arizona. He adds, "People are reacting to today's problems with yesterday's primitive responses. Rather than physically battle tigers, we must be subtly attuned to office politics. As a result, we end up pumping high-energy chemicals for low-energy needs. The price is high; over the long haul, we turn the energy inward and burn out."[6]

When we respond to daily annoyances such as a traffic jam or the computer crashing in the same physiological way we would to a life-threatening event, we gradually wear ourselves down and may seriously compromise our immune system's ability to combat illness.

Stress and the Immune System

Most of us are not surprised if we get a sore throat or indigestion when we're anxious about an approaching deadline. What we've know for years – anecdotally – about the effect that stress has on our body's ability to fight off illness is only beginning to be scientifically validated. While research is still very much in the preliminary stage, a plausible model is being developed in the field called psychoneuroimmunology (PNI), to explain how our thoughts, emotions, and experiences may influence our susceptibility or resistance to disease.[7] For example, in 1996, research at Johns Hopkins University showed that people who overreact to certain types of stress that we all experience (such as driving in the car) may be as much as twenty times more likely to have silent heart disease than people who react less dramatically.[8]

In his book *Love and Survival*, Dr. Dean Ornish cites research comparing the negative effects of isolation and loneliness with the positive effects of love and companionship on the health of the heart. A study of 10,000 married men with angina at Case Western Reserve University showed that those who felt loved by their wives had significantly fewer angina attacks than those who did not feel loved, even when risk factors were high. Research on ulcers found similar results; those in a close, loving relationship seemed to have a lower incidence of ulcers than those who did not, after other factors were accounted for.[9]

Today there is increasing evidence that managing stress helps to maintain good physical health. Many companies now fund stress-management courses for their employees as part of rehabilitative programs after serious illnesses. This is considered a good investment that helps reduce absenteeism.

The End of an Illusion: Work-Related Stress in Midlife
Remember the predictions in the 1960s that, in the coming decades, we would have so much free time that we would not know what to do with it? Technology would simplify our working lives and give us the leisure time we craved. The reality has turned out to be just the opposite. In the twenty-five years between 1969 and 1994, time at work for the average American increased by 158 hours per year. It is not uncommon for women and men in the high-tech industry and other fields to work 70 to 80 hours or more per week.[10]

A lack of employment security is another major stressor in modern-day midlife. In 1992, nearly half of all Americans worried about losing their jobs; in the latter half of the 1990s, job insecurity plagued both Americans and Canadians in all areas of employment.[11] The days are long gone when an employee could anticipate a predictable, orderly rise through the ranks of the company, a reward for twenty-five years' service, and a comfortable retirement. Gone also is the expectation of working nine to five, five days a week. An estimated 75 to 80 percent of all absenteeism from work can be linked to stress-related health problems.

Economic pressures, downsizing, restructuring, mergers, and business globalization are all part of an unprecedented era of change that has wreaked havoc with people's ability to cope. Electronic communication technology coupled with a global economy has made it almost impossible to slow down. We have laptops, cell phones, faxes, e-mail, voicemail, and world-wide, overnight courier services. David Shenk, in his book *Data Smog: Surviving the Information Glut*, writes, "In a society that has come to be so broadly defined by information technology, it is becoming increasingly clear that the information revolution sweeping us into a new realm of communications is also serving as one of our greatest stressors."[12]

Even a holiday is no longer a guaranteed time for relaxation and renewal. Now we can (and do) work anywhere and all the time – sometimes with disastrous consequences for ourselves and our families.

While the pressures have an impact on all workers in this culture, there are particular ways in which they affect men and women in midlife. The post-war baby-boomer generation moved into young adulthood and beyond with enormous expectations that they could do and have whatever they wanted. Many feel disappointed, trapped, bewildered, and angry that they are now faced with retraining or seeking new career paths in midlife.

One male interviewee said, "I was raised with work as a focus in life, and then I was declared redundant in 1992. I had to start a business in order to eat. Working seven days a week to survive is not enjoyable any more. There is no satisfaction."

As mentioned earlier, women may be especially susceptible to work stress, as they face multiple role conflicts and excess responsibilities both at work and at home. A large city law firm we know classifies women as part-time who opt off the partner track to spend more time with their young children and therefore work *only* nine to six, Monday to Friday. Companies' expectations of workers have increased, and people try to meet them in order to hold onto their jobs. As the gap widens between these unrealistic expectations and the ability to fulfil them, high levels of stress result.

This distress stems from "a poor fit" between the *capabilities* of the individual and the *demands* of the job; and between the *needs* of the individual and the *ability* of the job environment to meet those needs.

The two on-the-job factors that seem to increase stress the most are:

- *Responsibility without authority*, that is, being responsible for making a system work, without having the authority to implement changes. This is often the plight of middle managers who have programs and staff for whom they are responsible; yet higher-level managers to whom they report have the authority to make work changes. Nurses and teachers tend to face this type of stress. They see problems on the ward or in the classroom, but generally do not have the authority to change procedures.

- *Lack of control over workload or work flow* can both produce anxiety and demoralize people. In a recent Harvard study, nearly 55 per cent of shift workers said the pace of their work was the most common problem in job-related stress.[13] Because of layoffs, fewer people now do the same amount of work.

Some people are more prone to be negatively affected by work stress than others. An example is the well-known "Type A" personality, who exhibits an exaggerated sense of time urgency, aggressiveness, and competitiveness. Those who gain their sense of identity and self-esteem through work (and devalue their roles as partners or parents) are also vulnerable to work stress and eventual burnout. People who have a general sense of mastery over their lives are less likely to be debilitated by work stress than those who feel constantly at the mercy of external circumstances.

Burnout!

Hubert Freudenberger, an expert on burnout, suggests the following definition of burnout: "to deplete oneself, to exhaust one's physical and mental resources, or to wear one's self out by excessively striving to reach some unrealistic expectation imposed by one's self or by values of society."[14]

The early signs of work-related stress, which can lead to burnout, emerge in a gradual and unsuspecting way. Typically, you become less focused and efficient at work. You lose confidence and pleasure in what you do. Feelings of frustration, irritability, and anxiety increase, as do difficulties in relationships with co-workers. You may suffer from minor somatic complaints, such as stomach upsets, headaches, frequent colds, sleep disturbances, backaches, and constant fatigue.

Increasingly, you don't feel like going to work, until, as one woman put it, "It became harder and harder to get out of the bed in the morning, until finally I just couldn't."

Burnout results when you can no longer cope with the accumulation of work stress. It is closely linked with and shares many of the characteristics of depression. While depression affects every part of your life, burnout is specific to work. However, burnout can easily spiral into an episode of major depression, and often does.

Is Retirement Good for Your Health?

Because work is a primary way we define ourselves, the transition from full-time employment to retirement poses potential health risks. This was increasingly an issue of growing concern among our interviewees, all of whom were in or nearing their fifties. While most people like the idea of early retirement (with a pension), it is increasingly a notion of the past. Those under sixty-five are more and more threatened by unanticipated forced departure from employment through layoffs and downsizing. As might be expected, the research indicates that involuntary retirement can have negative effects on health, while voluntary retirement seems to have positive or, at worst, neutral effects. As in our general discussion of stress, the amount of control the individual has over the decision is a critical factor.[15]

Many people now start their own ventures in their fifties as a bridge to retirement. Others who are self-employed wonder if they will ever be able to retire. This too is a source of stress for many boomers.

Taking Stock: How Stressed Am I?

Most of the time, we don't realize how stressed we are. In fact, we usually don't want to know. It is just too stressful to contemplate how overwhelmed and sometimes helpless we feel! Yet understanding our stressors and how we react to them is exactly what we need to do. If we are to become more adaptable and resilient, and take charge of our responses, we must identify and understand the causes of our stress and know the things that replenish us. This section provides a simple exercise to help you do just that.

THE ENERGY TUB

1. Sit quietly. Close your eyes and take three deep breaths.
2. When you are ready, imagine a big, comfortable bathtub – perhaps an old-fashioned slantback or the bath from a favourite getaway.

3. Take a few moments, so that you have a clear picture of the bathtub in your mind, and then quickly sketch it on a piece of paper (Figure 1).

4. Sit back and close your eyes again. Image a water-line in the tub

Figure 1 Draw your Tub.

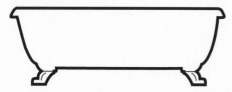

that indicates the amount of energy that you have right now – an empty tub indicates total depletion and a full tub signifies how you feel at your most robust and vital. Be honest. Draw the line as a depiction of how you really feel right now, not how you wished you felt or hope to feel tomorrow. Usually, the first image that comes to mind is the most accurate (Figure 2).

5. If your energy level is less than optimal, think about the stresses

Figure 2 Draw your present energy level.

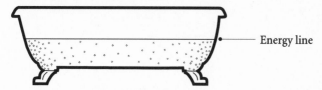

Energy line

that deplete you. For each of these things, draw a drain on the bottom of the tub and name it. Do it quickly, writing down whatever comes to mind. Examples could include the illness of a parent, a difficult loss, a chronically sore back, demands of teenagers, etc. (Figure 3). Be honest and specific. This is only for you. If the bottom of your tub looks more like a colander than a bathtub, don't give up!

6. Now think about the areas of your life that replenish you and give you energy. For each one of these, draw a faucet pouring

Figure 3 Draw the drains on your energy.

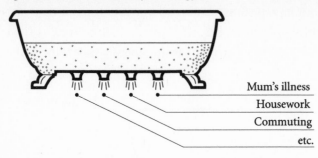

Mum's illness
Housework
Commuting
etc.

water into your tub and label it. Make note of which ones provide a flow and which ones trickle (Figure 4). Some examples include spiritual beliefs, a back rub from your partner, time with your best friend, snowshoeing, etc. Again, be specific. Don't dismiss anything. Many things can be both a source of stress and of renewal in different ways, so mark them as both (one example may be your relationship with your parents).

Figure 4 Add some things that restore your energy.

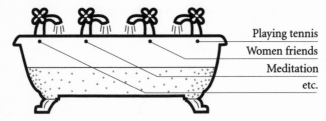

Playing tennis
Women friends
Meditation
etc.

7. Now take a good look at your energy tub. To the side of your tub or on another sheet, make a list of the drains and a list of what replenishes you. Are you surprised by any of them?

8. Go over these lists and see what you've left out. Write down any more emotional, physical, mental, spiritual, and social drains and energy restorers that come to mind.

9. Pick one or two of your energy drains and think about how to close them. Make these directions specific and give yourself a set length of time in which to carry them out.

10. Take a moment to appreciate the sources of renewal you have in your life. Choose one to do in the next week.

This is a useful exercise to return to, from time to time, to see if your energy tub is filling up. Remember that stress can be a positive force in motivating you to create and grow.

(Source: Personal communication about the "Energy Tub" exercise from adult educator LaDonna Smith, Vernon, BC, Canada.)

The Fine Art of Stress-Proofing

As we have seen, each of us deals with stress in a unique way that depends on our temperament, our past experiences, our current environment, and the severity of the stressors we are facing. You know you are feeling stressed when your mind races and you can't turn off your thoughts, when your back pains recurs, or when you feel very irritable. It's important to be able to identify your particular stress alarm.

The total picture of the stressors in your life can be overwhelming. We need to break down the situation into manageable components. Try following these steps:

- First, identify the stressors in your life. Do the Energy Tub exercise if you haven't already.
- Differentiate between the stressors you can change or modify and those you can't.
- Identify which are draining the most energy from you.
- For those that you can change, look at various options. Can you avoid or eliminate any of the stressors? Can you take a break from them or delegate them to someone who wouldn't find them stressful?
- For those you can't change, learn how to alter your responses.

Because everyone's stressors and stress responses are different, there is no one approach that works for everyone all the time. What does seem constant is that, in order to "de-stress" ourselves, we must learn to get in touch with our "relaxation response," a term coined by Dr. Herbert Benson.[16]

Getting in Touch with the Relaxation Response

In the late 1960s, Herbert Benson was conducting research on hypertension, using biofeedback techniques to train monkeys to control their blood pressure. He was approached by some practitioners of transcendental meditation, who claimed they could lower their blood pressure through meditation.

Benson initially dismissed their claims, but later agreed to measure their physiological responses. He found that by sitting quietly and giving their minds a focus they slowed their heart rates and metabolisms. Benson used the term "relaxation response" to describe what he saw in the laboratory. He realized that, with commitment and practice, everyone could learn to use this natural restorative.[17]

Inviting the relaxation response is a process of "letting go inside" – the kind of feeling you might have while lying in a hammock on a summer day or having a massage. The relaxation response is an effective and rejuvenating process, which is at the heart of all stress-proofing. There are a number of different ways of gaining access to the response, some of which are described below. Chapter 22, on complementary and alternative medicine, contains additional information on other effective mind-body relaxation techniques.

Diaphragm breathing occurs when you inhale slowly and deeply, so that you see or feel your belly rising and falling with your breath. This deceptively simple technique is a fundamental tenet of all Eastern meditation techniques, and demonstrably lowers blood pressure and releases stress. It is not the way we usually breathe. Indeed, the shallow breathing we use most often signals a condition of "red alert" to the body and keeps us in a state of chronic stress.

Biofeedback uses modern monitoring equipment to measure muscle tension, skin temperature, and pulse rate to signal changes in the autonomic nervous system's activity. Monitoring these changes helps people observe how and why they become stressed, and eventually to control their responses. This technique may be particularly helpful for people who are sceptical about how meditation works or concerned about their ability to get in touch with the relaxation response.[18]

Meditation has been practised for centuries in many ancient spiritual traditions. It consists of two elements:
* creating a mental focus, such as counting one's breaths or repeating a word, sound, or prayer;

- developing a passive attitude towards all distracting thoughts. This means allowing distracting thoughts to pass through your mind, while continually returning your awareness to your breathing or the word.

You can use meditation as a powerful way to relieve stress by practising it for as little as fifteen minutes a day. It is now used extensively in stress-reduction programs in North America and Europe.[19] To maximize the benefits, invest in a good book or a course in meditation. As Vietnamese Buddhist teacher Thich Nhat Hanh says, "Meditation is not evasion; it is a serene encounter with reality."[20]

Creative visualization The process of creative visualization is a way to consciously evoke positive images of safe, calm places, in order to relax our minds and bodies, and alter our self-defeating thought patterns.

Remember that a positive change in one area can have a ripple effect in other parts of your life.

Improving Your Relationship with Stress

Mentally

Our stress response is greatly affected by our negative assessment of situations. Under stress, we think globally and catastrophically. Sometimes, the thunderclouds on the horizon seem to signal the end of the world rather than just a passing storm. Too often, like Chicken Little, we run around crying, "The sky is falling!" What we need at this point is perspective. It is a good time to ask ourselves the question Richard Carlson poses in his best-seller, *Don't Sweat the Small Stuff*: "Will this still matter a year from now?"[21]

We also create more subtle forms of mental stress by undermining and criticizing ourselves constantly. If you become aware that you are doing this, work at stopping these negative thoughts and replacing them with an image of something positive you did that day. If you find yourself intensely self-critical, consider psychotherapy.

Physically

It is often when stress affects us physically that we sit up and pay attention. Backaches, indigestion, heartburn, headaches, and muscle spasms are a few of the ways that stress manifests itself. We can go a long way toward stress-proofing ourselves physically if we follow three basic rules of general health:

- Eat nutritiously. Fill up with foods that nourish and sustain you. Empty calories will leave you undernourished and vulnerable to stress.
- Exercise effectively. A vigorous walk or exuberant dance can do wonders in releasing the tension held in the body.
- Sleep adequately, and learn to rest. Learn what your body needs and provide it. Shortchanging yourself here is a direct path to illness or injury (see Chapter 15).

Emotionally

The two extremes of bottled-up unexpressed feelings and explosive temper tantrums can be equally harmful in terms of the toll stress takes on our bodies and psyches. It is very important to learn ways to vent your anger and frustrations creatively, to express your feelings appropriately, and then to let them go. The experience of releasing emotions facilitates a return to balance. Again, psychotherapy can be helpful in understanding and releasing long-held negative feelings.

Socially

When author Dean Ornish lectures, he sometimes asks his audience these questions:

- How many people still live in the same neighbourhood where they were born?
- Who has extended family nearby whom they see regularly?
- How many people have worked at the same job and attended the same church, synagogue, temple, or mosque for ten or more years?

Ornish reports that usually in an audience of three thousand, some ten or twenty people raise their hands. He then points out to the audience that loneliness and isolation are known to "increase the likelihood of disease and premature death from all causes by 200 to 500 per cent."[22]

Strong family ties, a circle of friends, and community involvement are very important in cushioning us from the ravages of stress. Volunteering and helping others are definitely good for your health.[23]

Spiritually

Research confirms that those with deeply held faith and spiritual beliefs are more protected from stress-related illness than those without beliefs. In addition, being part of a like-minded religious community can ease feelings of isolation and alienation. In his powerful book *Man's Search for Meaning*, Victor Frankl writes about his experience as a concentration-camp survivor. He found that those who had a strongly held purpose for living were able to withstand the horrors of the camp, while those without purpose or positive self-direction died quickly. He determined to live to write about his experience.[24]

STRESS-HARDINESS[25]

Stress-hardy people exhibit the four "C" characteristics:

Control: Stress-hardy people believe they can influence events. They are willing to act on that belief rather than be victims of circumstances.

Challenge: They view stress as a challenge and an opportunity for growth rather than a threat.

Commitment: They have an attitude of curiosity and involvement in whatever is happening.

Closeness: They have close personal relationships and a lively social network.

Tips to Shift Your Energy

Here is a list of suggestions to help you shift your focus and reframe your thoughts in a stressful moment. Please feel free to use these, create your own, and share them with friends. Post a few on the fridge, your computer, or the bathroom mirror.

- Stop and take three deep belly breaths. You can do this while you're driving, walking, or sitting in a meeting.
- Use technology to your advantage. If you're in the middle of a project, screen your calls. Hit automatic redial.
- Pick a spot for your keys and glasses and always put them there.

- Hire someone to come and help you get rid of clutter, to put those pictures in albums and recipes in a file.
- Allow yourself ample time to get places.
- Allocate some time for yourself each day.
- Turn off the computer. Turn off the television. Read a book or listen to music.
- Plan something to look forward to when you finish a project. Too often we don't congratulate and reward ourselves.
- Pace yourself. As David Posen points out, even Wayne Gretzky didn't play a whole game without a break.[26]
- Plan regular treats – a massage, tickets to a ball game, facial or pedicure, dinner and a movie, etc.
- Go for a walk. Get up from where you are, move and stretch.
- Ask yourself, "Will this matter in 100 years?"
- Find something to laugh or smile about every day.
- Learn to say no.
- Ask for support when you need it.
- Learn to differentiate between what you can and cannot control.
- Accept that you are not perfect and allow for mistakes.
- Stay away from excessive caffeine. It's a strong stimulant.
- Go to bed an hour earlier tonight.
- Sit down and meditate for five minutes right now.
- Love and touching are good for your health. Hug your child, mate, friend, or pet.
- Think of a current stress as a challenge rather than a burden.
- Try something new – watercolour painting, line dancing, rollerblading.

THE BOTTOM LINE

Develop a healthy relationship with stress. Pay attention to your body's stress alarm. Have fun, be silly, laugh. Stress-proof yourself with some of the techniques and tips suggested in this chapter.

Contacts and Further Information

Organizations

- American Psychological Association, 750 First St. N.E., Washington, DC 20002–4242; Tel.: (800) 374–2721.
- Canadian Mental Health Association, 2160 Yonge St., Toronto, ON M4S 2Z3. Tel.: (416) 484–7750; Fax: (416) 484–4617; E-mail: cmhanat@interlog.com (or contact a local office in your phone book).
- Canadian Psychological Association, 441 MacLaren St., Suite 260, Ottawa, ON K2P 2H8. Tel.: (613) 234–2815; Fax: (613) 234–9857.
- National Mental Health Association (U.S.), 1021 Prince St., Alexandria, VA 22314–2917. Tel.: (800) 969–6642.

Websites

- American Institute of Stress (U.S. government): http://www.nimh.nih.gov
- Canadian Mental Health Association: http://www.cmha.ca
- Canadian Psychological Association: http://www.cpa.ca
- National Mental Health Association (U.S.): http://www.worldcorp.com/dc-online/nmha

See list at end of Chapter 15 for additional websites.

Books

- *Full Catastrophe Living: Using the Wisdom of Your Body and Mind to Face Stress, Pain, and Illness* (The Program of the Stress Reduction Clinic at the University of Massachusetts Medical Center) by Jon Kabat-Zinn. New York: Delta Books, 1990.
- *Imagery in Healing: Shamanism and Modern Medicine* by Jeanne Achterberg. Boston: New Science Library, 1985.
- *Man's Search for Meaning* by Victor Frankl. Boston: Beacon Press, 1963.
- *Mastery: The Keys to Success and Long-Term Fulfilment* by George Leonard. New York: Plume Books, 1992.

- *Minding the Body, Mending the Mind* by Joan Borysenko and Larry Rothstein. Reading, MA: Addison Wesley, 1987.
- *The Miracle of Mindfulness: A Manual on Meditation* by Thich Nhat Hanh. Boston: Beacon Press, 1976.
- *Staying Afloat When the Water Gets Rough: How to Live in a Rapidly Changing World* by David B. Posen. Toronto: Key Porter, 1998.
- *Time Shifting: Creating More Time to Enjoy Your Life* by Stephan Rechtschaffen. New York: Doubleday, 1996.
- *The Wellness Book: The Comprehensive Guide to Maintaining Health and Treating Stress-Related Illness* by Herbert Benson and Eileen Stuart. New York: Fireside Books, 1992.
- *Your Money or Your Life: Transforming Your Relationship with Money and Achieving Financial Independence* by Joe Dominquez and Vicki Robin. New York: Penguin Books, 1992.

Related Chapters in This Book
- *Chapter 1: The Midlife Journey* will help you see current stress within the context of the midlife journey.
- *Chapter 2: Understanding the Female Menopause* and *Chapter 3: Is There a Male Menopause?* describe how hormonal changes can affect your stress level.
- *Chapter 5: Making Changes That Last!* provides some helpful suggestions on how to make positive lifestyle changes that help you manage stress.
- *Chapter 7: The Active Living Solution* and *Chapter 8: Food for Thought: Healthy Eating in Midlife* provide suggestions on exercise and healthy eating – which are essential stress-proofing tools.
- *Chapter 9: The Boomer's Drugs of Choice* suggests some practical ways to quit smoking and reduce alcohol intake – ineffective behaviours we often use to cover up or to manage stress.
- *Chapter 15: When Times Are Tough: Depression, Anxiety, and Insomnia* helps you determine when to seek professional help and provides some practical advice on getting a better night's sleep.
- *Chapter 23: Body, Mind, and Soul* reminds us that the spiritual journey is an integral part of well-being in midlife.

CHAPTER FOURTEEN

Now Where Did I Put Those Glasses?

> Last night, sailing off to sleep at last, I couldn't remember the name of the thing you use to strain spaghetti. Imagine that, I've used it thousands of times. I could visualize it. But I couldn't remember what the bloody thing was called.
> — Mordecai Richler, *Barney's Version*[1]

The other day a friend wandered into her bathroom and could not remember why she was there. A colleague told us she recently flew to Toronto with mismatched shoes. We all know the frustration of introducing our best friend and drawing a complete blank on his or her name. The great philosopher William James recounts the time he lost his bearings while getting ready for a dinner party. He undressed, washed up, and then climbed into bed.[2]

Whenever we begin to discuss midlife memory lapses in our seminars, there is a collective sigh of relief. Someone says, "Oh, I thought I was the only one with early Alzheimer disease." Inevitably, this is followed by nervous laughter, then an outpouring of stories and concerns.

During a menopause seminar at Ottawa's Carleton University, we were trying to reassure participants that some hormonal changes are transient and that their memory lapses would diminish after menopause. Suddenly we overheard a woman in her sixties whisper to her companion, "That's what they think!"

While the jokes abound, most of us are quietly terrified that our current bouts of forgetfulness foreshadow the onset of dementia that sometimes accompanies getting older. Psychologist Cynthia Green says in a 1998 *Newsweek* article that "memory [has become] the new life crisis issue."[3]

In her book *Getting Over Getting Older*, author Letty Cottin Pogrebin talks about why memory lapses are so frightening. She says, "Forgetting and remembering are critical issues of aging, partly because any sign of slippage triggers our fears of gerontic dementia, and partly because memory is the pathway to personal history wherein lies proof that we have lived and loved and made a difference in the world." The author goes on to take both a serious and light view of memory loss, punctuated by a quote from Gloria Steinem who said, "At this age, being able to remember something is as good as an orgasm."[4]

Both the medical establishment and the marketplace are quickly responding to the latest boomer crisis. Memory and aging are being studied by the U.S. National Institutes of Health, the drug companies are racing to develop a pharmaceutical solution, sales of gingko biloba have increased expeditiously, and "memory training centres" are sprouting up across North America.

This chapter explains how memory works and suggests the changes we can expect as we age and as our hormone levels change. It helps you differentiate between normal memory loss and a state of disease. Lastly, it provides advice on how to improve your memory and handle those annoying memory lapses we all encounter.

Understanding Memory

Despite our concerns about our mental fogginess, scientists who study the brain are amazed that we remember as much as we do. Even basic day-to-day tasks such as getting to work in the morning or preparing a meal involve a complexity of components that we must remember. When you combine this with the daily bombardment of information and stimulation we receive from colleagues, newspapers, radio, television, billboards, the telephone, and the Internet, it is nothing short of a miracle that our memories perform daily and as well as they do.

How does the memory work? The analogy of the memory as computer is one of the simplest and most useful. We have three basic types of memory:

- *Sensory memory* controls that very brief stage of perceiving what is important and what needs to be saved in short-term memory. For example, your sensory memory registers or does not register the lunch-menu options posted in the cafeteria for a particular day of the week. If you know you will not have lunch there that day, sensory memory is likely to perceive the information as not important enough to store in your short-term memory.

- *Short-term, or "working," memory* manages information in the present. It is like the RAM in your computer: what we perceive registers briefly here for its usefulness in the moment and then evaporates.
- *Long-term memory* stores things for extended periods of time. Long-term memory is like the computer's hard drive: past experiences are recorded in the cerebral cortex of the brain, just as data are recorded on your hard drive.[5] New information is stored in the long-term memory in association with other relevant information that is already there. Thus, hearing a specific voice may retrieve memories of a certain conversation you had with that person.

The more often a memory is activated, the more deeply embedded the pattern of connection becomes – hence, the value of repetition in learning. The decision to store or discard a piece of information is made in a part of the brain called the hippocampus. The decision to save or discard is based on two key questions:

- Does the information have emotional significance? For example, we will remember the face of someone we are attracted to more readily than the face of someone we feel neutral about.
- Does the information relate to things we already know?

So, the more associations there are to a piece of information, the more likely we are to remember it.

What Causes Memory Loss?

A number of factors contribute to memory loss:

- *Aging and Heredity.* Our overall brain mass decreases by 5 to 10 per cent in our sixties and seventies, causing the memory to be a little slower and less detail-oriented.[6] However, these changes are relatively minor and do not affect everyone. People vary greatly in their ability to recall at any age. Heredity also appears to play a significant role in memory loss. In his book *The Midlife Man*, Art Hister quotes a Swedish study of twins which concluded that 38 per cent of our ability to acquire and process information is due to the environment. The remaining 62 per cent is the result of our genes. It is important to keep in mind the impact of both aging and heredity when looking at the research on estrogen in the following section.[7]

As we get older, it seems to take longer to recall and retrieve information, and it takes more effort to learn new tasks. This is manifested in poorer performances on tests such as recall and the recognition of listed words. Immediate tasks that do not require the retrieval of information from the short-term memory show little change with age, and memories of the distant past appear to remain intact. These age-related changes in memory function affect both men and women and do not seem to relate to hormone fluctuations.[8]

- *Illness.* Hypertension, diabetes, obesity, stroke, and heart disease all increase the risk of mental decline. Alzheimer disease (which is discussed in more detail later in this chapter) gradually destroys the hippocampus and the ability to form new memories.

- *Sleep Deprivation.* Not getting enough sleep can disrupt memory formation. Some of the common causes of sleep deprivation such as excessive drinking, depression, and anxiety may exacerbate the problem.

- *Information Overload.* As we struggle to keep up in the Information Age, it is easy to overlook the significance of this factor. Both the volume of information and the speed with which it comes to us today are much greater than they were fifty years ago. In *Data Smog: Surviving the Information Glut*, David Shank writes, "Our brains have remained structurally consistent for over 50,000 years, yet exposure to processed information in this country has increased by a factor of thousands (lately, the volume and speed of information have been increasing as much as 100 per cent each year)."[9] Something has to give. When we are bombarded with more than we can absorb, we not only can't remember much of it, but, more important, we sometimes have trouble taking in anything at all.

- *Chronic Stress.* Persistent stress affects memory in a number of ways. When the "fight or flight" response is activated for longer than the brief time for which it was intended, stress hormones lower the energy in the brain. Trying to juggle many tasks can impair your concentration and affect your ability to remember multiple details. For example, if you are worrying about a sick child at home while you are setting up a meeting, you may remember the day of the meeting, but not the time or place.

- *Low or Fluctuating Levels of Estrogen.* Estrogen is important to the healthy functioning of the brain, especially in the areas related to mood and memory. As mentioned earlier, memory lapses are a common concern among women in the menopausal period, who have lowered or fluctuating estrogen levels. Before we all rush out for estrogen therapy, however, it is important to consider the benefits and risks of HRT and to see this menopausal complaint as part of a bigger picture. For a midlife woman who is sleep-deprived because of hot flashes, stressed by a demanding job and home life, and depressed because of the recent loss of her mother, it is a wonder that she does not suffer more serious memory lapses more often than she does. Is memory loss the problem or really only the symptom for boomer women of how stressful their lives have become? This is discussed in greater detail later in this chapter.
- *Medications.* Memory function is also influenced by certain medications, including beta blockers used to treat heart disease and high blood pressure, anti-anxiety drugs, some sleeping pills, stomach medications, anti-Parkinson drugs, and some antidepressants.

Estrogen and the Female Brain

Are memory lapses basically due to estrogen fluctuations? Are they likely to be temporary or long term? As with other areas of estrogen research, considerable controversy exists about the answers to these questions.

Barbara Sherwin of Montreal's McGill University Menopause Clinic has spent the last decade meticulously researching the effects of estrogen on memory in menopausal women. According to Sherwin, there is now sufficient evidence that estrogen does help maintain certain aspects of long- and short-term verbal memory in women. And while estrogen was originally believed to have no effect on visual memory, research now indicates some relationship. Sherwin believes that the effect of estrogen is specific, rather than global, and that improvements resulting from estrogen therapy may be modest. She also stresses the importance of remembering that the aging process itself may account for some cognitive decline, independent of any hormonal effect.[10]

Her research does give a physiological justification to menopausal women who are baffled and frightened by these memory losses. Until recently, most physicians have been largely unaware of how distressing cognitive difficulties are for midlife women, and thus have not inquired about them. Many women who see memory loss as evidence of declining competence or a source of shame remain silent about their concerns.

In her recent book, *Menopause and the Mind*, neuropsychologist Claire Warga makes a strong case, based on recent research, that the forgetfulness, verbal slips, lessened concentration, and other cognitive difficulties that are so common in midlife do result from estrogen depletion. She states that the effects of this "hormone-deficiency state" are likely to be long term without intervention.[11]

On the other side of the debate, menopause and breast-cancer specialist Dr. Susan Love says that it is hard to separate any effects of hormones on your ability to think clearly from the effects of the stresses of midlife. She goes on to point out that the current research is based mostly on studies comprised of small numbers of women or conducted over short periods of time (three to six months).

She cites one study in which half of a group of female monkeys who had their ovaries removed were given replacement estrogen, while the other half were not. In a series of memory tests, the monkeys given the estrogen performed much better than the other group, up to the three-month mark. At that point, the untreated group caught up. She says that surely we can do as well as the monkeys! "We may not be able to avoid the toll the years take . . . ," she adds, "but as with puberty and pregnancy, we do get back on an even keel."[12]

This is a rapidly evolving field of research in which we may expect to know much more about estrogen's effect on the brain in the next few years. For the present, Robert Josse, chief of the division of Endocrinology and Metabolism at the University of Toronto, put it well at a recent conference when he said, "The data on estrogen and the memory is still soft."[13]

Memory and Midlife Men

There is relatively little research about gender differences and memory, but we do know that, while men start out with more brain cells than women, they lose them three times as fast as women as they age.[14] This clearly affects cognitive functioning and memory. Numerous male interviewees spoke to us about the frustration and embarrassment of fuzzy thinking and mental lapses. One fifty-year-old man said, "My memory is going. I have a young son from my second marriage and I don't want to be a decrepit old dad for him. I got so worried that I even talked to my doctor, who said he has problems too. It didn't make me feel much better." It seems that memory lapses are just as disturbing for men in midlife as for women; clearly more research needs to be done.

Alzheimer Disease and Other Dementias

The term "dementia" refers to a syndrome of progressive, irreversible changes in the brain. It is characterized by severe dysfunctions, including the loss of cognitive abilities that allow a person to carry out his or her usual daily activities. Alzheimer disease (AD) is the best known and most common of the many forms of dementia. People may develop other forms of dementia resulting from circulatory problems, such as stroke, Parkinson disease, alcoholism, head injury, or lack of oxygen during an operation. Women are more likely than men to develop dementia, primarily because they live longer.

To diagnose dementia, or more specifically AD, a number of tests are used, including a blood test to rule out B12 deficiency and thyroid disease, and (when indicated) a brain scan to rule out a tumour or multiple small strokes. More specific tests are then used. Since older people who are depressed may appear confused, forgetful, and withdrawn, they can easily and incorrectly be labelled with dementia. Depression needs to be ruled out before further tests are conducted. It can still be difficult to say with certainty that a person has AD. Only an autopsy and a microscopy of the brain can absolutely confirm the diagnosis.

Usually, people with AD are physically healthy, but they decline in cognitive function in a relatively short period.[15] The disease erodes not only their memories but also their personalities and self-awareness. They have impaired insight: they may put a book in the refrigerator and believe it belongs there. They have impaired judgement: they may go out in their socks in winter and get lost, or act inappropriately, such as laughing when they hear someone has died. Usually, the disease is more painful to the family than to the sufferer.

There is no cure for AD at this time and there are few effective treatments, although many new drugs are emerging to slow the progression of the disease and to help manage it. The role of estrogen supplementation in women is currently being studied seriously. Preliminary evidence suggests that estrogen is, to some degree, relevant in both preventing and treating Alzheimer disease. More extensive and long-term studies are necessary to see if hormone replacement therapy could really help prevent the disease.[16] At this point the only identified risk factors are age and heredity.

GINGKO BILOBA

Recent claims that gingko biloba can improve memory and concentration have largely arisen from a study showing that gingko seemed to slightly delay the progression of dementia in patients with mild forms of Alzheimer disease. While gingko dilates the arteries and sends more blood to the brain, it is no Viagra for the mind. There is no scientific evidence that the herb can improve memory and concentration in healthy people.[17]

Is It Alzheimer Disease?: Ten Warning Signs

It is important to be able to differentiate between "normal" memory loss and a state of disease. These facts from the U.S. Alzheimer Society help to distinguish between the two.[18]

1. *Memory loss that affects day-to-day functions.* It's normal to occasionally forget appointments, a colleague's name, or a friend's phone number and remember them later. A person with AD may forget things more often and not remember them later, especially things that have happened recently.

2. *Difficulty performing familiar tasks.* Busy people can be so distracted that occasionally they may leave the carrots on the stove and only remember them when serving dessert. A person with Alzheimer disease may be unable to prepare any part of a meal or forget she even ate it.

3. *Problems with language.* Everyone has trouble finding the right word sometimes, but a person with AD may forget simple words or substitute inappropriate words, making her sentences difficult to understand.

4. *Disorientation of time and place.* It's normal to forget the day of the

week or your destination for a moment, but a person with AD can become lost on his own street, not knowing how he got there or how to get home.

5. *Poor or decreased judgement.* People may sometimes put off going to their physicians if they have an infection, but eventually seek medical attention. A person with AD may not recognize the infection as a problem, or may not seek help at all. They may also dress inappropriately, such as wearing heavy clothing on a hot day.

6. *Problems with abstract thinking.* From time to time, people may find balancing a chequebook difficult. Someone with AD could forget completely what numbers are and what one does with them. A person with AD may not just forget a birthday but not understand what a birthday is.

7. *Misplacing things.* Anyone can temporarily misplace a wallet or keys. A person with AD may put things in inappropriate places: an iron in the freezer or a wristwatch in the sugar bowl.

8. *Changes in mood or behaviour.* Everyone becomes sad or moody sometimes; a person with AD can exhibit rapid mood swings – from feeling calm to sad to angry – for no apparent reason.

9. *Changes in personality.* People's personalities can change somewhat with age, but someone with AD may change dramatically, becoming extremely confused, suspicious, or withdrawn. Changes may also include apathy, fearfulness, or acting inappropriately.

10. *Loss of initiative.* It's normal to tire of certain business activities or social obligations from time to time, but most people regain their initiative. A person with AD may become very passive, requiring cues and prompting to become involved in a simple conversation.

This list was adapted with permission from the Alzheimer Society of Canada. See the end of this chapter for how to contact the society for more information.

What Helps

What can help with the annoying and sometimes embarrassing memory lapses of midlife? Here are some suggestions.

• *Reduce your levels of stress.* Look at the big picture, and determine what you can change and what you can't change. Take one small step to minimize the stress in your life. It is only when you reduce stress and distractions and get enough sleep that you will be best able to use your full memory.

- *Keep things in perspective.* A workshop participant told us how mortified she was during a class discussion when she was unable to recall the name of a film she had seen the night before. A few minutes later, a woman half her age got up to talk about a novel she was reading and simply laughed when she couldn't remember the title. Some forgetfulness is normal, no matter what our age. Our fears and expectations are what get us into trouble!
- *Be informed.* Understand the differences between memory lapses and cognitive impairments that signify illness.
- *Do aerobic exercise regularly.* This will enhance the brain's oxygen supply.
- *Eat a healthy diet.* Include foods that mimic the effect of estrogen in the body – phytoestrogens and antioxidants. Eat regularly to keep your blood-sugar levels constant.
- *Develop and practise co-ordination skills.* Musicians and conductors often maintain memory, precision, and mastery well into old age.
- *Make use of technology.* Use computers, personal recording devices, day-planners, and other aids to help you remember birthdays, appointments, telephone numbers, and people's names.
- *Know that you are not alone.* As with many situations, knowing you're not the only one who is forgetful helps you to relax.
- *Maintain a sense of humour.* We know a group of women friends who joke that each will be responsible for several crucial words when they're older, in order that they can all function together. Think about taking yourself more lightly.
- *Use it or lose it.* Challenge yourself with new learning. Play Scrabble or bridge, do crosswords, join an investment club, or learn a new language. Remember to pay attention, repeat what's worth remembering, and link what you're trying to remember with what you already know.
- *Education helps.* Research shows that advanced education is associated with good mental activity in old age.
- *Remember that you are aging.* Like it or not, some of the memory

lapses are age-related. However, not everyone is debilitated by memory problems. Think of the many "sharp as a tack" seventy-year-olds you know.

- *Make lists and use them* (if you can find them, that is!). The act of writing things down can help you remember, even if you do not refer back to the list.
- *Shift the emphasis.* Dr. Patricia Allen of the New York Menopause Research Foundation says, "At twenty-six, you may be very quick to find the right word, but when you're fifty you don't have to cram for exams any more – if you've done your work right, you've got wisdom. You can mentor. You know what's important and what's not. It makes sense that, when you give up one thing, with a little luck, you're going to find something else."[19]

Men also spoke of the shift they started to experience in midlife, realizing that they had something to give to younger people. A forty-eight-year-old choreographer said, "The things that really mattered in the past don't matter so much any more. I don't feel the same sort of struggle. I'm more comfortable with myself and I am calmer. I feel I have gifts and experiences that I want to pass on. That's a good feeling."

Current research offers hope about the regenerative possibilities of our brains. Where once it was believed that a dead brain cell was gone forever, new research suggests that the brain can regrow some cells. What we can do for ourselves now is to practise the suggestions listed above and to continually challenge our assumptions that memory loss is inevitable as we age. It is all too easy to become so anxious about forgetting that we don't keep our focus on remembering.

THE BOTTOM LINE

Learn the difference between "normal" midlife memory problems and the cognitive impairment of Alzheimer disease. Your anxiety about your memory problems can make the situation much worse than it really is. As always, choose a healthy lifestyle. Remember to use it or you will lose it. Keep a sense of humour when you can't remember something! Even children and young people forget.

Contacts and Further Information

Organizations
- Alzheimer Society of Canada: contact your local branch (in telephone book) or call 1–800–616–8816.
- The Alzheimer's Association (U.S.), 919 N. Michigan Ave., Suite 1000, Chicago, IL 60611–1676. Tel.: 1–800–272–3900; Fax: (312) 335–1110.

Websites
- Alzheimer Society of Canada: http://www.alzheimer.ca
- The Alzheimer's Association (U.S): http://www.alz.org

Books
- *Committed to Memory: How to Remember and Why We Forget* by Rebecca Rupp. New York: Crown Publishers, 1998.
- *Improving Your Memory: How to Remember What You Are Starting to Forget* by Janet Fogler and Lynn Stern. Baltimore: Johns Hopkins University Press, 1994.
- *The Memory Book* by H. Lorayne and J. Lucas. New York: Ballantine Books, 1996.
- *Menopause and the Mind* by Claire Warga. New York: The Free Press, 1999.
- *Searching for Memory: The Brain, the Mind, the Past* by Daniel Schacter. New York: HarperCollins, 1997.

Related Chapters in This Book
- *Chapter 2: Understanding the Female Menopause* and *Chapter 3: Is There a Male Menopause?* provide more information on the hormone changes that are part of midlife.
- *Chapter 4: The Search for the Fountain of Youth* gives you more information on normal aging and what to expect.
- *Chapter 7: The Active Living Solution* contains helpful hints on how to get active, which may improve your cognitive performance.
- *Chapter 8: Food for Thought: Healthy Eating in Midlife* gives you information about the foods you need to feed your brain.

- *Chapter 9: The Boomer's Drugs of Choice* reminds you that smoking, drinking, and taking drugs can impair your intellectual functioning, and gives you some common-sense ideas on quitting or cutting down.
- *Chapter 13: Stress-Proofing in Midlife* helps you reduce midlife stress that may affect your memory.
- *Chapter 15: When Times Are Tough: Depression, Anxiety, and Insomnia* gives you information on these common problems, all of which can affect your memory and cognitive abilities.
- *Chapter 21: Hormone Replacement Therapy (HRT): The Big Decision* will help you decide whether HRT is right for you.

When Times Are Tough: Depression, Anxiety, and Insomnia

The lowest ebb is the turn of the tide.
— Henry Wadsworth Longfellow[1]

Midlife Blues

We all feel depressed and anxious and have sleepless nights from time to time. But women and men in midlife may be particularly vulnerable to more serious and long-lasting bouts of depression, anxiety, and insomnia because of the accumulation of stresses at this time. These may include the death of a parent, the serious illness of a partner or close friend, living with a chronic health problem, financial difficulties, and career changes that may involve job loss or retirement. The accumulation of stress may activate vulnerability to depression that has been ignored or denied until now.

The physical changes of midlife – especially hormonal changes for women – can increase the likelihood that you will suffer periods of insomnia. And, in spite of earlier research to the contrary, there is now evidence that these changes may also contribute to the onset of anxiety and depression during menopause.[2] Amid nervous laughter, many menopausal women have told us that they fear they may be going crazy, because they feel so anxious about everyday events or start to cry for no apparent reason. They are so exhausted from sleepless nights that they do not know how they keep functioning. For men, the physical signs of aging that begin to appear in midlife can sometimes exacerbate feelings of anxiety or depression. Temporary impotence, feeling exhausted, or suffering from angina can send them into a tailspin.

While insomnia is a major symptom of depression, it can also be a disorder in its own right that may or may not lead to depression. Sleep problems can occur as a result of worries about work or family life, night sweats, poor sleep hygiene, too much food and alcohol at bedtime, or too little exercise. Whatever the reasons, sleeplessness can become a chronic problem that intensifies our reactions to other difficulties.

In this chapter, we explore depression, anxiety and sleep disorders. The chapter is designed to help you gain a basic understanding of these complex and difficult issues and to feel more comfortable discussing these problems with your partner, friends, and family physician. Most important, it is designed to help you recognize when you or someone you love needs to seek professional help.

Understanding Mood Disorders

Mood disorders are powerfully destabilizing illnesses that affect not only the mood of a person but also his or her thoughts, judgement, perspective on life, physical health, family relations, and work life. They fall into two main categories:

- Unipolar disorders (commonly called depressive disorders), which can increase in severity from mild depression (dysthymia) to major depressive disorder and include seasonal affective disorder (SAD).
- Bipolar disorders (formerly known as manic-depressive disorder), which consist of fluctuations between depressive and manic episodes. They increase in severity from the milder version, called cyclothymia, to major manic and depressive episodes.

Unipolar (Depressive) Disorders

Depression knows no boundaries in terms of age, race, religion, sex, or socio-economic class. It is the most common of the mood disorders. Depression causes untold suffering for those who have it and for those who care about them. Sir Winston Churchill, a long-time sufferer, called it "the black dog." King Saul had it; so did Virginia Woolf, William Styron, Margot Kidder, Leonard Cohen, and probably someone you know. In fact, 10 to 15 per cent of North American men and 25 per cent of women will experience depression at least once in their lives.[3]

In spite of new and effective treatments, depression remains a very misunderstood, underdiagnosed, and undertreated illness. This is at least partly because of the tremendous stigma still attached to illnesses that affect our emotions and thoughts, and the profound sense of shame that many sufferers experience. Socio-economics also play a part. Because psychotherapy is not usually covered by health insurance, people with lower incomes are less likely to seek and receive adequate diagnosis and treatment.

Depression is an illness that does require treatment. It is vastly different from the sporadic bouts of "the blues" that we all feel from time to time, when we are disappointed, our hormones are raging, or the weather is gloomy. It is also very different from grief over a significant loss, such as the death of a friend or relative. Feelings of grief are part of the ebb and flow of human experience that also allow us to relish the joys of being alive. It is only when these normal feelings of grief remain unresolved for a long period of time that grief can develop into depression.

Because the phrase "I'm depressed" is used to describe a range of experiences, it is useful to think of depression as a continuum of increasing severity.

THE DEPRESSION CONTINUUM

➤ increasing severity

"A Bad Day" ➤	"The Moody Blues" ➤	Dysthymic Disorder ➤	Grief Reaction➤	Major Depressive Episode
• Passing feelings and moods	• More persistent moodiness	• Long-term loss of pleasure • Low self-esteem • Low energy	• Sad, time-limited feelings of loss in response to a specific event	• Impaired functioning • Disturbed eating and sleeping • Intense loss of pleasure • Thoughts of death

Source: Adapted with permission from *The Complete Book of Menopause* by C. Landau, M. G. Cyr, and A. Moulton (New York: Grosset/Putnam, 1994), p. 176.

Dysthymia **Carol**, a forty-eight-year-old working mother suffers from dysthymia, the medical term for chronic, low-grade depression. She describes it this way: "I just don't feel any joy in my life. I do my job. I look after the kids. We see our friends, but nothing seems to give me any pleasure. Maybe I'm just lazy – I feel so tired all the time. I guess I should just pull up my socks and get on with things. But if one more person wants something from me, I think I'll scream."

People with dysthymia manage to function but feel burdened, exhausted, and inadequate. They experience a marked lack of pleasure in daily life. "I'm just kind of going through the motions," one woman said. Dysthymia is "the common cold" of the depressive disorders. In contrast to major depression, it comes on gradually and waxes and wanes over time.

People diagnosed with dysthymia tend to be intensely self-critical, blaming themselves for their illness, and often struggling with feelings of worthlessness and hopelessness. Like Carol, they find getting through the day is an effort, and lack a sense of pleasure and joie de vivre. They do their work but often do not live up to their potential. They often suffer from sleep and/or eating disturbances, have trouble concentrating and making decisions. They may have a lot of physical complaints of a rather vague nature. Unfortunately, their negative, glass-half-empty view of themselves and the world has usually existed for so long that, on questioning, they often say, "This is just the way I am" or "I'm not naturally a cheerful person."

Before you decide that this fits you or your partner, remember that this is not a short-lived experience of a few days or weeks. It is medically described as "a chronically depressed mood for most of the day, more days than not, for at least two years."[4] We certainly advise you *not* to wait that long to seek help.

Because people with dysthymia see their illness as "normal" for them, it can be difficult to diagnose. Once diagnosed, however, it seems to respond best to psychotherapy alone or in combination with antidepressant medications such as selective serotonin reuptake inhibitors (SSRIs). These include the familiar names of Prozac, Paxil, and Zoloft.

Major Depressive Disorder A fifty-two-year-old male high-school teacher described his experience with major depression like this: "It was like being in an altered state. Nothing could reach me. Nothing mattered. The pain was so great I felt I couldn't go on any more. I felt numb. I felt so utterly worthless and hopeless."

If dysthymia is like the common cold, major depression is akin to an acute and potentially life-threatening episode of pneumonia, which seriously impairs your ability to function in normal ways. Very often, the family has to take over very basic activities. For example, the sufferer may, for a time, be unable to make the most simple decisions, such as what to wear in the morning. Major depression is characterized by many of the same symptoms as dysthymia, but to a more intense and serious degree.

The following traits are characteristic of major depression:
- intense loss of pleasure and interest in life
- extremely sad, despondent feelings beyond the norm, which last at least two weeks and are a change from previous functioning
- disturbed sleep patterns, including early-morning waking, insomnia, and sometimes hypersomnia (sleeping all the time)
- disturbed eating patterns, ranging from feeling unable to eat to overeating
- significant weight loss or gain
- overwhelming feelings of fatigue
- a sense of restlessness or unease that nothing seems to alleviate, difficulty concentrating, indecisiveness
- unwarranted feelings of worthlessness, self-blame, and guilt
- decreased interest in sex or in being with others
- recurrent thoughts of death, self-harm, or suicide, and, more seriously, a specific suicide plan or attempt.

A major depressive episode would be diagnosed if four of the above symptoms in addition to depressed mood were identified for at least two weeks, causing serious impairment in functioning at work or home – and if these traits were not the result of substance abuse, a medical condition, or a bereavement during the previous two months.[5]

Certain illnesses such as thyroid imbalance, heart disease, stroke, cancer, Alzheimer disease, and chronic pain caused by conditions such as arthritis can trigger depression. It can also be a side-effect of certain prescribed drugs, as well as some over-the-counter pain relievers and antihistamines. Depression can also complicate recovery from an illness. For example, people who suffer a major depression following a heart attack are more likely to die within six months than those who are not depressed.[6]

In William Styron's powerful memoir of his journey through a crippling and almost suicidal depression, he writes, "the pain of severe depression is quite unimaginable to those who have not suffered it." He goes on to say that, during the worst phase of this depression, "despair came to resemble the diabolical discomfort of being imprisoned in a fiercely overheated room. And because no breeze stirs this cauldron, because there is no escape from this smothering confinement, it is entirely natural that the victim begins to think ceaselessly of oblivion."[7]

Suicide   Whether contemplated, planned, or acted upon, suicide is an extremely complex issue, determined by many factors. When someone talks seriously about suicide it is an urgent cry for help. The most important thing to remember is never to ignore or devalue suicidal thoughts or comments.

There are significant differences between the sexes when it comes to suicide. Seventy-eight per cent of all suicides are committed by men. The rates for men are highest in the twenties, thirties, and teen years, followed by men aged sixty-five and older. While fewer women actually complete suicide, the highest rate of suicide for women in Canada is between the ages of forty-five to fifty-four.[8] This is clearly a finding that requires more study.

Studies show that those who attempt suicide (usually women) and those who complete the act of suicide (mostly men) are very different. "Attempters" are more likely to be desperately calling for help, while "completers" are truly determined to end their lives. Male-female differences in reaching out for help, the nature of the underlying problems, and learned responses to stress all seem to play a part in determining these different profiles.[9] These differences suggest that North American society's admiration for the macho male hero can have very dire consequences.

For the severely depressed, the risk of suicide increases during the first couple of weeks to a month of treatment, when a person still suffers from mental and emotional distortions, but has more energy for taking action against themselves.

Seasonal Affective Disorder (SAD)   Many of us who live in Canada or the northern United States find ourselves feeling glum as the days shorten in the autumn. We may feel less energetic and a little blue as we adjust to the early darkness, compared to our high energy and good spirits in the long summer days. For sufferers of seasonal affective disorder (SAD), the shorter hours of sunlight can have debilitating effects.

To be diagnosed with SAD, a person has to meet the criteria for major depression identified earlier, with the following additional provisions:

- a clear seasonal onset of the disorder in the fall and a full recovery by late April;
- symptoms that cannot be attributed to a seasonal psychosocial stressor, such as winter unemployment;
- the ratio of seasonal to nonseasonal episodes is at least three to one and the episodes recur seasonally.

Most people with SAD come to medical attention when they describe symptoms of increased appetite, weight gain, carbohydrate craving, profound fatigue, psychomotor slowing, and difficulty initiating activities, especially early in the day. Inexplicably, 80 per cent of sufferers are women between the ages of eighteen and forty-five. While there is no research available at this time, one certainly wonders about the role of hormones, as this group of women is of child-bearing age. As with dysthymia, many people suffering from SAD come to view it as just the way they are in the winter months and so for years may not recognize it as an illness that can be treated.

The first line of treatment is bright-light therapy. The atypical symptoms of carbohydrate craving and prolonged sleeping are the best predictors of a sufferer's positive response to light. The treatment consists of spending a half hour each day, preferably starting early in the morning (before 8 a.m.), sitting in front of a portable light box in a relaxed setting. Light therapy works well for 50 to 68 per cent of the people who try it.[10]

If the light is not sufficient, it can be augmented with L-tryptophan, an amino-acid precursor to serotonin, to increase the brain serotonin levels. The next step would be standard antidepressant medication, slowly discontinued in the spring, when the symptoms resolve, in order to avoid a mild manic episode. Many chronically depressed people find their symptoms worsen in winter and the adjunct of light therapy to their medication/psychotherapy regimen is beneficial.

Bipolar Disorders (formerly manic-depressive illness)
Bipolar disorders are not nearly as prevalent as depressive disorders. They consist of chronic, fluctuating cycles between the two poles of depression and elation or mania. The mood switches can be dramatic and rapid, but

more often they are gradual. In the depressed part of the cycle, some or all of the symptoms of major depression will occur. In the manic phase, the following symptoms appear:

- inflated sense of self and grandiose ideas
- inappropriate elation and irritability
- radically reduced need for sleep, or excessive sleep
- disconnected and racing thoughts, quicker and louder speech
- inappropriate and often embarrassing social behaviour
- poor judgement and impulsive activity, loss of touch with reality
- increased sexual drive

Like the depressive disorders, bipolar disorders exist on a continuum of increasing severity and intensity. Cyclothymia is the milder version. It consists of alternating periods of relatively mild mania and mild depression (dysthymia). This mild mania is characterized by an "abnormally and persistently elevated euphoric or irritable and expansive mood that lasts for at least four days."[11] Behaviour tends not to be as bizarre or extreme as it is in a true manic episode. In the early stages, this illness is difficult to recognize, because people in the manic stage may simply appear more social and creative than usual. This may be a welcome relief to their families, friends, and co-workers, and to themselves if they have been depressed. Because people tend only to seek treatment in the depressed phase, a misdiagnosis can be made and inappropriate treatment prescribed. If antidepressants are prescribed during the depressed phase, they can seriously exacerbate the manic phase.

Some Answers to Key Questions

What Causes Depression?
Most often, a combination of genetic, psychological, and environmental factors is involved in the onset of a depressive or bipolar disorder. Both these disorders have a significant genetic component, the physiological cause being low levels of the chemical serotonin in the brain. At the same time, not everybody with the genetic predisposition has the illness. One's general psychological makeup plays a part as well. People who have low self-esteem or are easily overwhelmed by stress may be more prone to depression. Environmental factors are also enormously important. These

include relationship problems such as separation and divorce, children leaving home, financial insecurity, unemployment, a lifestyle that includes alcohol and/or drug abuse, and overwork, to name a few.

Significant loss and bereavement leave everyone more vulnerable to the possible onset of depression. For people in midlife, loss can be a key factor. In addition to the loss of parents, friends, and partners, there is the loss of youth and the increased awareness of mortality to accept. We live in a culture that largely does not support the grieving process, so many people end up becoming depressed rather than experiencing their grief. It is important, when we feel depressed, to ask ourselves if we are ignoring some significant loss.

How Is Depression Diagnosed?
The following quiz will help you determine if you need to seek help.

SHOULD I SEEK HELP ABOUT DEPRESSION?
If you answer Yes to two or more of these questions, you may be depressed and should see your family physician as soon as possible. **Throughout the last two weeks:**

1. Have you been having trouble going to sleep, staying asleep, or sleeping too much?
2. Have you been waking early, feeling tired, and finding it difficult to return to sleep?
3. Have you lost interest in everyday pleasures, such as sex, hobbies, and being with friends?
4. Have you been feeling tired and down most of the day and finding everything an effort to do?
5. Have you lost or gained more than five pounds? Have you been eating more or less than usual? Have you been craving certain foods?
6. Have you had serious trouble concentrating or making decisions?
7. Have you been feeling worthless and blaming yourself a lot when things go wrong?
8. Have you been crying and feeling weepy, or getting angry easily?

9. Have you had a lot of physical complaints, such as recurrent headaches, backaches, and stomachaches, which are not part of an identified medical condition?
10. Do you have a gloomy view of the future?
11. Have you been thinking about death and/or suicide?

(This questionnaire was designed by the authors, using ideas from a variety of sources.)

A good diagnostic evaluation will first rule out the possibility that your symptoms are a result of certain prescription drugs or an existing medical condition. It will include a detailed description of your symptoms – their inception, severity, and frequency of occurrence, as well as any previous treatment you have received. It will also include a personal history, especially related to possible depressive illness among other family members, and contain information about possible substance abuse, suicidal thoughts, and your current level of functioning.

What Are the Gender Differences in Depression?

At all ages, women are more likely to be diagnosed with depression than men, except late in life, when male depression and suicide rates increase rapidly. Men in midlife may be particularly vulnerable to depression at two stages: in early midlife, when overworking tends to be at its height, and in late midlife, when they are confronted with retirement. In their early and mid-forties, some men feel overwhelmed by chronic stress on the job; some feel saddened by a recognition that the future no longer holds unlimited promise. They may feel trapped in unsatisfying careers in order to meet their financial obligations and raise their children. As one man we interviewed said, "At fifty, society sees you as disposable and replaceable by younger workers. I felt a disturbing lack of achievement. I was confused about the values I had accepted until then, and panicky about where I was going. I was floundering – emotionally and physically." At retirement, men are more prone to depression, in part because they no longer have the busyness and recognition of work to help them keep their feelings at bay.

Terrence Real, in his recent book about male depression, suggests that men consider feelings of helplessness and neediness unmanly, so they tend to deny and hide them. When they are no longer able to do this, their descent into depression can be much steeper. He also points out that depression in men can look quite different from depression in women. It may appear in a more agitated form, with symptoms of rage, self-destructive behaviour, and drug and alcohol abuse.[12] Hospitalization for alcohol and drug dependency is particularly high in males in the age group of forty-five to sixty-four.[13] Men need, and too often do not have, a trusting relationship with a physician who enables them to discuss their feelings, rather than act on them in a negative way.

As previously discussed, midlife women often find themselves sandwiched between caring for children and elderly parents, while holding down full-time jobs and managing the family home. Cultural and social factors can play a part, as women see themselves aging in a society that places so much value on youth.

As one woman put it, "My mother had a stroke, my youngest child was having trouble at school, and my husband's company was downsizing, all at the same time. I started getting severe headaches, which I tried to ignore, and my periods were all over the place. One day I just couldn't get out of bed. I just cried and cried. I really didn't know that I had gotten so low."

High stress levels, little if any personal time for renewal, coupled with the hormonal upheaval of menopause, can leave midlife women very vulnerable to depressive illnesses. The relation of hormones to depression in midlife women remains controversial. Many studies indicate that the incidence of depression at midlife is associated only with psychosocial problems; however, a recent article in *Menopause*, the journal of the North American Menopause Society, states: "while retrospective and prospective studies demonstrate that depression does not occur specifically during menopause, . . . in the minds of many clinicians, the incidence of depression seems to increase during the menopausal years."[14] Also, in the perimenopause, women report particularly intense premenstrual mood changes.

While menopause itself does not cause depressive disorders, there is no question that women's moods and psychological well-being are profoundly affected by fluctuations in hormones. In the case of a surgically induced menopause, the effect of such a dramatic drop in hormone production is clearly a factor. A woman with a history of depression is more vulnerable during menopause. So, the diagnosis of depression for midlife women is very complex.

How Is Depression Treated?

Developing a treatment plan requires a frank and thorough discussion between you and your physician or psychotherapist. The plan you will devise will most likely consist of either psychotherapy or psychotherapy combined with antidepressant medication. It should entail an assessment of your psychosocial stresses and menopausal symptoms, as well as looking at your support system.

With the advent of Prozac in the mid-1980s, the treatment of both dysthymia and more severe forms of depressive disorders changed radically. Unlike the previous generation of drugs, which produced severe side-effects, the selective serotonin reuptake inhibitors (SSRIs) have enabled many people previously incapacitated by their illness to function at a more acceptable level. Even the disturbing possible side-effects of decreased libido and inability to achieve orgasm are being addressed by an ever-increasing availability of newer and more effective medications. The side-effects of SSRIs should be minimal and should markedly decrease within four to six weeks.

Well, why isn't everybody on SSRIs if they make you feel so great? First of all, if you are not depressed, they won't improve your mood. Aging hippies in search of a prescription high to remind them of the good old days should look elsewhere. Second, SSRIs don't erase problems. If you are so depressed that you are barely functioning, the SSRIs, in the right form and correct dosage, can turn down the thermostat of your intensified emotions and give you some breathing room, freed of the worst extremes of your symptoms. This enables you to address personal difficulties more effectively through psychotherapy. The SRRIs are also beneficial when used cyclically to treat perimenopausal premenstrual mood changes.

ALTERNATIVE TREATMENT FOR DEPRESSION

A 1996 analysis of twenty-three controlled scientific studies showed that the herb St. John's wort has been proven as effective in

alleviating mild depression as traditional antidepressant medications – and with fewer side-effects. It also appears to relieve nervous
unrest and sleep disturbances. Again, the use and dosage are best
determined in consultation with your health care provider.

There are several forms of psychotherapy that effectively help depressed
individuals. Two of the most commonly recommended are psychodynamic
therapy and cognitive/behavioural therapy. Psychodynamic therapy may
be short term or it may focus on resolving long-term internal psychological conflicts. The latter is often recommended when short-term therapies
do not work. Cognitive and behavioural therapies focus on changing negative styles of thinking and negative behaviour patterns that have become
habitual to a person in a depressed state. These tend to be shorter term and
specific. Whether psychotherapy alone or in conjunction with medication
is indicated for treatment will depend on a number of variables, best
addressed through evaluation and consultation. See Chapter 16 for more
information on psychotherapy.

For many sufferers, the biggest obstacle to treatment is a sense of shame
and the negative stigma that is still associated with depression. In spite of
many efforts by public health organizations to educate the public, many
people still believe that a person becomes depressed through some weakness of character, some personal failing, or an unwillingness to apply
oneself. Unfortunately, because the illness erodes self-esteem, depressed
people often believe that they are weak or lazy. Repeated attempts to "snap
out of it" inevitably fail. Depressed people feel demoralized and defeated
and take this as reinforcement of the negative impression they already have
of themselves.

The interplay of depression and hormone changes can further complicate treatment for women. Too often, we have heard stories of women who
were clinically depressed being dismissed with "It's just your hormones," or
women who were going through hormone-related changes being incorrectly diagnosed with depression. The best antidote to this problem is open
and honest communication with your family physician and thoughtful,
sensitive referrals to other licensed health care providers, such as psychologists, social workers, and psychiatrists, for treatment.

What Can I Do for Myself?

There are a few fundamental dos and don'ts when you feel depressed for longer than a couple of weeks. While we recognize that expending any extra effort when you are depressed may feel impossible, we include this list nonetheless. Often, the smallest change can begin to lift the sense of gloom and remind you that feeling helpless and desperate is a part of the illness, not the total reality of your life.

- Do get help as quickly as you can.
- Do not remain isolated. Tell someone how you really feel.
- Do not medicate yourself with alcohol and drugs. Many people who say that they would of course take insulin if they were diabetic baulk at the idea of taking antidepressant medication. Further discussion sometimes reveals that they are, in fact, self-medicating with drugs and alcohol and making their depression worse.
- Do not set yourself difficult goals or make major life decisions at this time.
- Don't expect yourself to just suddenly recover. People rarely do.
- Do get a little physical exercise, if you can. It will help.
- Do try to be kind to yourself and, for the time being, lower your expectations of yourself.

How Can I Help Someone Who Is Depressed?

The most important thing you can do is help a depressed person get appropriate treatment. Depending on the person and the severity of the illness, this may mean encouraging him or her to see a psychotherapist, to possibly try medication, and to stick with treatment long enough to see if it helps. Offer as much reassurance, affection, and understanding as you can. One woman said that her partner's reminders that she had an illness and that she would recover helped her enormously on the days when she couldn't remind herself of this. Being able to listen to someone's feelings, without giving advice or problem-solving, is very important. Another woman told us, "It was so much easier to deal with the depression after I told my partner how I was feeling, and he said it was okay, he still loved me." Even the smallest suggestion that, if you just tried a little harder, you might not feel depressed, can discourage a person tremendously. And of course, never ignore remarks about suicide.

Being the primary support person for a friend or family member suffering from depression can be draining and frightening. Because we want our partner or friend to be better, it is easy to find the illness frustrating in its duration and intensity. We may feel guilty about having fun or enjoying ourselves in the face of their misery. Just as when you care for someone with a physical illness, it is critical that you take good care of yourself. Schedule time to do things that replenish you, and be willing to reach out to friends.

Anxiety Disorders

A professional midlife woman described her anxiety this way: "Ever since my three kids left for university, I have been a nervous wreck. I am constantly worried that they will either not eat, or not study, or get some kind of sexually transmitted disease. I know it is totally irrational, but I can't seem to stop. My husband says I am driving him crazy and now he's mad at me."

We all worry from time to time. To a certain extent, anxiety is a normal part of life and protects us by alerting us to danger. Only when it increases to such an extent that we are debilitated and when it is clearly out of proportion to our current circumstances do we need to seek help. As with depression, being in a chronic state of anxiety can feel so familiar and "normal" that it does not occur to us that we may need help.

Anxiety disorders are defined medically as a group of quite different conditions that all share anxiety at their core. They include (among others) panic attacks, phobias, generalized anxiety disorder, obsessive-compulsive disorder, and post-traumatic stress disorder. In this section, we focus on panic disorders and generalized anxiety disorder, which are most common in midlife.

Panic Disorders

A fifty-one-year-old third-grade teacher described her first panic attack this way: "I was walking down the hall to the classroom where I have taught for several years, when suddenly I was overcome with a feeling of abject fear about going into my room to teach. I was short of breath; my heart was beating wildly and I felt weak all over. The feeling passed quickly, but now I am really scared that it will come back."

Panic attacks are truly terrifying. An overwhelming sense of fear sweeps over us suddenly, intensely, and for no apparent reason; it can leave the sufferer wondering if she or he is having a heart attack or going crazy. The typical symptoms of chest pain, shortness of breath, and a choking sensation send many people to emergency wards or physicians' offices. Usually, the attack lasts less than ten minutes and consists of some combination of the following: trembling, sweating, unsteadiness, depersonalization (feeling outside yourself), nausea, chills or hot flashes, and a fear of dying. Because the attacks recur, sufferers feel intense anxiety anticipating when the next one will occur. In trying to understand why it happened, many incorrectly attribute the cause of the panic to the situation within which it occurred. Thus one can become phobic about certain situations that really have nothing at all to do with the onset of the panic attack.

To diagnose a panic disorder, the following criteria must be met:
- You must have one or more panic attacks per week for four weeks *or* one or more panic attacks followed by persistent fears of panic.
- The attacks have to be spontaneous and unexpected.
- The attacks cannot be triggered by a specific event, such as an examination.[15]

Many women suffer panicky feelings and panic attacks for the first time in the menopausal years. A female university professor in her early fifties told us, "I've always been so level-headed. Now I get so much more panicky and anxious, and for no real reason. I find it very disturbing." A recent small study indicated that HRT may somewhat diminish anxiety in the menopausal period, implying that either the lessened amount of estrogen or the fluctuations in estrogen levels are related to the degree of anxiety a woman feels.[16] More studies are needed to arrive at any conclusive results.

Fortunately, there are now effective medical treatments that can ease the panic quickly by acting on biochemical transmitters in the brain. Usually, the antidepressant paroxetine, sold under the trade name Paxil, is prescribed. Since it takes three to six weeks for the medication to become effective, benzodiazepine is usually prescribed to abort the panic attack should it occur. As the paroxetine takes effect, the benzodiazepine can be decreased or stopped, and used only when needed. Cognitive behaviour therapy may be recommended at the same time to try to break the negative cycle. This is done by working to replace the fearful and illogical thoughts (that something catastrophic is about to happen) with more appropriate, reality-based thinking.

ALTERNATIVE TREATMENT FOR ANXIETY

Kava-kava is an alternative medicine that has shown some promise in calming anxiety. Kava-kava, which is made from the pulverized roots of a large shrub found in the South Pacific, contains active components that can affect the central nervous system, reducing anxiety and improving sleep. German studies have shown promising results with kava-kava for these patients, with few side-effects.[17] Excessive use of kava-kava can lead to a puffy face, muscle weakness, red eyes, and skin rashes, and alcohol can increase its toxicity.[18]

Generalized Anxiety Disorder (GAD)

Whereas panic attacks are short and debilitating and phobias are linked to some particular object or situation, generalized anxiety disorder (GAD) is diffuse and all-encompassing. It is characterized by excessive, chronic worry, free-floating anxiety and jitteriness. GAD can sometimes present itself as a physical symptom, such as breathlessness or hyperventilation. Our mind and body are so interconnected that many physical conditions, such as Irritable Bowel Syndrome, can be mixed with anxiety or depression as part of the syndrome. People with GAD often worry about issues such as finances, or a loved one's safety, even though there may be no real cause for concern. Usually, people suffering from generalized anxiety know that they are reacting completely out of proportion to their circumstances. They feel terribly ashamed and embarrassed by this.

Rapid heartbeat, shakiness, sweating, dry mouth, sweaty palms, tightness in the chest, and sleeping problems are all symptoms of GAD. For a diagnosis to be made, sufferers must have these symptoms most days for six months or longer. We recommend that no one wait that long to seek help. A thorough assessment should rule out the possibility that such symptoms relate to medications or specific medical conditions such as heart disease and hyperthyroidism. Treatment usually consists of psychodynamic or cognitive/behaviour therapy combined with medication, as well as a consideration of possible lifestyle changes. For example, reassurance based on factual data about the state of one's physical health can sometimes be helpful for highly anxious people.

When Bette Midler said, "So much to worry about, so little time," she must have been talking about midlife. For so many women that we talked with, midlife is a time when they wake early each morning, hit the floor running, and don't stop until they collapse back into bed at night. This level of stress can lead to chronic anxiety. One fifty-year-old woman, who has a parent with Alzheimer disease, three children under the age of ten, and is going through a major work transition, said, "I feel constantly anxious, which I know doesn't do a bit of good. I worry about everyone and everything. It's not fair to my family or to me, but I don't know what to do."

It is essential to know when to seek professional help for anxiety. It is just as important, if not more so, to take some positive steps before you find yourself in dire straits. For example, you might assess your current life circumstances to determine what your stressors are and how you might ease or eliminate them. It is also helpful to create a plan for monitoring and looking after your own physical and emotional well-being. If you find yourself unable to do this, remember that it is just as legitimate to seek professional help to stay well as it is to seek help to recover once you have hit bottom.

Now I Lay Me Down to Sleep (I Hope!)

Exhaustion and chronic sleeplessness are two of the most frequent complaints that women bring to our clinics. They feel profoundly weary, trapped in a never-ending cycle as they get fewer and fewer nights of deep, uninterrupted sleep. One woman said, "It's an unfair trick of nature. First, I couldn't sleep because my young children woke me up. Then I stayed awake waiting for my teenagers to come home. Now I am up and down, awake because my husband gets up a few times, or because I have to pee, or I'm having night sweats and have to change my nightgown. It sounds funny, but it's not. I wake up more tired than when I went to bed and wonder how I will drag myself through another day."

Sleep Disorders

Sleeping, like eating, is one of those essential, bottom-line functions. If you are not sufficiently well-rested, you simply cannot work efficiently and creatively, and your experience of pleasure is greatly diminished. You become more easily confused and irritable and more prone to accidents, illnesses, and to serious problems of depression and anxiety. Most of us need a minimum of seven to eight hours of sleep each night – and few of us get it. Recent research on primates who sleep as long as sixteen to eighteen hours a day implies that we humans, their close relatives, are chronically sleep-deprived.[19]

There is also controversy about whether a "sleep debt" can ever be repaid. As we age, it seems less likely that a longer sleep on the weekend can really compensate for shortened hours of sleep during the work week. If you get just one hour less sleep per night for a week, you miss a whole night's sleep! "I'm just too old to pull off one of those all-nighters we used to do in university," said one man we interviewed.

The two most common sleep disorders are insomnia and sleep apnea. The medical diagnosis of **insomnia** is applied when:

- a person has difficulty falling asleep or maintaining sleep or has non-restorative sleep for at least a month.
- these disruptions are significant enough to cause distress or impairment in daily functioning.
- the sleeping problem is not the result of other emotional/mental disorders (such as depression) nor a result of medication.

Usually, people with insomnia report difficulty falling asleep and intermittent waking during the night. In depression, the most common complaint is early-morning waking. The distress about not being able to fall asleep becomes a preoccupation ("Am I going to sleep tonight?") that can lead to a vicious cycle. The harder you try to sleep, the more frustration builds and the less likely it is that sleep will come.

Sleep apnea is a potentially serious and life-threatening condition that affects men primarily. The person briefly stops breathing while asleep and may not resume respiration for between ten seconds and two or three minutes. An occasional episode of apnea is quite common, and is not significant. See your family physician if you are having more than 15 to 20 episodes of apnea per hour or more than 100 a night, especially if you are struggling with excessive sleepiness in the daytime. Look for symptoms of snoring coupled with times when you seem to struggle to breathe. A visit to a sleep laboratory can help arrive at a diagnosis.

Because sleep is such a basic cornerstone of well-being, it is critical to find ways to improve sleep, before much else can change. A thorough physical and emotional investigation, as well as a lifestyle assessment are necessary in order to understand the particular nature of a person's sleep difficulty. Most important in alleviating the problem is helping the apnea or insomnia sufferer practise better sleep hygiene. Be patient. Chronic sleep problems do not change over the course of one night or a week.

How to Get a Good Night's Sleep

Treatment for insomnia needs to be tailored to fit the person's sleep problems. As mentioned, these need to be carefully determined through a physical exam, a detailed history of the problem, and, sometimes, a visit to a sleep laboratory. When you are having a lot of trouble sleeping, think about what your body may be trying to tell you. Are you sitting at your computer until midnight, and then falling into bed wound up and exhausted? Do you have financial or family problems that you are trying to ignore? Listen to the message your body is sending you.

The experts' recommendations – called improvements in "sleep hygiene" – are sensible suggestions for helping all of us achieve a good night's sleep:

- Establish a regular time for going to bed and getting up (even on weekends). A routine that helps you unwind (such as taking a bath or listening to music) can also help.
- Get to know your unique sleep needs and rhythms. They may be quite different from those of your partner.
- Don't just lie there. If you can't sleep, don't fight it. Get up and go to a different room. Read, sip warm milk, until you feel sleepy.
- Be active. Exercise can effectively curb sleep problems, if done at least three hours before bedtime. Exercising immediately before going to bed may have the opposite effect!
- Practise a mind-body discipline that calms the nervous system, such as hatha yoga, tai chi, or mindfulness meditation.
- Do not use alcohol to help you sleep. While it might seem to help initially, alcohol actually interferes with your sleep patterns later in the night.
- Avoid heavy meals late at night and stimulants such as caffeine and nicotine in the evening.
- If you have the urge to urinate in the night, do not drink any fluids after 7:00 p.m.

- Most people sleep best when the room is 15 to 18 degrees Celsius (60 to 65 degrees Fahrenheit). If you have hot flashes or night sweats, be sure to use a cotton sheet under your duvet or blanket so that you can change it if you need to – or consider investing in a dual-control electric blanket. If night sweats are seriously disturbing your sleep, talk with your physician about the use of hormone replacement therapy or alternative remedies.

- See a doctor if you snore. This is not a trivial problem. Laser-assisted palate surgery done in a physician's office can fix obstructed breathing and has a success rate of 90 per cent.

- Be very cautious about using sleeping pills. While prescribed sleeping medication can sometimes help hardcore insomniacs break the sleeplessness habit, the body can quickly develop a tolerance for them and become dependent on them. Sleeping pills should be used in acute situations of stress, and never for longer than two weeks. There are two new sleeping pills on the market, zeleplon (marketed as Sonata) and zopiclone (Imovane) that help to induce natural sleep stages. They do not cause next-day drowsiness as the old hypnotics did.

- Reserve your bedroom for relaxation, sleep, and sex. Looking at a desk full of work as you lie in bed will inhibit your ability to fall asleep!

- If you try all of the above and still find yourself awake most of the night and dragging during the day, consult a professional.

ALTERNATIVE SLEEP SUPPORTERS

Alternative therapies may be helpful for occasional bouts of insomnia.

Try gentle music, relaxation audio tapes, creative visualization, progressive muscle relaxation, gentle therapeutic massage, or the old standby of warm milk and honey.

Valerian. Controlled studies have shown that people with sleep problems benefit from taking valerian, a natural herb sedative. The recommended dosage is 150 to 300 mg of valerian extract thirty minutes before going to sleep.[20]

Melatonin. Used in small doses (0.3 to 1 mg), melatonin can help people who have difficulty falling asleep. Higher doses (5 mg) may be needed to maintain sleep through the night. As with any sleeping medication, do not use daily. Because melatonin is a hormone, use it only under the guidance of a health practitioner familiar with it. It is particularly effective for time adjustments related to jet lag.[21]

The Shared-Bed Sleeping Quiz[22]

Men and women sleep differently. See how you do on the following quiz.

1. When a man and a woman sleep together, who sleeps more deeply?
2. Who dreams in more vivid colours?
3. Who is more likely to have nightmares?
4. Who is more likely to snore, and who is more likely to be disturbed by snoring at night?
5. Who is more likely to live longer – a woman who sleeps eight hours a night or a man who sleeps ten hours a night?

Answers

1. The man. Women are lighter sleepers and tend to be disturbed more when a bedmate changes position.
2. The woman. Studies show that women consistently report more colour in their dreams.
3. Women report more nightmares up to about age fifty, when both sexes seem to experience them equally.
4. The man on both counts. Most snorers (there are an estimated 35 to 40 million snorers in the United States) are male, middle-aged, and overweight. And while it may seem to many bleary-eyed women that their partners' snoring has kept them awake most of the night, many snorers suffer from sleep apnea, associated with snoring. Although most people with sleep apnea are unaware they have it, they almost never get a good night's sleep.
5. The woman, for two reasons. First, because sleeping between seven and eight hours a night correlates in studies with optimum longevity and because women, in general, tend to live slightly longer than men.

THE BOTTOM LINE

If you think that you, your partner, or a friend may be suffering from depression, anxiety, or insomnia, get help right away. Don't self-medicate, don't isolate yourself, and don't give up. There are safe and effective treatments available.

Contacts and Further Information

Organizations

- American Psychiatric Association, 1400 K St. N.W., Washington, DC 20005. Tel.: (202) 682–6000.
- American Psychological Association, 750 First St. N.E., Washington, DC 20002–4242. Tel.: (800) 374–2721; Web: http://www.apa.org
- American Sleep Disorder Association, 6301 Bandel Road, Suite 101, Rochester, MN 55901. Tel.: (507) 287–6006; Fax: (507) 287–6008; Web: http://www.asda.org
- Canadian Mental Health Association, 2160 Yonge St., Toronto, ON M4S 2Z3. Tel.: (416) 484–7750; Fax: (416) 484–4617; E-mail: cmhanat@interlog.com; Web: http://www.cmha.ca (or contact a local office in your phone book).
- Canadian Psychological Association, 441 MacLaren St., Suite 260, Ottawa, ON K2P 2H8. Tel.: (613) 234–2815; Fax: (613) 234–9857; Web: http://www.cpa.ca
- Mood Disorders Association of Canada, 1000 Notre Dame Ave., Suite 4, Winnipeg, MB R3E 0N3. Tel.: (204) 786–0987; Fax: (204) 786–1906.
- National Center for Sleep Disorder Research, 2 Rockledge Center, 6701 Rockledge Dr., Suite 7024, Bethesda, MD 20892–7920. Tel.: (301) 435–0199; Fax: (301) 480–3451.
- National Institute of Mental Health (U.S.), 5600 Fisher's Lane, Room 7C02, Rockville, MD 20857–0001. Tel.: (800) 421–4211; (301) 443–4513; Fax: (301) 443–4279; Web: www.nimh.nih.gov
- National Mental Health Association (U.S.), 1021 Prince St., Alexandria, VA 22314–2917. Tel.: (800) 969–6642; Web: www.worldcorp.com/dc-online/nmha

- National Sleep Foundation, 729 15th St. N.W., Floor 4, Washington, DC 20005. Tel.: (202) 347−3471; Fax: (202) 347−3472; Web: http://www.sleepfoundation.org
- Sleep/Wake Disorders Canada, 3080 Yonge St., Suite 5055, Toronto, ON M4N 3N1. Tel.: (416) 483−9654; Fax: (416) 483−7081; Web: http://www.geocities.com/~sleepwake

Books

On Depression
- *Darkness Visible: A Memoir of Madness* by William Styron. New York: Vintage Books, 1992.
- *Feeling Good: The New Mood Therapy* by David Burns and Aaron Beck, New York: Avon Books, 1992 (rev. and updated, 1999).
- *I Don't Want to Talk About It!: Overcoming the Secret Legacy of Male Depression* by Terrence Real. New York: Scribner, 1997.
- *Listening to Prozac* by Peter Kramer. New York: Penguin Books, 1993.
- *Natural Alternative to Prozac* by Michael T. Murray. New York: William Morrow, 1996.
- *You Mean I Don't Have to Feel This Way?: New Help for Depression, Anxiety, and Addiction* by Colette Dowling. New York: Bantam Books, 1993.

On Anxiety
- *Don't Panic: Taking Control of Anxiety Attacks* by R. Reid. New York: HarperCollins, 1996.
- *Feel the Fear . . . and Beyond* by Susan Jeffers. New York: Fawcett Columbine, 1998.
- *Feel the Fear and Do It Anyway* by Susan Jeffers. New York: Fawcett Columbine, 1987.
- *How to Control Your Anxiety Before It Controls You* by Albert Ellis. New York: Birch Lane Press, 1996.

On Bereavement
- *Grace and Grit* by Ken Wilber. Boston: Shambala, 1991.
- *A Grief Observed* by C. S. Lewis. London: Faber & Faber, 1963.

- *Midlife Orphan: Facing Life's Choices Now That Your Parents Are Gone* by Jane Brooks. New York: A Berkeley Book, 1999.
- *Who Dies?: An Investigation of Conscious Living and Conscious Dying* by Stephen Levine. New York: Anchor Books, 1982.

On Sleep Disorders
- *No More Sleepless Nights* by Peter Hauri and Shirley Linde. New York: John Wiley, 1990.
- *Say Good Night to Insomnia* by Gregg D. Jacobs. New York: Henry Holt, 1998.

Websites
- American Self-Help Clearinghouse (sponsored by CMHC Systems): http://www.cmhc.com/selfhelp
- Bereavement Site (sponsored by Administration on Aging, U.S. Department of Health and Human Services): http://aoa.dhhs.gov/jpost/gr.death-dying.html
- The Emotional Support Guide: Internet Resources for Physical Loss, Chronic Illness and Bereavement: http//asa.ugl.lib.umich.edu/chdocs/support/emotion/html
- Mental Health Net (sponsored by CMHC Systems): http//www.cmhc.com
- Psych Central: Dr. John Grohol's Mental Health Page: http://www.coil.com/~grohol/
- Sleep Disorders (sponsored by National Sleep Foundation): http://www.sleepfoundation.org/disorder.html
- Sleep Medicine: http://www.users.cloud9.net/~thorp
- The Sleep Site (sponsored by Columbus Community Hospital): http://www.thesleepsite.com
- Mental Health Server (sponsored by Internet Mental Health): http://www.mentalhealth.com

Related Chapters in This Book
- *Chapter 1: The Midlife Journey* explores midlife as a time of reckoning, turbulence, and regeneration.

- *Chapter 2: Understanding the Female Menopause* and *Chapter 3: Is There a Male Menopause?* provides more information on the body-mind connection and the physical changes of midlife that can affect mental and emotional well-being.
- *Chapter 7: The Active Living Solution* gives you guidance on how to be more active in midlife.
- *Chapter 9: The Boomer's Drugs of Choice* discusses moderate drinking and how much is too much. Many people erroneously use alcohol to treat depression, anxiety, and sleep problems.
- *Chapter 10: Growing Apart and Together: Relationships in Midlife* explores the ingredients of a healthy relationship and the importance of social support in hard times.
- *Chapter 13: Stress-Proofing in Midlife* helps you assess your stress level and provides common-sense ways of dealing with midlife stressors.
- *Chapter 16: Partners in Health Care* provides additional information about psychotherapy.
- *Chapter 23: Body, Mind, and Soul* discusses how your spiritual beliefs can improve your overall well-being.

PART THREE

An Ounce of Prevention
Is Worth a Pound of Cure

CHAPTER SIXTEEN

Partners in Health Care

> One of the most powerful tools for your healing is to develop
> a relationship with a health care team in which all members
> respect the body's ability to heal and maintain health, and are
> willing to facilitate this process.
>
> — Christiane Northrup, author of
> *Women's Bodies, Women's Wisdom*[1]

In today's world, health care is about more than physicians and hospitals. It's about prevention, self-care, mutual aid, and becoming partners with a variety of competent health care providers. These may include a dentist, a social worker, a naturopath, a chiropractor, an ophthamologist, a psychologist, a family physician, and many others.

Evidence suggests that people do better and are more satisfied with their care when they act as partners with their health professionals. But this is not always easy to do. For example, it takes chutzpah to question a physician when you are sitting there wearing only a paper gown. Some physicians, too, remain slow to embrace this approach. They prefer patients who are compliant and defer to their recommendations.

This chapter gives you some practical advice on how to be a partner in your own health care by being assertive and responsible, and building ongoing two-way communication with all of your other health care providers. It offers a male and female midlife health-assessment checklist, so that you know what kind of tests and screening should be part of good preventive care in midlife. Finally, it suggests some guidelines for using the Internet to find more information on a variety of health problems.

Who's in Charge Here Anyway?

In the last two decades there has been a major shift in the practice of medicine. As educated consumers have demanded more control and input into their care, the medical profession has responded with what it calls patient-centred care. This approach encourages physicians to see patients as partners in their own care. It encourages patients to ask questions and share the responsibility for medical decisions affecting them. It also acknowledges the emotional and psychological aspects of illness.[2]

Here are some tips on how to develop a partnership with your family physician and other health care providers:

- Remember, your input is vital to your physician's ability to treat you effectively and respectfully.

- Educate yourself about your own health problems. Seek out some of the resources recommended in this book and others. Surf the Net, looking for reliable sites, such as those sponsored by universities, government health departments, and well-established nongovernmental health organizations, such as the Cancer Society, the Heart and Stroke Foundation, or the Arthritis Society.

- Share what you learn with your health care provider. If you are reading an article or book about your health concern, bring it along to your appointment.

- Consider joining a support group. People share their stories and solutions and provide support that only others with similar problems can give. These groups most often meet face to face, although increasingly they are available on-line as well. There are support groups for every issue you can name: from diabetes to depression, gambling addiction, parenting teenagers with drug problems, and caring for elderly parents with Alzheimer disease.

- Take prescribed medications as directed. Report any side-effects to your physician and discuss alternatives. The modern cornucopia of pharmaceuticals offers many variations on the same drug. You and your physician may try several different ones before you find the one that is best for you.

- Tell your physician and alternative practitioners whether you are using over-the-counter medications, vitamins, herbs, or other complementary and alternative medicines. These may react with prescription drugs.

The Doctor Will Hear You Now

The quality of your care depends on your ability and that of your health care provider to work together effectively. Central to this partnership is two-way communication. Research has shown that you are likely to do better if you have a physician with whom you can communicate. When your physician listens and presents you with options for care, you are more likely to feel in control, to tolerate symptoms well, and to assume responsibility for improving your health. More important, you may be diagnosed more accurately, respond better to treatment, and recover more quickly.[3]

A 1995 survey of more than 70,000 *Consumer Reports* readers found that, while most people felt that their physicians were competent and concerned, a significant number were unhappy with their physicians' communication skills. Men scored male and female physicians about the same. Women found female physicians were better than males in terms of communication, caring, and thoroughness.[4]

The days of Hippocrates, who advised physicians not to discuss the nature of the disease or treatment with a patient, are long gone. In today's medical environment, you need someone who is good at both listening and interacting.

Two-Way Communication

Here are some of the things you can do to promote a positive relationship with your health care provider.

- Notice your physician's communication skills. Does he listen to you? Is she open to questions? Do you get "cut off" or interrupted often? Does he explain how a medication works and what side-effects to expect? Is she open to your ideas about looking after your problem?
- Take a few minutes before your appointment to review the things you want to discuss, either by writing them down or organizing them in your mind. Decide which are most important, as the visit may not cover all your concerns. Get to the point as quickly as you can.

- Be knowledgeable about your family history and past health history. Bring previous records if you have them.
- If you need to talk about some personal or emotional issues with a physician, book extra time to give both of you the chance to have an uninterrupted, relaxed visit.
- Maintain eye contact. It encourages a practitioner to deal more directly with you.
- Ask questions and make sure you understand what you are being advised to do. Don't be embarrassed to ask for clarification of medical terms. If you are getting a lot of information all at once, ask the practitioner to take five minutes at the end of the appointment to summarize the key points. Studies show that patients are more satisfied with their care and more likely to remember key information when it is summarized at the end of their appointments.
- If you are unsure or uncomfortable about a recommendation for treatment, ask for information about alternative approaches. State your concerns and ask for a referral to a specialist if necessary.

What about Psychotherapy?

It is not unusual for men and women in midlife to find that they require or might greatly profit from psychotherapy. Navigating the rough waters of the midlife passage can mean being confronted again with earlier traumas or losses that were never addressed. It can also be a time of feeling overwhelmed by too many stresses and too few inner resources. Psychotherapy can be a means of dealing with current distress, and can also be good preventive medicine. When you address emotionally troubling issues, they are much less likely to make you physically ill.

When it comes to psychotherapy, it is important to be a good consumer, just as when you choose a family physician or alternative practitioner. Finding the right psychotherapist can be challenging at the best of times, let alone when you feel emotionally distraught and vulnerable. In this section we will look briefly at how to find a good psychotherapist, different approaches to psychotherapy, and what you can expect from the process.

A visit to your family physician is a good place to start. If the physician knows you, your family, and personal history well, he or she is usually in a good position to make a referral. Unless you need to see someone immediately, it is better to have several names and invest some time in interviewing different therapists.

During the initial consultation, ask about the psychotherapist's training, years of experience, and orientation. While many therapists belong to professional organizations with strict ethical guidelines and rules of professional conduct, this is not a requirement. In Canada, anyone can advertise as a psychotherapist without a licence or educational qualifications.

So many different health care professionals provide psychotherapy that the various designations can be very confusing. Psychiatrists, family physicians, and general practice (GP) psychotherapists are the only ones who are medical physicians, and therefore the only mental health practitioners who can prescribe medication. If your family physician offers psychotherapy, check to see if she or he has upgraded therapy skills through educational courses, or belongs to an organization of GP psychotherapists.

Clinical or counselling psychologists (Ph.D.s) are registered in the province or state in which they practise. They are trained in the diagnosis and treatment of many emotional and mental disorders, and may work with individuals, couples, families, or groups, depending on their orientation and training. Clinical social workers work in agencies or in private practice, also treating individuals, couples, and families. Marriage and family therapists specialize in issues relating to couples, parents, and children, and the extended family.

While the words "psychotherapy" and "counselling" are often used interchangeably, generally counselling refers more to a problem-solving, here-and-now approach and psychotherapy implies a more in-depth, longer-term approach. There are many different kinds of psychotherapy and different ways of categorizing them. There are short-term and long-term therapies; supportive and insight-based, cognitive-behavioural, psychoanalytic, and bioenergetic therapies, to name a few. The approach suggested will depend on the nature of your problems.

At your first meeting, find out what the therapist's rates are and what his or her policy is regarding billing and charges for missed appointments. The cost of psychotherapy will vary, depending on the therapist's years of experience and additional training. You can check with his or her professional organization to find out the recommended fee structure. In most Canadian provinces, the services of psychiatrists and family physicians practising psychotherapy are covered by provincial health plans. Private health-insurance plans usually cover a limited number of sessions with a licensed psychologist. Large organizations often have employee-assistance programs (EAPs), which provide a limited number of sessions with a specified mental health professional for employees and their families.

Once you have this information, the most important issue is whether there is a good fit between you and the psychotherapist. Do you feel comfortable with the therapist's personal style and approach to your concerns? Positive rapport and a feeling that the two of you will be able to work well together are critical to your progress. Research shows that therapy is most successful when the expectations of the client and the therapist match, regarding the goals and method of treatment.[5]

The length of the therapy will vary according to a complex group of factors, including the nature, duration, and severity of your problems and the connection or "working alliance" between you and your therapist. Short-term therapies will focus more on addressing a specific problem. Cognitive-behavioural therapies are often recommended for phobias, and have an educational component – you "learn" new behaviours. Insight-based, dynamic therapy, such as psychoanalysis, addresses longer-term problems, believed to originate in unresolved conflicts from childhood.

If you have difficulty finding someone with whom you have a good fit, ask your family physician for another referral. Friends or relatives who have had successful psychotherapy can also be a good referral source. While less personal, most provincial and state psychology and social-work organizations have reliable referral lists. (See the Contacts and Further Information at the end of Chapter 15.)

Many people find that self-help and support groups, such as Alcoholics Anonymous, are good sources of both counselling and support. Being with others who are going through the same difficulties can be very healing.

An Ounce of Prevention

As we get older and struggle to find the right care for our aging parents, it is hard not to be concerned about the state of our health care system. Will there be enough money for the operations, tests, therapy, and care that a growing population of older citizens will need?

The answer is a qualified yes. There will be a health care system to help us in old age, but only if two things come to pass. First, we need to make some fundamental changes in the ways health care is administered in Canada and the United States. As the massive baby-boom population hits midlife and older, chronic diseases such as arthritis, diabetes, and heart disease will preoccupy the health care system. These problems are best dealt with outside acute-care hospitals. As we age, we will need more community health care and homecare services to help us remain independent in our own homes. This is especially important for women, who carry out most of the informal care for family members who are ill. In the new century, hospitals will become places primarily for high-tech procedures. Home will be where we recover and, increasingly, where we will die.

Getting ready to care for each other in old age is on the minds of many boomers, especially those who have decided not to have children. One group we know, whose members live in Nova Scotia, have already started to plan a communal kind of arrangement they call a "Care Club." Everyone will have a role – someone to cook, someone to act as a nurse and as a physician, someone to do the accounting for the group. Ironically, we may see communal living experiments in the new millennium as we did in the 1960s.

The second change that is required is a greater focus on health promotion and preventive medicine. As we age, our needs for testing, vaccinations, and screening change. Healthy lifestyles, healthful, supportive environments, and effective preventive care can help us live longer and healthier. Yet, in our current system, it is estimated that only 2 to 3 per cent of our annual health care expenses go to health promotion and preventive care.

Medical experts agree that improving health requires improved access to preventive medicine. How to deliver preventive medicine in a system wrestling with enormous cost constraints is another question.

In 1976, the Canadian government established the Canadian Task Force on Periodic Health Examinations to review the scientific evidence for and against the effectiveness of various interventions, such as screening tests and specific examinations, to prevent disease in healthy people. In 1980, the U.S. government formed a similar task force, and the two groups decided to collaborate in their work. They examined the scientific literature and made recommendations as to who should be tested for high blood cholesterol, diabetes, and many other conditions.

These two groups regularly publish their findings, and governments use their recommendations in setting guidelines for preventive care in Canada and the United States. Each intervention is rated according to the evidence found to support its effectiveness.

Many physicians are frustrated by the large number of interventions for which experts claim there is insufficient evidence. For several medical conditions, the Task Force confronted a dilemma: would early detection and intervention cause more anxiety and harm or make possible a better outcome? A typical example of this is PSA (prostate-specific antigen) testing for prostate cancer. Urologist groups are still arguing the Task Force recommendations about whether or not the PSA test is cost-effective and whether early detection saves lives.

At the same time, new tests to determine whether you have the gene for breast cancer and other diseases are raising many ethical questions. One woman who is attending an ovarian cancer clinic for people with a family history of ovarian cancer said recently, "I am so scared each time I go to the clinic, I cannot sleep for a few days. I am always wondering if it is worth it. I decided not to be tested for the breast-cancer gene. I couldn't handle living with that information. What could I do? Have my breasts cut off? This is scary stuff!"

Genetic research is opening up new and unknown territory for us all. Those considering genetic testing face two key questions:

- Will a positive result require radical action I am not ready for?
- Could the information prove more hazardous to my health than the disease itself?

In a recent study evaluating psychological issues associated with hereditary breast cancer, the investigators found that the risks of testing include anxiety, depression, altered self-image, and insurance and employment discrimination.[6]

We all need to address two other important questions:

- Should we be testing for diseases we can't yet cure?
- What are the psychological and social implications of such testing?

These and many other questions will have to be answered before we can fully accept genetic testing as an essential part of our health services. At the same time, we do know that heredity plays an important role in how long we will live and, in some cases, from what we will die.

THE MALE CHECK-UP CHALLENGE

"In their twenties, men think that they are too strong to go to the physician; in their thirties, they think that they are too busy; and in their forties, they are too worried about what their physician may find," says Ron Henry, co-founder of the Men's Health Network, an advocacy group in Washington, DC.[7] Studies repeatedly show that men are far less likely than women to go to physicians and to establish relationships with family physicians. The result can be prolonged (and sometimes unnecessary) suffering and a danger that men's health problems will not be diagnosed until they are at an advanced stage. Remember, men, nine of ten cancers are curable if discovered before they spread. So read the next section and make your appointment now!

Testing, Testing: What to Expect at Your Midlife Check-Up

As emphasized, if your physician is to provide good preventive care, he or she must know your family history of disease, your past health history, your current lifestyle practices, and what your work and home environments are like. Good preventive medicine focuses on your specific age and needs, so you are responsible for making sure that your physician has the information he or she needs to deal with you in a holistic manner. This means taking time to talk about your anxieties and mental health, as well as about your physical health.

It also means taking a pro-active stance: talk with your physician about lifestyle changes and holistic ways that you can prevent disease and illness. For instance, if you still smoke, ask for help with quitting. Don't hide problems with gambling or recreational drugs. Discuss daily habits such as coffee intake, alcohol use, and diet. Ask about exercise and what is best for you at your stage of life. If you are having sexual problems, your check-up is a good time to raise your concerns. As we have seen in previous chapters, you may discover physical causes that can be quickly corrected.

Only after your physician assesses all of these factors can you both decide what kind of preventive medicine and lifestyle changes you have to make. The kinds of tests you require, for example, are strongly related to your age, medical history, and levels of risk for a particular problem.

Many of what used to be routine screening tests in healthy people (such as chest X-rays and complete blood tests) are now reserved for people with symptoms or risk factors. However, there is general agreement that several screening tests are good preventive medicine in midlife:

THE MIDLIFE HEALTH-ASSESSMENT CHECKLIST

For men and women (unless otherwise indicated)

Test	How Often?
Blood pressure	Every 1 to 2 years.
Heart-health electro-cardiogram (ECG)	Men: Baseline ECG around age 40 and repeat every two years. Women: Baseline ECG around age 50, and repeat every two years.
Blood lipids	Every 5 years if normal.
Screen for diabetes	Repeat every 2 to 3 years, depending on risk. Higher risk with family history, obesity. African-American ancestry. Women who have delivered a baby weighing more than 9 lb (5 kg) are also at higher risk.
Vaccination updates (Hepatitis B, Td-tetanus and diphtheria, Hepatitis A)	On a regular basis.
Influenza vaccine	Annually for anyone with lung disease, heart disease, cancer, or diabetes, or at high risk for flu.
Pneumonia vaccine	Given once in a llifetime for anyone with lung disease, heart disease, cancer, or diabetes, or at risk for pneumonia.

Skin check	Every 2 to 3 years; more often if you have abnormal lesions or moles, or a family history of melanoma.
Vision screening, including glaucoma	Every 2 to 3 years. Remember, midlife is the time when vision starts to change.
Dental care	Every 6 to 12 months. Discuss with your dentist – gum problems often become more prevalent in midlife.
Testing for STDs	As required.
Hearing tests	As required.

For Men Only:

Digital rectal examination plus PSA (for prostate cancer)	Annually after age 50 or sooner if you have symptoms or a family history. African-American men have a 30-per-cent higher risk; they should start screening at age 40. (See Chapter 18 for more information on the PSA test.)
Stool test (for colorectal cancer)	Every 1 to 2 years.
Learn self-examination of testicles	Once with a physician or nurse, then practise it yourself.

For Women Only:

Pap smear	After 3 normal annual tests, repeat every 2 to 3 years.
Digital rectal examination plus stool test (for colorectal cancer)	Every 1 to 2 years.

Learn self-examination of breasts	Once with a physician, or nurse, then practise regularly.
Clinical breast examination	Annually after age 40.
Mammography	In Canada, every 2 years between ages 50 and 69, if test is normal and you are not at high risk. In the United States, annually, after age 40. (See Chapter 19 for information.)
Bone density test	At menopause or earlier if at high risk for osteoporosis. (See Chapter 17.)
TSH: thyroid testing	Every 5 years.

Additional Tests You Might Require
- Colonoscopy/sigmoidoscopy (use of lighted tube-like instruments to directly inspect the bowels and remove tissue for biopsy if necessary). If you have two or three relatives with a history of colon cancer, or if you have one or two positive tests for blood in the stool, a rectal examination, stool testing, and a sigmoidoscopy or colonoscopy may be recommended every three to five years, starting at age forty.
- Additional immunization. Before travelling, visit a travel medical clinic or your family physician to discuss your need for vaccines such as those for Hepatitis A and Hepatitis B, medication for malaria, etc. A pneumonia vaccine is useful if you have asthma or chronic bronchitis.

Using the Internet to Learn More[8]
There are millions of health sites on the Internet. Much of it is useful, some of it is not, and some of it is downright quackery. Here are some tips to help you find the useful ones.
1. Look for sites that are sponsored by non-profit organizations dedicated to a particular problem (e.g, the Cancer Society) or by

professional organizations and universities. The last part of the domain name or URL may give you some of this information:

- "com" often refers to commercial sites;
- "org" is for non-profit organizations;
- "edu" is for educational institutions;
- "ca" is a country code for Canada; many sites originate in the United States unless otherwise specified;
- "gov" is a U.S. government site.

2. While some commercial sites provide excellent information, be wary of those that are trying to sell you something.

3. Look for a "last-updated date" on the site to see if the information is current. Some sites are also certified as providing trustworthy information, such as the Geneva-based Health on the Net Foundation's certification (HONCODE).

4. We have checked all the sites listed in this book, and we recommend them as a good place to start. Sites appear and disappear regularly, however, so some of the URLs listed here may no longer exist.

5. A number of general-health sites offer extensive links to other sites on more detailed topics. Some of the best are listed at the end of this chapter. The Internet books listed here also contain other key health sites. You can "bookmark" these sites, so you can return to them easily.

6. Remember to enter the URL carefully. One error in a space or symbol means that your computer will not be able to find the site.

7. Support organizations and self-help groups on the Web differ from those that are designed primarily to provide information. They provide "chat rooms," where people with similar problems can share experiences and solutions. Be sure to read the "Frequently Asked Questions" before you post a question, so that you are not repeating a query that is already answered on-line. It is a good idea to "lurk," or listen in, for a while so you get a sense of group norms for participating. Then feel free to express yourself. Most good support websites have a monitor who follows the conversation and handles any problems that arise.

8. Some people set a timer when they start to "surf" the Web. You'll be amazed how quickly three hours can pass!

9. Don't abandon libraries. Reference librarians are great allies in your search, and there is still something special about turning the pages of a book.

THE BOTTOM LINE

Search out the information you need to be an informed consumer. Find a good family physician and a reliable alternative practitioner when you need one. Learn to communicate effectively and become an assertive and responsible partner in your health care. Think prevention: adopt a healthy lifestyle and talk with your health care providers about preventive strategies and monitor your mental as well as your physical health. Reach out to others with similar problems and enjoy the support you will receive in return.

Contacts and Further Information

Organizations

- American Institute for Preventive Medicine, 30445 Northwestern Highway, Suite 350, Farmington Hills, MI 48334. Tel.: (800) 345–2476; Fax: (810) 539–1800.
- The Canadian Women's Health Network, Suite 203, 419 Graham Ave., Winnipeg, MB R3C 0M3. Tel.: (204) 942–5500; Fax: (204) 989–2355.
- National Institute on Aging (U.S.) Information Center, P.O. Box 8057, Gaithersburg, MD 20898–8057. Tel.: (800) 222–2225.
- National Self-Help Clearinghouse (U.S.), 25 W. 43rd St., Room 620, New York, NY 10036. Tel.: (212) 642–2944.
- National Women's Health Network (U.S.), 514 10th St. N.W., Suite 400, Washington, DC 20004. Tel.: (202) 347–1140; Fax: (202) 344–1168.

Websites

- The American Council on Science and Health: http://www.acsh.org
- American Public Health Association: http://www.apha.org

- Canadian Health Network: http://www.canadian-health-network.ca
- Canadian Public Health Association: http://www.cpha.ca
- Canadian Women's Health Network: http://www.cwhn.ca
- Centers for Disease Control and Prevention (U.S.): http://www.cdc.gov
- Family Internet: http://www.familyinternet.com
- Health Answers: http://www.healthanswers.com
- Health Canada Online: http://www.hc-sc.gc.ca
- Healthfinder (U.S. government): http://www.healthfinder.gov
- The Health Information Resource Database: http://nhic-nt.health.org
- Healthy Way Canada: http://www.healthyway.sympatico.ca
- Help Yourself to Health Information (sponsored by Ontario Prevention Clearinghouse): http://www.opc.on.ca/healthinfo:
- National Women's Health Network (U.S.): http://www.womenconnect.com/or20550g.htm
- *New England Journal of Medicine*: www.nejm.org
- Quackwatch: Your Guide to Health Fraud, Quackery, and Intelligent Decisions (reports misleading websites and questionable advertising on the Net): http://www.quackwatch.com
- Self-Help Sourcebook: http://www.cmhcsys.com/selfhelp

See Chapter 22 for websites about alternative and complementary care.

Books

- *The Black Woman's Health Book: Speaking for Ourselves* by Evelyn White (ed.). Seattle: Seal Press, 1990.
- *Good Health Online* by Jim Carroll and Rick Broadhead. Toronto: Prentice Hall Canada, 1997.
- *Health Online* by Tom Ferguson. Reading, MA: Addison Wesley, 1996.
- *Ourselves, Growing Older: Women Aging with Knowledge and Power* by Paula Worters and Diana Siegal. Boston: Boston Women's Health Collective, 1994.
- *Taking Care by Taking Charge* by Marilyn Linton. Toronto: Macmillan, 1996.

Newsletters
- *Harvard Women's Health Watch: Information for Enlightened Choices from Harvard Medical School*, P.O. Box 420234, Palm Coast, FL 32142–0234. Tel.: (800) 829–5921.
- *The Johns Hopkins Medical Letter: Health After 50*, 550 North Broadway, Suite 1100, Johns Hopkins, Baltimore, MD 21205–2011. Tel.: (904) 446–4675.
- *Midlife Issues*, 11215 Juniper Mesa Rd., Juniper Hills, CA 93543.
- *University of California at Berkeley Wellness Letter*, c/o Health Letter Associates, 632 Broadway, New York, NY 10012. Tel.: (212) 505–2255; Fax: (212) 505–5462.
- *University of Toronto Health News*, 109 Vanderhoof Avenue, Suite 200, Toronto, ON M4G 2H7. Tel.: (416) 696–8818; Fax: (416) 696–5075.
- *Women's Health Matters*, The Health Letter of Women's College Hospital, 76 Grenville St., Toronto, ON M5S 1B2. Tel.: (416) 323–7322.

Related Chapters in This Book
- *Chapter 5: Making Changes That Last!* describes health as more than health care and provides some practical advice on how to make lifestyle changes that last.
- *Chapter 17: Keep Your Bones Strong* will help you assess your risk for developing osteoporosis and gives you more details on screening tests for bone density.
- *Chapter 18: Prostate Health* provides a self-test for prostate problems and further explores the dilemmas associated with PSA testing.
- *Chapter 19: Breast Health* will help you assess your risk for breast cancer and supplies more detailed guidelines on mammography.
- *Chapter 20: You Gotta Have Heart!* will help you assess your risk for heart disease and gives you more detailed guidelines on preventive screening tests for heart health.
- *Chapter 21: Hormone Replacement Therapy (HRT): The Big Decision* will help you decide whether HRT is right for you, as well as informing you of the important ways your physician should monitor your health while you are taking hormones.

- *Chapter 22: Complementary and Alternative Medicine Is Coming on Strong* provides more information on complementary and alternative therapies that help in the healing process.

CHAPTER SEVENTEEN

Keep Your Bones Strong

In many cases, osteoporosis is preventable. Diet, exercise, and appropriate medical treatment can reduce your chances of suffering from this devastating disease.

— Osteoporosis Society of Canada[1]

Cynthia had always thought of her seventy-two-year-old mother, **Moira**, as a strong, active, and capable woman who would never grow old. It did not seem real to watch her now, stooped and frail, nervously holding the railing as she made her way down the steps of the building that housed her physician's office. The diagnosis had been clear. Moira was suffering from osteoporosis, a painful, sometimes disfiguring bone disease. Cynthia had noticed that her mother had not stood up as straight in the last few years, and she knew that her back had been bothering her a lot, especially at night. But it had been a shock to learn that her mother, once taller than she, was now several inches shorter owing to small fractures or collapsed vertebrae in her spine. Moira's physician had explained the necessity of immediate treatment to prevent further bone loss and to improve her bone strength. Without treatment, Moira was at very high risk of breaking her hip or other bones.

At age fifty, Cynthia was fair-skinned and slender like her mother. She knew about osteoporosis and had heard that her own risk for the disease escalated around menopause. Now she knew it was time to take action – both in terms of her mother's treatment and in assessing the state of her own bones.

Moira and Cynthia's story is a common one. Osteoporosis – an exaggerated loss of bone tissue that leaves the bones abnormally thin and porous – affects one in four women over age fifty and greatly increases their risk of breaking a bone. Fortunately, a variety of treatments can now help Moira, and it is not too late for Cynthia to prevent the same thing happening to her.

This chapter is designed to help you understand how bones are formed and remodelled throughout life, as well as how to prevent and treat osteoporosis.

Bone Basics

Think of your skeleton as a mineral bank in which the body stores its calcium. Up until age twenty, you "deposit" your bone mass. This peak bone mass remains relatively stable for the next fifteen years. Then, after age thirty-five, you begin to "withdraw" or lose bone mass (a process called resorption) as a natural consequence of aging. Like a bank account, your total bone mass remains constant when the rate of deposits equals the rate of withdrawals.

Deposits are encouraged and withdrawals are discouraged by several factors including hormones (estrogen, testosterone, and others), physical activity (such as walking, dancing, and strength training), growth, fluoridated water, and optimal calcium intake. Other factors, such as chronic dieting, excessive alcohol use, smoking, a lack of physical activity, some chronic diseases, and the decline in estrogen levels at menopause, inhibit the formation of new bone-tissue deposits and encourage more withdrawals.

Osteoporosis is diagnosed when bone-tissue withdrawals exceed bone-tissue deposits. Over time (without our realizing it) osteoporosis can lead to a loss of 30 to 40 per cent of bone tissue. When this happens, bones eventually become so weak that minor falls – and even normal activities such as sneezing – can cause the bones to break. Collapsed vertebrae can cause chronic pain, a hump in the upper back, and a loss of height of ten or more cm (four or more inches) over a lifetime.

People who have a lot of bone in their bank when they reach midlife and begin to gradually lose bone mass are the least likely to develop osteoporosis. This is why it is so important to build bone mass in the early years. Young women and men who build up their bone banks before the age of twenty with healthy eating and active living, and by not smoking, reduce their risk for osteoporosis in later life. As an eighty-year-old woman

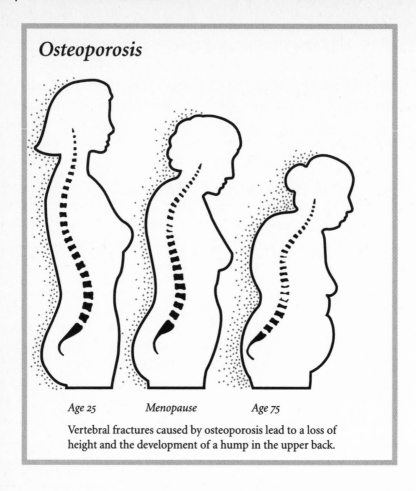

Osteoporosis

Age 25   Menopause   Age 75

Vertebral fractures caused by osteoporosis lead to a loss of
height and the development of a hump in the upper back.

in our practice who has severe osteoporosis said, "Women today are lucky
to know about this. If I had known how to prevent osteoporosis when
I was younger, I wouldn't have this pain and I'd be free to do the things I
want to do."

Gender Differences in Bone Health[2, 3, 4]
The pattern of bone loss after the mid-thirties is different for women and
men. With age, calcium absorption decreases in both sexes. Generally,
however, men begin with a greater bone mass than women do. They tend
to lose bone with age in a slow, gradual way, while women experience accelerated bone loss during the five to ten years following menopause. It is possible for a woman to lose as much as 30 per cent of her bone mass during

this period. After age seventy-five, men and women tend to lose bone at about the same rate. Those women who have a small bone mass to begin with and then experience an accelerated loss in menopause may already be in the minus position, called osteopenia, or low bone mass.

Estrogen in women and testosterone in men protect the bones by keeping resorption in check. The overwhelming majority of older men have adequate levels of testosterone to accomplish this. In rare cases of severe testosterone deficiency, men may experience bone loss just as severe as that of postmenopausal women. Women, on the other hand, are eight times more likely to develop osteoporosis than men.

GENDER DIFFERENCES IN BONE MASS

Women	*Men*
• less bone mass at peak	• greater bone mass at peak
• estrogen decline at menopause	• testosterone production maintained
• over age 50, 1 in 4 women have osteoporosis	• over age 50, 1 in 8 men have osteoporosis
• by age 65, 1 in 2 women have osteoporosis	• by age 70, 1 in 5 men have osteoporosis

---

Should Men Be Concerned about Their Bone Health?

Most men are unaware that bone strength is a health issue for them as well as for women. In a recent Gallup survey reported in *Executive Health's Good Health Report*, more than half of the men interviewed thought that they couldn't develop osteoporosis.[5] Although osteoporosis is much more common in women, in Canada 20 to 30 per cent of osteoporotic fractures occur in men. These fractures can lead to significant physical disabilities and emotional problems.[6] One fifty-nine-year-old man we interviewed said, "One day I was walking in a store, when my hand caught on a piece of material and my back twisted. I felt sudden pain; I never dreamt it would be a fracture due to osteoporosis. I thought only women got that."

There are a number of reasons men develop osteoporosis:

- low peak bone density, due to genetics, delayed puberty, very low calcium intake, smoking, etc.;
- prolonged immobility and lack of weight-bearing exercise, usually as a result of a childhood illness;
- the long-term use of glucocorticoid medications, (e.g., prednisone, cortisone) for treating conditions such as asthma, rheumatoid arthritis, and Crohn disease;
- low levels of male hormone;
- heavy use of alcohol or tobacco;
- 50 per cent of men develop osteoporosis for unknown reasons (idiopathic osteoporosis).[7]

Osteoporosis and Menopause

After menopause, one in four women is at risk for developing osteoporosis. Natural aging and the hormone changes in menopause combine to exaggerate an imbalance in the normal process of calcium deposits and withdrawals. Lowered estrogen levels accelerate bone resorption at the same time that aging decreases the amount of calcium a woman absorbs from her food. Thus, a woman loses bone mass faster for eight to ten years after her last period.

Premenopausal women who have oophorectomies (removal of the ovaries), female athletes who cease to menstruate, and women with anorexia are at increased risk because of estrogen deficiency. When young women lose so much fat that they stop menstruating, estrogen production is disrupted. This leads to a reduced peak bone mass and increases their risk for osteoporosis in later life.

In the United States, seven to eight million people already have osteoporosis and 17 million more have low bone mass to begin with. Osteoporosis accounts for 1.5 million hip, wrist, and spine fractures.[8] One in three white Canadian women over age fifty will fracture a hip in her lifetime. Up to 20 per cent of older women who break their hips die within twelve months due to complications. Some 34 per cent of men who fracture a hip die within less than one year. Among those who survive, 50 per cent will be incapacitated, many of them permanently.[9] Collapsed fractures of the vertebrae can cause chronic, debilitating pain that interferes with one's ability to remain active and independent. It is possible to have osteoporosis and never suffer a fracture. However, the condition greatly increases your chance of fractures.

Are You at Risk for Developing Osteoporosis?

Fill out the Osteoporosis Risk Checklist that follows to assess your own risk. Some of the risk factors you cannot control, such as your family history and race; other factors, such as diet, weight, muscle mass, and exercise patterns, you can influence.

We have added a factor to the list that is not commonly found in risk assessments. We call it the "Ideal" Body Syndrome – smoking, chronic dieting, and over-exercising in pursuit of society's thin, unrealistic, so-called ideal body shape. This behaviour and the relentless pursuit of slimness are prevalent among young North American women. At age fifty, they face the strong possibility of developing serious and painful disability because of this earlier and continuing obsession. Male marathon runners who do not consume enough calories are also at risk.

Women with large frames who are at the heavier end of the healthy weight range are less likely to develop osteoporosis. (see Chapter 8). The extra weight stresses the bones and the fat pads serve as sites for the synthesis of estrogen. For bone protection, some extra weight may be an advantage.

OSTEOPOROSIS RISK CHECKLIST

Check off the risk factors that apply to you. The more boxes you check, the more likely you are to develop osteoporosis.

[ ] Female

[ ] Age 50 or over

[ ] Prolonged sex-hormone deficiency (menopause in women, testosterone deficiency in men)

[ ] Excessive use of certain medications (cortisone, prednisone, thyroid hormone, anticonvulsants, aluminum-containing antacids)

[ ] Ovaries surgically removed or early menopause (before age 45)

[ ] Family history of osteoporosis

[ ] Low intake of calcium throughout life

[ ] Limited exposure to sunlight or insufficient vitamin D in your diet
[ ] History of little or no regular exercise; or over-exercise (in women, to the point that periods stop)
[ ] Prolonged immobilization and/or sedentary lifestyle
[ ] Thin with small bones
[ ] White or Asian (osteoporosis is less likely in black women)
[ ] History of anorexia or bulimia
[ ] "Ideal" body syndrome
[ ] Smoker (or ex-smoker)
[ ] Heavy alcohol user (2+ drinks per day)
[ ] Heavy caffeine consumption (3+ cups per day)

There are not yet enough scientific data to rank these factors; however, some are stronger predictors of bone loss than others. These include a strong family history of osteoporosis, prolonged use of glucocorticoids or thyroid medication, early menopause, amenorrhea, and decreased levels of sex hormones. If you have one or more of these strong predictors, the Osteoporosis Society of Canada advises you to discuss further assessment with your physician.[10]

Testing for Osteoporosis

The first outward signs of osteoporosis are those that Moira experienced at the beginning of this chapter: a reduction in height, curving of the spine (kyphosis), and persistent back pain. It is possible to assess the state of your bone mass well before you notice these physical signs.

A bone mineral density test (bone densitometry) can measure bone thickness far more precisely than standard X-rays. It is a painless and safe procedure that takes from ten to twenty minutes. The amount of radiation exposure is much less than a standard chest X-ray. Your results are generated by computer and then compared with healthy bone in the average young woman or man. You must be referred by a physician to get a bone densitometry test. Because bone densitometers (the machine that performs the test) are available on a limited basis across Canada, people who are at high risk are generally given priority for the test.

WORLD HEALTH ORGANIZATION GUIDELINES
FOR INTERPRETING THE BONE DENSITY MINERAL (BMD) READING

Bone mass	BMD reading	Fracture risk
Above normal	+1, +2	
Normal	0 to −1	
Low bone mass (osteopenia)	−1 to −2.5	2 times increased fracture risk
Osteoporosis	−2.5 to −4.0	4 to 5 times increased fracture risk
Severe osteoporosis (presence of 1 or more fragility fractures)	−2.5 to −4.0 plus 1 or more fragility fractures	20 times increased fracture risk

In addition to bone densitometry, new technologies for assessing bone health are currently being evaluated. One of these is the heel ultrasound. You immerse your foot in warm water that allows high frequency sound to pass through your heel. Radiologic absorptiometry of phalanges (RAP), which measures bone density in one finger, is another new technique.

Should I have a Bone Mineral Density Test (BMD)?
If you are middle-aged or older and have several of the risk factors in the Osteoporosis Risk Checklist or one of the strong predictors of osteoporosis, request a bone mineral density test. A BMD will
- detect low bone density and help you decide whether or not to consider using preventive treatments;
- predict your risk of fracturing;
- confirm a diagnosis of osteoporosis;
- help you and your physician monitor your rate of bone loss and the effectiveness of treatment.

Maintaining Bone Health

To maintain strong bones in midlife and later life, both women and men need to

- enjoy healthy eating that includes a diet rich in calcium;
- enjoy an active lifestyle that includes weight-bearing activities and resistance exercises;
- refrain from smoking and limit alcohol intake.

Those at high risk for developing the disease, or who already have a low bone mass, should talk with their physicians about the advisability of taking medication (described later in this chapter) as an adjunct to these healthy lifestyle practices.

Eat a Diet Rich in Calcium

The skeleton contains about 99 per cent of the body's calcium. The other 1 per cent is essential for the proper functioning of the heart, nerves, and muscles, and for normal blood clotting. Since the bones act as the bank for calcium, they pay a high price when the body withdraws calcium for use in other parts of the body.

A well-balanced diet with plenty of calcium-rich foods is one of the best ways to maintain the optimal calcium reserve in your bones. The average adult needs about 1,000 milligrams of calcium each day; however, the Osteoporosis Society suggests that men and women over age fifty should consider consuming up to 1,500 milligrams per day, especially if their risk for osteoporosis is high.[11]

Dietitians advise women and men to get their calcium first from foods (mainly milk and milk products), because they contain other nutrients as well, such as vitamin D and magnesium, which help the body absorb and use calcium. People with milk intolerance can consume lactose-reduced milks, yogurt (the live bacterial culture helps break down the lactose sugar), and other foods that contain calcium. Vegetarians will have to work harder at getting the required amount of calcium through alternatives such as seaweed, beans, nuts, tofu, and certain vegetables, and other foods that contain calcium (see chart that follows).

In response to the demand for more calcium, food producers are beginning to make foods that are supplemented with calcium. One company has introduced a mineral water with 300 mg of calcium; another

Milk and Other Sources of Calcium

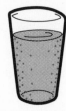

$= 315 \ mg$

1 cup of milk (1%, 2%, whole, chocolate)

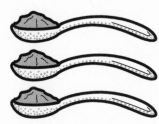

$= 262 \ mg$

3 tablespoons of parmesan cheese

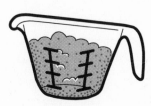

$= 200 \ mg$

1 cup of cooked dried beans or lentils

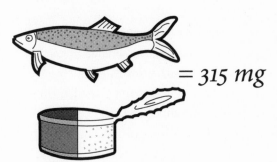

$= 315 \ mg$

11 sardines or 1/2 can of salmon with bones

produces a super-charged milk that has 33 per cent more calcium than regular 1-per-cent milk. Calcium has also been added to soy beverages and some orange juices.

THE VITAMIN D CONNECTION

One of the advantages of milk as a source of calcium is that it is fortified with vitamin D, which increases calcium absorption by as much as 30 to 80 per cent. In fact, vitamin D deficiency may increase bone resorption, thereby causing or aggravating osteoporosis.[12] The Osteoporosis Society of Canada recommends that Canadians in midlife receive 400 IUs of vitamin D per day.[13] Exposing your face and hands to ten to fifteen minutes of sunshine each day will also enable your body to make enough vitamin D. There is no vitamin D in yogurt or cheese.

Calcium Supplements[14]

Vegetarians and others who find it difficult to obtain the recommended amount of calcium from their diets alone may require a calcium supplement combined with a calcium-rich diet. When choosing a supplement, consider the amount of calcium per dose, the price, absorbability, lead content, and suitability for you. If a particular type causes stomach upset or constipation, experiment with different forms, such as chewable or effervescent tablets.

Products made from calcium carbonate are most often recommended, because they contain the highest percentage of calcium per mg; they are more slowly absorbed than other kinds of calcium and are inexpensive. Supplements made from dolomite, oyster shell, or bone meal are likely to have high levels of lead, and should be avoided.

To maximize the absorption of the calcium in supplements:
- take your supplement with food or immediately after eating;
- take calcium with plenty of water;
- take two smaller doses instead of one large one; and
- take calcium at bedtime (except for calcium carbonate), as it may be better utilized by the body at night.

CALCIUM CONTENT OF SOME COMMON FOODS

Choose and enjoy at least three calcium-rich foods each day.

Milk and milk products	*Portion*	*Calcium*
Milk (whole, 2%, skim)	1 cup/250 ml	315 mg
Fortified soy beverage	1 cup/250 ml	325 mg
Buttermilk	1 cup/250 ml	301 mg
Milk powder, dry	3 tbsp/45 ml	159 mg
Cheese – Swiss, Gruyère	1.75 oz./50 g	493 mg
– brick, Cheddar, Colby, Edam, and Gouda	1.75 oz./50 g	353 mg
– mozzarella	1.75 oz./50 g	269 mg
– cottage	½ cup/125 ml	87 mg
– Brie	1.5 oz./45 g	83 mg
Yogurt, plain	1 cup/175 ml	292 mg
Ice cream	½ cup/125 ml	87 mg

Meat and alternatives	*Portion*	*Calcium*
Sardines, with bones	8 small	153 mg
Salmon, with bones	½ can/213 g	242 mg
Almonds, dry roasted	½ cup/125 ml	200 mg
Sesame seeds	2 tbsp./25 ml	176 mg
Tofu, firm, with calcium sulphate	¼ cup/60 ml	430 mg
Soybeans, cooked	1 cup/250 ml	90 mg
Beans, cooked (kidney, navy, pinto, garbanzo)	1 cup/250 ml	175 mg
Chicken, roasted	3 oz/90 g	13 mg
Beef, roast	3 oz/90 g	7 mg

Breads and cereals	*Portion*	*Calcium*
Bran muffin	1/35 g	50 mg
Whole-wheat and white bread	1 slice	30 mg

Fruit and Vegetables	Portion	Calcium
Hijiki seaweed, dry	¼ cup/60 ml	162 mg
Wakame seaweed, dry	¼ cup/60 ml	104 mg
Amaranth (cooked)	1 cup	276 mg
Broccoli (cooked)	1 cup/250 ml	178 mg
Orange	1 medium/180 g	56 mg
Banana	1 medium/175 g	8 mg
Lettuce	2 large leaves	10 mg
Figs, dried	10	270 mg

Combination dishes	Portion	Calcium
Homemade lasagna	1 cup/250 ml	286 mg
Soup made with milk	1 cup/250 ml	189 mg
Baked beans (canned)	1 cup/250 ml	163 mg

Sources: Health Canada: *Canadian Nutrient File*, 1991, and *Becoming Vegetarian* by Vesanto Melina, Brenda Davis, and Victoria Harrison. Toronto: Macmillan Canada, 1994.

Maximizing Your Calcium Intake

Here are some ways to maximize the calcium you take in through foods:

- Consult a reliable food chart to make sure you are getting an adequate amount of calcium every day.
- Eat foods from which the calcium is easily absorbed. Best foods are dairy products. Vegetables such as broccoli, collards, kale, turnip, greens, and bok choy and the bones in fish are also easily absorbed.
- Know which foods contain calcium that is *not* readily available to the body. These include foods containing oxalates (found in many green vegetables such as spinach, chard, and rhubarb).
- Reduce your consumption of food products that cause calcium loss through urine. The most important are excess sodium (salt) and caffeine. Do not consume more than three cups of coffee per day. Excessive protein intake can also increase the amount of calcium you

lose in urine. Follow Canada's Food Guide to Healthy Eating, which recommends two to three servings of protein each day (one serving is two to three ounces of meat, fish, or poultry, one-third of a cup of tofu, or one to two eggs). Dairy foods need not be limited, as any calcium loss is offset by the high amount of calcium they provide.

Active Living and Osteoporosis

Regular physical activity is essential for maintaining bone health. In fact, many studies have confirmed that weight-bearing activities (i.e., those in which you carry your own weight, such as walking, dancing, mowing the grass, and tennis) reduce the rate of age-related bone loss and improve the bone density of individuals with osteoporosis on drug therapy.[15]

In contrast, an inactive lifestyle can accelerate osteoporosis. It is not the lack of movement so much as it is the lack of mechanical stresses on the bone that do the damage. Astronauts demonstrate this. They experience rapid skeletal bone loss when suspended weightless in space, despite vigorous physical activity. Prolonged bed rest owing to illness or injury can have a similar dramatic effect on your loss of bone. That is why it is important to resume weight-bearing activities, such as walking, as soon as possible.

Exercise specialists now advise us to add twenty to thirty minutes of resistance (or strength) training with weights three times a week to complement aerobic activities. Studies have shown that weight training (with weights ranging from half a pound to five pounds) can help prevent osteoporosis by building both muscle and bone strength.[16]

Supervised, individualized strength training is also becoming part of treatment programs for very old people with osteoporosis. As well as building bone strength, exercise can improve overall strength and balance, which are crucial for independence and the prevention of falls. So don't be surprised if you find an eighty-year-old pumping iron on the weight machine beside you at the gym!

Swimming and cycling, because they support your weight and cause less pull of the muscle on the bone, do not offer the same benefits as weight-bearing activities. Walking is probably the most enjoyable and the simplest way to build bone strength. A daily thirty- to forty-minute walk exposes you to the sun for vitamin D at the same time that you're improving your heart health and helping manage your weight. Walking, combined with strength training for the upper body, two or three times a week is an ideal, no-drug prescription for healthy, strong bones. Tai chi (an ancient form of Chinese exercise) is also a useful activity, since it promotes flexibility and balance, and thus helps to prevent falls.

Therapies for Osteoporosis

Hormone Replacement Therapy

Studies have shown that hormone replacement therapy (HRT) can cut fracture risks by as much as 50 per cent. Bone protection appears to be greatest when estrogen replacement begins immediately after a woman's last period and continues for at least ten years;[17] however, therapy that is started at age sixty and continued into later life still appears to be beneficial.[18] Bone loss resumes at an accelerated pace once therapy stops. When used to prevent and treat osteoporosis, the intent is not to replicate premenopausal hormone levels, but to provide the lowest levels required to protect the bones. New studies suggest that lower doses of estrogen than have been traditionally prescribed, combined with adequate calcium intake, may prevent bone loss as well.[19]

Women who are considering the use of HRT to prevent or manage osteoporosis should be fully informed of all the personal risks and benefits before making the decision to use it on a long-term basis. Chapter 21 "Hormone Replacement Therapy (HRT): The Big Decision" provides additional information on HRT as well as a chart to help you in making your own decision. Fortunately, there are also new options for women who cannot or do not want to take HRT (described below). Premenopausal women who are taking oral contraceptives to relieve menopausal symptoms will be happy to know that their use of them can improve their bone health as well.

Most men continue to produce enough testosterone as they age to keep their bones healthy. Testosterone may be prescribed to those men with osteoporosis who also have a below-normal hormone level.

Additional Therapies

In addition to HRT, a number of other drugs are being studied or used to control osteoporosis. These include:

- *Alendronate* (a biphosphonate marketed as Fosamax) is a non-hormonal, anti-resorption drug that has been approved for the prevention and treatment of osteoporosis. Clinical trials have shown that alendronate can prevent bone loss in the spine, hip, and total body as effectively as HRT in 85 per cent of women, if started within five years after menopause.[20, 21] *Etidronate*, another biphosphonate (sold as Didrocal or Didronel), can increase spinal bone density. Sometimes a combination of biphosphonates and HRT may be used.
- SERMs (Selective Estrogen Receptor Modulators) are the new "designer estrogens," which provide the benefits of estrogen to the bones and heart without stimulating the breast and uterus. This opens up another important choice for women who are at risk for breast cancer and have osteoporosis or low bone mass. Raloxifene (sold as Evista) has been shown to decrease bone loss, increase bone density, and decrease fractures by 52 per cent.[22]
- *Calcitriol*, the active metabolite in vitamin D, promotes the absorption of calcium.
- *Calcitonin*, which is sometimes used in the form of a nasal spray or injection in treating osteoporosis, has the advantage of relieving pain in women who have vertebral fractures.

Women and men at risk for developing osteoporosis who choose not to use HRT or the above therapies should work to strengthen their bones, consider consulting a dietitian and naturopath about nutrition and alternative therapies, and ask their physicians to closely monitor their bone density.

THE BOTTOM LINE

Healthy habits make strong bones. To prevent osteoporosis and related bone fractures, women and men in midlife need to:

- eat plenty of calcium-rich foods.
- stay active: walk regularly and practise strength training two or three times a week;
- quit smoking;
- have a bone mineral density test if you are at risk. The information you get from the results can help you be more pro-active in preventing or slowing bone loss.

While we can't stop the aging process that includes the loss of bone density, we can do a great deal to help ourselves walk with strength and dignity into the future.

Contacts and Further Information

Organizations
- National Osteoporosis Foundation (U.S.), 1150 17th St., N.W., Suite 500, Washington, DC 20036–4603. Tel.: (202) 223–0344; Fax: (202) 223–2237.
- Osteoporosis Society of Canada, 33 Laird Dr., Toronto, ON M4G 3S9. Tel.: (416) 696–2663 or 1–800–463–6842; Fax: (416) 696–2673.

For information on support groups, call the Osteoporosis Society of Canada.

Websites
- International Osteoporosis Foundation: http://www.effo.org
- National Osteoporosis Foundation (U.S.): http://www.nof.org
- National Resource Center (U.S.): Osteoporosis and Related Bone Diseases (sponsored by the National Institutes of Health): http://www.osteo.org
- Osteoporosis Society of Canada: http://www.osteoporosis.ca

Books
- *Better Bones, Better Body: Beyond Estrogen and Calcium* by Susan E. Brody. New Canaan, CT: Keats Publishing, 1996.
- *Preventing and Reversing Osteoporosis* by Alan Gaby. Rocklin, CA: Prima Publishing, 1994.
- *Strong Women Stay Young* by Miriam Nelson. New York: Bantam Books, 1997.
- *Understanding Calcium and Osteoporosis* by Carol Rudoff. Menlo Park, CA: Allergy Publications Group, 1991.
- *Understanding Osteoporosis: Every Woman's Guide to Preventing Brittle Bones* by Wendy Cooper. London, U.K.: Arrow Books, 1990.

Related Chapters in This Book

- *Chapter 2: Understanding the Female Menopause* contains more information on menopause and how it affects bone health.
- *Chapter 7: The Active Living Solution* provides information on how to start and stay on a physical-activity program that will enhance the health of your bones.
- *Chapter 8: Food for Thought: Healthy Eating in Midlife* gives you more information on planning and enjoying a healthy, varied diet that will enhance your bone strength and overall well-being.
- *Chapter 9: The Boomer's Drugs of Choice* provides practical advice on quitting smoking and cutting down on alcohol use.
- *Chapter 16: Partners in Health Care* provides some useful information on how you can use the Internet to find out more about bone health.
- *Chapter 21: Hormone Replacement Therapy (HRT): The Big Decision* will help you understand the pros and cons of using HRT and provides a decision-making guide that takes your personal risk for developing osteoporosis into account.

CHAPTER EIGHTEEN

Prostate Health

Most men think an enlarged prostate is a disease of the elderly. So for them, admitting that you have it is admitting that you're old.   – Dr. John Trachtenberg, urologist[1]

Bill was fifty-five years old. Over the last two years he had become increasingly anxious about urinary problems he was having; he had to get up two or three times each night and felt a sense of urgency that made him nervous when he was not near a bathroom. Bill thought that he might have a prostate problem, but he was embarrassed to discuss it with his partner or his doctor. He believed that a prostate problem is an old man's disease, and he was afraid that treatment would interfere with his sex life.

Finally, Bill's discomfort and his wife's urging pushed him to see his family doctor. A physical exam revealed that Bill had benign prostatic hypertrophy (BPH) – a non-malignant enlargement of the prostate gland. To Bill's relief, his physician assured him that this was a common condition in men his age and that there was no reason to anticipate sexual problems. After an open discussion of his treatment options, Bill and his doctor opted for a wait-and-see approach. Bill decided to make some lifestyle changes that might improve his symptoms – losing weight, reducing his intake of alcohol and coffee, and refraining from drinking liquids in the evening. They agreed to meet again if the condition worsened and to consider drug therapy at that time.

Bill's story is typical of how many men over fifty feel about prostate problems. They are frightened; they deny the problem and delay discussing it with their spouses or doctors, which often causes them unnecessary worry and anxiety. Indeed, a 1991 Gallup poll in the United States found that more than 60 per cent of men were reluctant to discuss the symptoms of prostate problems with their doctors because of the attached stigma of old age.[2] It also points to the emotional distress that often accompanies prostate symptoms. What middle-aged man has not been frightened by the increasingly dramatic coverage of prostate cancer in the popular media?

In this chapter, we describe the changes in the prostate that are part of the aging process for all men. The prostate is sometimes called "the gland that always goes wrong," because it is likely to cause a problem for most men as they get older. Indeed, evidence that men in ancient Egypt had difficulty with urination because of enlarged prostates has been found in papyri dating back to the fifteenth century B.C.[3]

Prostate Problems and Aging

Understanding changes in the prostate that are part of normal aging and learning all you can about how to keep your prostate healthy are important in midlife. The three most common prostate problems are:

- benign prostatic hypertrophy;
- prostatitis (inflammation of the prostate);
- prostate cancer.

Since early detection of problems can make a difference, it is important to know the symptoms of these three problems and to understand your treatment options.

If you have symptoms, talking with your partner and your physician is the first step. In the large majority of cases, prostate problems are non-cancerous. About half of the time prostate problems do not become severe enough to warrant drug or aggressive surgical treatment until late in life. And while the lifetime risk of getting prostate cancer is about 10 per cent (slightly higher for African Americans), only about 25 per cent of those men who do develop prostate cancer actually die of it. Most men diagnosed with prostate cancer will die from other, unrelated causes, such as heart disease, before they become ill from prostate cancer.

The Prostate Gland: Growing Pains

The prostate gland is a male sex organ that sits beneath the bladder and circles the urethra – the channel that carries semen and urine into the penis. The prostate's job is to assist in ejaculation by contracting and supplementing

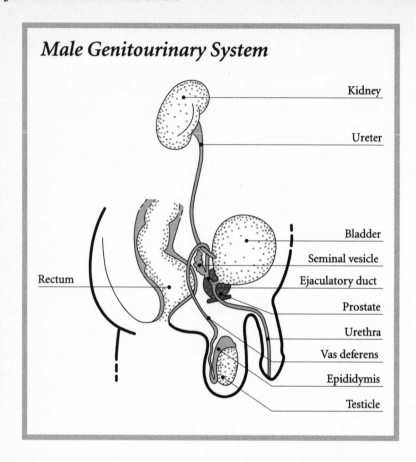

Male Genitourinary System

Kidney

Ureter

Bladder

Seminal vesicle

Ejaculatory duct

Rectum

Prostate

Urethra

Vas deferens

Epididymis

Testicle

the volume of fluid semen propelled through the urethral channel and out of the penis.

Boys are born with a prostate about the size of a pea. When a man reaches age twenty-five or so, the prostate starts to grow again slowly, but it does not become large enough to cause a problem until the man is forty or fifty years old. At the same time, the smooth muscle around the urethra starts to tighten. Because the prostate is located directly below the bladder, an enlarged prostate squeezes the urethra and increases pressure on the bladder.

The most common consequence of these changes is an increased need for visits to the toilet. This can create a lot of anxiety. One man said, "I hate the fact that I worry about going out for a pint of beer with friends after work. I get anxious about making it home in time to have the next leak." Another forty-nine-year-old man working in Toronto told us he had become a "downtown bathroom expert," because he knew the locations of all the bathrooms in the downtown area where he took his lunchtime walk. A frequent need to urinate also disrupts sleep patterns. Like the hot flashes that disturb a menopausal woman's sleep, night visits to the toilet can eventually force tired men to do something about problems with their prostates.

Diagnosing Prostate Problems

Most men are familiar with a standard part of a physical examination to detect prostate problems – the digital rectal examination or DRE (sometimes known as the "dreaded rectal examination"). While no one likes this part of a physical exam, it is painless and should not deter you from going to the doctor when you are experiencing symptoms of prostate problems. Since the prostate cannot be felt through the thick abdominal wall, the DRE is the only way to feel, or "palpate," the prostate. When an experienced family doctor or urologist inserts a finger into the rectum, he or she can feel the size and consistency of the prostate and whether or not there is any tenderness caused by an inflamed gland. Forty to 50 per cent of the time, he or she may be able to detect the early stages of prostate cancer.

Most of the time, the DRE, abdominal palpation, and an examination of the genitals are standard tests in physical exams of men over age fifty. Some physicians use other tests to support the DRE, including a blood test for prostate cancer called the PSA (prostate-specific antigen) and urinalysis. If there is suspicion of prostate cancer, a transrectal ultrasound of the prostate and additional tests may be used.

If there are any questions about the results of these baseline tests, a consulting urologist may perform additional procedures:

- A cystoscopy: Under local anesthetic, a long, telescope-like device is inserted through the penis and prostate into the bladder. The bladder is then inflated with warm water. This allows the urologist, who looks through the end of the instrument, to identify the specific location of an obstruction and to identify any other problems at the same time.

- Uroflowmetry (a urine-flow study) or other similar tests: These assess the flow rate of urine or detect the presence of an obstruction.
- A needle biopsy: A thin needle inserted into the suspected area is used to withdraw a small piece of tissue that is sent to the lab for examination under a microscope.

All of these tests can be performed in a urology clinic without hospitalization. A local anesthetic ensures that there is little physical discomfort. The psychological trauma of seeing the size of the cystoscopy instrument is another matter!

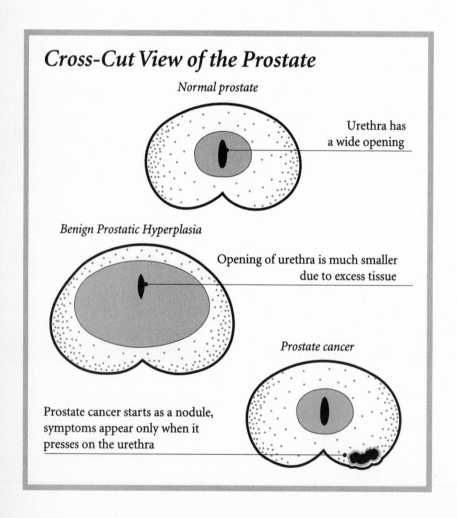

Cross-Cut View of the Prostate

Normal prostate

Urethra has
a wide opening

Benign Prostatic Hyperplasia

Opening of urethra is much smaller
due to excess tissue

Prostate cancer

Prostate cancer starts as a nodule,
symptoms appear only when it
presses on the urethra

Do I Have a Prostate Problem?

The Prostate Symptom Questionnaire, which is adapted from a World Health Organization questionnaire that many physicians use, can help you identify early symptoms of prostate problems.

THE PROSTATE SYMPTOM QUESTIONNAIRE[4]

If you answer Yes to any of these questions, talk with your physician.

1. Do you feel that your bladder is not completely emptied after you finish urinating?
2. Do you need to urinate more frequently than every two hours?
3. Does your stream stop and start again several times when you urinate?
4. Do you find it very difficult to postpone urinating?
5. Do you need to strain or force yourself to pass urine?
6. Do you need to urinate more than once during the night?
7. Do you ever experience urinary incontinence (accidentally passing urine)?

Adapted from the World Health Organization International Prostate Symptom Score, published in Nickel, J. C.; Norman, R. W. (CMA), *A Prostate Problem: Benign Prostatic Hyperplasia.* Montreal: Grosvenor House Press, 1993.

Benign Prostatic Hypertrophy

Benign prostatic hypertrophy (BPH) – a non-malignant enlargement of the prostate gland – can occur in all men regardless of education or social class. Ronald Reagan had prostate surgery for BPH during his term as president. Football legend Johnny Unitas was diagnosed with BPH when he was sixty-three. One interviewee put it this way: "You know you have an aging prostate when you go out behind the cottage and pee beside your nine-year-old grandson."

Doctors describe two types or categories of symptoms:

- **obstructive symptoms:** weak urine flow, dribbling, hesitancy, intermittency (the flow stops and starts), incomplete voiding, straining, and retention (not able to go); and
- **irritative symptoms:** frequent urination, night urinating, urgency, and incontinence.

In addition, urinary infection is a common complication of BPH.

Treating BPH

Most men with an enlarged prostate will need treatment at some point. At age fifty, 30 per cent of all men experience symptoms of an enlarged prostate, by age sixty about half experience some degree of BPH, and at age eighty, some 75 to 90 per cent of men are affected.[5] When and how you treat BPH is your decision, in consultation with your physician. Many men opt for a wait-and-see approach, with regular monitoring by their physicians. If symptoms become intolerable, they then talk with a urologist about other ways to deal with the problem. Currently, there are five common treatment options:

1. *Watchful waiting:* Keeping the condition under observation (the option Bill chose in our opening story) makes sense for men with mild to moderate symptoms. While BPH symptoms are likely to worsen over time, some recent studies suggest that, for some men, the symptoms stabilize or even improve over time. Once you are sure that your condition is benign, you decide when your discomfort level demands further treatment. Never ignore blood in your urine, painful ejaculations, or a complete inability to urinate, as these are signals that the condition needs treatment urgently. Lifestyle changes are recommended for mild cases of BPH during the watchful waiting. Exercising, losing weight, and cutting down on caffeine and alcohol can help.
2. *Herbal remedies:*[6, 7] The use of herbal remedies, particularly saw palmetto, is popular in Europe and a growing trend in North America. Some well-designed studies have shown that extracts of the saw-palmetto berry relieve symptoms and increase urinary flow rate within three months by blocking the effect of testosterone on the prostate. If you decide to try saw palmetto, avoid water-soluble extracts such as teas, as they are unlikely to contain any active

ingredients. Many products contain saw palmetto, zinc, pumpkin seeds, and pygeum bark, another herb used to reduce prostatic inflammation. Tell your physician whether you are taking any of these herbal remedies. Stop using it if you notice any unusual effects or a worsening of your symptoms, or if you notice no benefits within three months.

3. *Drug therapy:* As new, improved drugs emerge, the use of prescription medications is becoming more acceptable and often the treatment of choice. Drugs have proven useful in dealing with the symptoms of BPH without treating the actual obstruction. Sometimes, improvement may even come simply from taking action. A recent two-year multicentre trial in Canada reported that men taking a placebo had reduced their symptoms and improved urinary flow, and that 80 per cent of the participants in the trial reported side-effects to medication that was, in fact, a placebo.[8]

   Currently, three types of drugs are generally prescribed. The first group is alpha blockers (terazocin, doxazocin, and tamsulosin). These improve urine flow by reducing tension in the smooth muscles in the prostate, bladder neck, and urethra. Tamsulosin, the newest drug in this group, has been shown to have less severe side-effects, such as dizziness due to low blood pressure.[9] The second group of drugs (antispasmodic drugs such as oxybutynin chloride and flavoxate hydrochloride) is used to treat symptoms such as urgency and frequency of urination, because they reduce irritation and spasm of the bladder. The third type of drug (finasteride) blocks the effect of testosterone, the hormone that makes the prostate gland grow. The use of finasteride, however, has been limited by side-effects that may include lowered libido, ejaculatory problems, fatigue, and headaches. A recent analysis of the literature suggested that finasteride is most effective in men with "larger" prostates, and should be used only in such cases.[10]

4. *Surgery:* If the symptoms warrant it and you and your urologist decide on surgery, the surgeon is most likely to suggest a transurethral resection of the prostate, or TURP, which is still the gold standard for alleviating BPH. During a TURP, the urologist relieves

the pressure on the urinary system by removing excess tissue that is blocking urine flow. About two months after TURP surgery, 97 per cent of men report voiding with a good stream. About 70 per cent of men report losing the ability to ejaculate; others report less ejaculate. It goes to the bladder instead of being released at orgasm, and is eliminated with the urine later. Some men (about 5 to 10 per cent) develop impotence following surgery. Despite this, recent studies have found no difference in sexual dysfunction between men who had undergone surgery and others who were using the watchful-waiting technique.[11, 12]

5. *Non-surgical techniques:* Canadian and American studies are currently evaluating other non-surgical procedures. These techniques will not cure BPH, but will improve symptoms such as frequency, urging, and straining.

   • A transurethral needle ablasion (TUNA) has fewer side-effects and can be performed in a physician's office under local anesthetic. The procedure involves inserting a catheter through the urethra to the prostate side, then deploying a needle into the lobe of the prostate and releasing radio-frequency (RF) energy, which creates heat, reducing the excess tissue. Unlike other heat treatments, the RF energy is localized and controlled.

   • A similar technique uses a variety of lasers to vaporize excess prostate tissue.

   • Balloon urethroplasty uses a high-pressure balloon to dilate an enlarged prostate. This technique is often used with younger men who have moderately large prostates.

   • Transurethral microwave therapy (TUMT) uses microwave therapy to heat and destroy excess prostate tissue, while a cooling system protects the urinary tract.

For older men who are unable to undergo surgery, a catheter can be used to drain the bladder of urine. Temporary or permanent stents (they look like coils) that relieve obstruction because of BPH may be installed in the ureter as an alternative to a catheter.

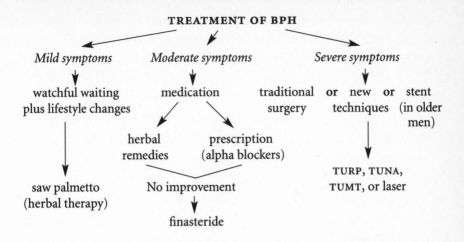

Source: Adapted with permission from BPH Management Algorithm by Andrew J. Portis and David A. Mador, "Treatment Options for Benign Prostatic Hypertrophy" in *Canadian Family Physician* 43 (August 1997): 1, 395–404.

Prostatitis

Infection of the prostate is called prostatitis. It is most commonly caused by Escherichia (E.) coli – the same bacteria that causes bladder and kidney infections in both men and women. There are three different types of prostatitis, which are usually treated successfully with antibiotics:

- *Acute bacterial prostatitis*: Symptoms come on quickly. They include fever, chills, low-back and very-low-abdominal pain, and painful, problematic voiding.
- *Chronic bacterial prostatitis*: Symptoms are less severe and include irritation on voiding and pain in the lower abdomen and groin area.
- *Nonbacterial prostatitis*: The symptoms are similar to chronic bacterial prostatitis, and although no specific bacteria can be found there will be evidence of infection in prostate secretions.

Prostatodynia, which means painful prostate, is sometimes called pelvic-floor myalgia (PFM). It exhibits symptoms similar to other forms of prostatitis, but no infection can be detected. Because of this, it is a very frustrating condition. A change in diet sometimes helps (eliminating alcohol, caffeine, and spices). Biofeedback and medication may help ease this condition; compassion and caring are also important.

Prostate Cancer

Prostate cancer is rarely seen before age fifty, but the older you get, the more likely you are to develop it. Men with a family history of prostate cancer are at higher risk, particularly if relatives were diagnosed with prostate cancer at a relatively young age. Some studies show that men with benign prostatic hyperplasia – the abnormal increase of normal cells – are more likely to develop prostate cancer. Race is also a factor: prostate cancer is more common in African Americans/Canadians and less common among Asian men.

The lifetime risk of getting prostate cancer has been estimated as one in eight.[13] An estimated 25 million American men over age fifty have prostate cancer; many of these men remain healthy and unaffected by the disease. As a quote in the August 1993 *University of California at Berkeley Wellness Letter* says, "Growing older is invariably fatal; prostate cancer is only sometimes so."

As the graph opposite shows, the incidence (number of new cases) of prostate cancer increased dramatically in Canada from 1969 to 1997. Two factors are likely responsible: the introduction of PSA testing and the fact that more and more men are living into very old age (75+). At the same time, however, death (mortality) rates for prostate cancer rose only very slightly over the same time period. Nevertheless, prostate cancer is the second leading cause of cancer deaths for Canadian and American men aged sixty-five and over – after lung cancer. Death rates from prostate cancer are higher in the United States than Canada, mainly because mortality from prostate cancer among African-American men has been found to be at least double that of Caucasian men.[14]

While the precise causes of prostate cancer are unknown, some studies have linked it to the consumption of a high-fat diet, and exposure to pesticides and sexually transmitted diseases. More research is needed, however, to confirm these links. There is some evidence that prostate cancer is linked to high testosterone levels – eunuchs do not develop cancer of the prostate.[15]

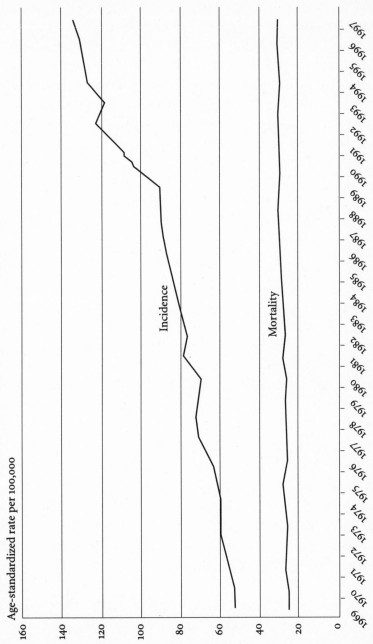

Age-standardized prostate cancer incidence and mortality rates for Canadian men, 1969-1997

Age-standardized rate per 100,000

Incidence

Mortality

160   140   120   100   80   60   40   20   0

1969 1970 1971 1972 1973 1974 1975 1976 1977 1978 1979 1980 1981 1982 1983 1984 1985 1986 1987 1988 1989 1990 1991 1992 1993 1994 1995 1996 1997

Source: National Cancer Institute of Canada, *Canadian Cancer Incidence and Mortality Rates for Canadian Men, 1969–1997*, Toronto: NCIC, 1997.

Studies examining the link between vasectomy and prostate cancer have not shown any clear relationships.

Detecting Prostate Cancer[16, 17, 18]

The signs and symptoms of prostate cancer may be the same as those for benign prostatic hypertrophy (difficulty urinating) or there may be no symptoms. The most commonly used tests are the DRE (discussed earlier) and the PSA test, which measures the level of total prostate-specific antigen (PSA) the prostate produces. A higher-than-normal level of PSA suggests prostate problems; however, it may not always be cancer.

PSA READINGS INCREASE WITH AGE	
Age range	*Upper Limit of* PSA *in ug/ml in*
40–49	2.5
50–59	3.5
60–69	4.5
70–	6.5

The PSA test is routinely used with men who have prostate symptoms. However, there is a great deal of disagreement between urologists and epidemiologists about using the PSA test as a routine screening tool for a healthy man with no symptoms. Some researchers and physicians also question whether the test does more harm than good to individuals (because of a high number of false positive results) and whether the costs to the taxpayer are justified when screening of men with no symptoms is done on a massive scale. The Canadian and American task forces on Periodic Health Examinations, who stringently analyse the costs and benefits of medical procedures, have recommended against PSA screening with healthy men, primarily because of its relatively low specificity and the possibility of detecting tumours that may never progress. On the other hand, the Canadian Urology Association Task Force on Prostate Cancer Screening and sister medical associations in the United States have recommended that the digital rectal exam (DRE) and PSA be performed annually on all men between the ages of fifty and seventy. They also recommend that men who are at high risk (men whose fathers, brothers, or uncles had prostate cancer) should be assessed on a regular basis, beginning as early as age forty.[19]

One must question whether PSA screening benefits those who undergo the test. False negative tests may miss cases of cancer. There are also false positives. False positive results can lead to a great deal of needless anxiety and invasive biopsies. However, a more specific test called Free PSA, which rules out false positives, is now available.

The use of the PSA (and the newer Free PSA test) is particularly important for African-American men or men who have a family history of the disease and are past age forty. The DRE and PSA together can make possible the early detection of significant prostate cancers that might be missed through the DRE alone.

Ultimately, each man must weight the pros and cons of PSA testing in his particular case and make his own decision in consultation with his physician.

Diagnosing Prostate Cancer

Following an abnormal digital rectal exam or an abnormal PSA test, transrectal ultrasound and a needle biopsy are used to diagnose prostatic cancer.

A positive diagnosis means running several more tests, including X-rays, a bone scan, and ultrasound to see if the cancer has spread. A pathology examination determines whether the prostate cancer cells are slow- or fast-growing.

If you are diagnosed with prostate cancer, talk with your physician about all of your treatment options, taking into consideration your age and overall state of health. Deciding upon the best course of treatment is not easy, since removing the prostate and undergoing follow-up radiation (sometimes combined with hormone therapy) may result in temporary (and in some cases, permanent) impotence and/or incontinence. Younger men are most likely to benefit from this kind of aggressive treatment.

In men over age sixty, the cancer may be the slow-growing kind that manifests few symptoms and will not lead to an early death. In this case, watchful waiting or watchful waiting combined with hormone therapy may be the most prudent course. Your physician will continue to monitor the disease with the PSA and other blood tests. If the PSA results continue to rise, changes in treatment or further tests are called for.

Keeping Your Prostate Healthy

Maintaining a healthy weight, regular exercise, eating a low-fat, healthy diet, and not smoking may help prevent prostate problems.

Exercise is good for all parts of the body. Your prostate is no exception. General exercise and regular sexual activity improve your overall fitness and health. There are also some specific exercises that you can easily do at home. These exercises, including Kegeling, squatting, yoga exercises, and exercises to strengthen the abdominal muscles, may be helpful.

KEGELING

Kegel exercises, long recommended for women with bladder problems, can also help men improve muscle tone in the prostate area. Kegel exercises are performed by tightening the pubococcyglus muscle near the rectum, which controls urine flow. Sitting or standing, pull your anal area inward, as if you were trying to postpone a bowel movement. Hold for 10 seconds, then relax. Repeat 10 times (this is one set). Perform 10 sets a day.

Diet and Prostate Cancer

Diet plays a role in both preventing and slowing the progression of prostate cancer. The Canadian Cancer Society recommends that men follow Canada's Food Guide to Healthy Eating (see Chapter 8). This means enjoying a low-fat, high-fibre diet, a moderate intake of caffeine, and food that delivers adequate amounts of vitamins and minerals. Antioxidants, including vitamins A, C, and E, beta-carotene, selenium, and lycopene (found in tomatoes, especially cooked), as well as zinc (highly concentrated in pumpkin seeds), may be particularly important to prostate health.

Antioxidants prevent oxidative damage to the cells, which may trigger cancer development (see Chapters 4 and 8 for information on this), although to date there is little clear evidence that a man's prostate-cancer risk varies with his consumption of dietary antioxidants. Lycopene, which is currently being studied at the U.S. National Institutes of Health to determine its protective properties, is the possible exception. Zinc appears to be important for the immune system, and has been shown to help the absorption of lycopene. It has been recently hypothesized that vitamin D deficiency may be a risk factor for prostate cancer; however, further investigation into this relationship is required.[20]

It has also been suggested that soy products may protect against prostate cancer. It appears that genistein in soy products inhibits androgen-dependent cancer cells in the prostate. Currently, there is not enough evidence to state that eating soy can help prevent prostate cancer for all men; nonetheless, the link seems promising. More research on the links between nutrition and prostate cancer is under way.[21]

Although the findings in scientific investigations of diet and prostate cancer have been contradictory in some cases, most of them suggest that a diet high in total fat may increase your risk. One study of 47,000 men showed that those who ate red meat as a main course five or more times per week were 2.6 times more likely to develop advanced prostate cancer than those who consumed red meat once a week or less. Fibre-rich eating may also help protect against prostate cancer. So enjoy lots of vegetables, fruits, cereals, and whole grains – a healthy prostate diet also protects against heart disease and diabetes.[22]

Foods and medications that can irritate the prostate (and therefore should be avoided or consumed sparingly) include alcohol, caffeine, highly spiced dishes, antihistamines, and some medications for gastrointestinal problems. If you develop prostate problems while taking a prescribed drug (e.g., antidepressant), contact your physician immediately. Early detection means checking with your doctor if you notice any signs of prostate problems.

Your sexual behaviour may also have a bearing on whether you develop a prostate infection. Urologists report that they find more cases of prostatitis in men with multiple sexual partners.[23]

In summary, lifestyle practices may be a significant factor in preventing prostate problems. And when you look after your prostate with common-sense lifestyle habits, you benefit in many other ways at the same time: you reduce your risk of heart disease and sexually transmitted diseases, increase your energy, increase your feeling of well-being, and even increase your interest in sex.

THE BOTTOM LINE

Expect the normal changes in the prostate that accompany aging. Evidence suggests that you may be able to delay or prevent prostate problems with a healthy diet, regular exercise, and healthy sex practices. If you do experience symptoms such as frequent or difficult urination, don't ignore them. See your physician. Most prostate problems are non-cancerous and easily treated. If you are between the ages of fifty and seventy, talk with your physician about having an annual DRE and PSA test. If you are an African American/Canadian or have a history of prostate cancer in your family, talk with your physician about having an annual DRE and PSA test beginning at age forty.

Contacts and Further Information

Organizations

- American Cancer Society: Contact your local office for information on prostate screening and prostate cancer.
- American Foundation for Urologic Disease, 1128 North Charles St., Baltimore, MD 21201. Tel.: (800) 242–2383 or (410) 468–1800.
- Canadian Cancer Society: Contact your local office for information on prostate screening and prostate cancer.

Websites

- Canadian Prostate Cancer Network (sponsored by the National Association of Prostate Cancer Support Groups, Lakefield, ON): http://www.cpcn.org
- Canadian Urologic Oncology Group (an affiliate of the Canadian Urologic Association, sponsored by Pharmacia & Upjohn): http://is.dal.ca/~bellorol/cuog.html
- Chronic Prostatitis: http://www.parsec.it
- The Male Health Center (founded in 1989 by Dr. Kenneth Goldberg, a certified urologist in Dallas, Texas): http://www.malehealthcenter.com

- Prostate Cancer Homepage (University of Michigan): http://www.cancer.med.umich.edu/prostcan.htm/
- Prostate Cancer Information Center (sponsored by Hoechst Marion Roussel Inc.): http://www.prostateinfocenter.com
- The Prostate Cancer Info Link (sponsored by Comed Communications Internet Health Forum): http://www.comed.com/prostate/
- University of Toronto Prostate Centre: http://www.library.utoronto.ca/www/medicine/prostate/
- Virginia Urology Center – BPH: http://www.uro.com/bph.htm

Please see Chapter 3 for additional websites on men's health.

Books
- *The Complete Prostate Book: Every Man's Guide* by Lee Belshen. Rocklin, CA: Prima Publishing, 1997.
- *Midlife Man* by Art Hister, MD. Vancouver: Greystone Books, 1998.
- *Private Parts: An Owner's Guide to the Male Anatomy* by Yosh Taguchi. Second edition. Toronto: McClelland & Stewart, 1996.
- *The Prostate: A Guide for Men and the Women Who Love Them* by Patrick Walsh and Janet Farrar Worthington. Baltimore: The Johns Hopkins University Press, 1995.
- *Prostate Cancer: A Guide for Women and the Men They Love* by Dr. Barbara Rubin Wainrib and Dr. Sandra Haber. New York: Dell Publishing, 1996.
- *The Prostate Sourcebook* by Steven Morganstern and Allen Abrahams. Chicago: Contemporary Books, 1993.

Related Chapters in This Book
- *Chapter 3: Is There a Male Menopause?* explains the relationships between hormonal changes and well-being in midlife.
- *Chapter 7: The Active Living Solution* gives you more information on how to stay active and fit in midlife.
- *Chapter 8: Food for Thought: Healthy Eating in Midlife* provides eating guidelines that may help prevent prostate problems.

- *Chapter 11: Enjoying Sex in Midlife* discusses the changes in sexuality you can expect with aging and provides some tips on keeping the spark alive. Some researchers believe that frequent ejaculations may help prevent prostate problems!
- *Chapter 12: Dealing with Impotence* helps men and their partners find the cause of erection problems and provides an introduction to treatment options for men who have impotence as a side-effect of prostate surgery.

CHAPTER NINETEEN

Breast Health

Knowledge is power, and most women have been denied real knowledge about their own breasts.   – Dr. Susan Love[1]

Aging and Your Breasts

The breast is a universal symbol of nurturing and abundance, as well as of sexual pleasure and beauty. From the budding of the breast in puberty to the sexual pleasure of love-making, to breast-feeding babies, the breast is fundamental to female identity. In North American culture, where the ideal has come to be a perfectly matched pair of firm eighteen-year-old breasts, women easily feel deficient or defective because they do not meet this impossible standard. Women tend to judge their bodies harshly, saying their breasts are too small, too big, or not the right shape.

So, when a midlife woman finds a lump in her breast, she is not only warned that something is awry with her body. She also feels that something may be fundamentally wrong with her as a woman. While the statistics repeatedly tell us that we are much more likely to die of a heart attack, the spectre of cancer of the breast fills us with dread. If a midlife woman has also had the difficult experience of supporting her mother or a friend, colleague or favourite aunt during a painful struggle with breast cancer, she is likely to be even more overwhelmed if she feels something suspicious during her breast self-examination.

Sometimes, it seems that the prominence given by the media to the statistics surrounding breast cancer adds to our fear. While we wholeheartedly support the media attention that results in greater funds for research and treatment, we also want to draw attention to the preventive importance of loving and knowing our bodies well, exactly as they are.

The focus of this chapter is on ways to maintain breast health and prevent cancer of the breast. It begins with a description of normal breasts, including those that are lumpy, dense, or painful. From there it helps you understand and assess your personal risk factors for breast cancer. It then discusses the importance of healthy lifestyle practices in maintaining breast health and the impact of new drugs that may help prevent breast cancer. We also review the standard early-detection techniques and the various ways you need to follow up a suspicious lump.

Readers looking for more information on the treatment of breast cancer are encouraged to review the contacts, books, and websites we recommend at the end of the chapter. All of these will give you more information and lead you to more detailed sources that deal with breast-cancer treatment.

Breast Anatomy

Some women have small, compact breasts, while others have large, pendulous breasts. Some breasts feel "lumpy," while others are "dense," because they have a higher proportion of breast tissue and smaller amounts of fat. Some women have one breast that is bigger than the other. Although it looks round, the breast is actually shaped like a tear: breast tissue extends to the armpit, or axilla (hence, the need to examine under the arm as well as the breast itself). As shown in the illustration below, the breast itself contains the nipple, areola, milk ducts, milk lobules, and fat. Some women's breasts can feel like a sack full of split peas or grains of rice; others feel soft and smooth.

The glands in the breast respond to the ebb and flow of the hormones estrogen and progesterone. Sometimes, this causes swelling and aching before the menstrual flow. Women with lumpy breasts sometimes develop non-malignant lumps that come and go during the cycle. Sometimes, a swelling of the duct behind the nipple causes a slight milky discharge at midcycle. All of these changes are normal and require a physician's attention only if they persist, cause serious discomfort, or if the nipple discharge is bloody.

As we age, some of the glandular tissue in the breast shrinks and is replaced by fat, usually after menopause. This is why women over age fifty have better results with mammography. Because their breasts are not as "dense," it is easier to detect any abnormality.

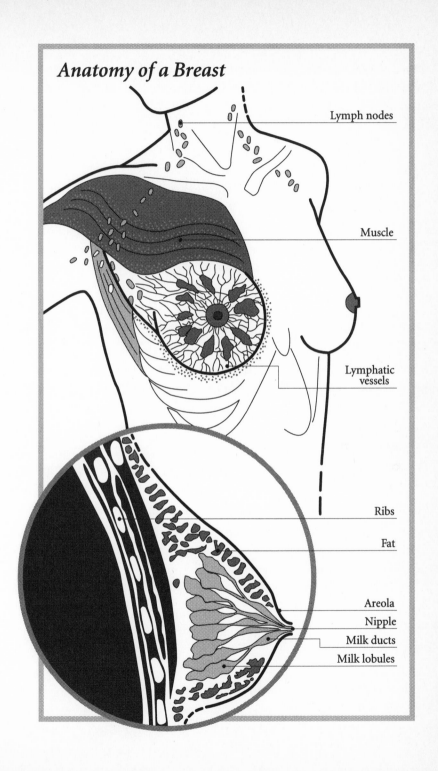

Anatomy of a Breast

Lymph nodes

Muscle

Lymphatic
vessels

Ribs

Fat

Areola

Nipple

Milk ducts

Milk lobules

When Your Breasts Are Lumpy and Painful

About 70 per cent of women have painful and tender breasts at some time in their lives, usually before menstruation or when other hormone fluctuations occur.[2] One woman told us, "At certain times of the month, I cannot stand my partner to hug me or even get close to my breasts." This condition usually disappears completely one to two years after menopause, unless the woman is on hormone replacement therapy (HRT).

Unfortunately, there is no cure for breast pain, but there are things you can do to relieve the discomfort. Reduce the amount of caffeine (e.g., in coffee, tea, and colas) you drink and the fat you eat. Other helpful changes include increasing the amount you exercise, taking vitamins E, C, A, B6, and evening primrose oil, and wearing a firm bra. Different forms of iodine supplements are used with varying degrees of success. Molecular iodine seems to work the best, with the fewest side-effects. More trials are needed before it can be used routinely. Sometimes, anti-inflammatory, over-the-counter drugs such as ibuprofen can help. If the pain is severe enough that it interferes with your daily activities, talk with your physician about it. There are some prescription medications (such as danazol and bromocriptine) that are used to treat severe breast pain, but these need to be closely monitored by you and your physician.[3]

Fibrocystic breast disease – the tendency to have abnormally lumpy breasts – is quite common, especially during the reproductive years and the perimenopause. It affects about 50 per cent of women between the ages of thirty and fifty. Lumpy breasts can be frightening; however, most of the lumps found by women with lumpy breasts are non-cancerous cysts, or solid benign tumours called fibromas. These lumps may vary in size from one millimetre to many centimetres.

Women with simple fibrocystic breast syndrome do not have an increased risk for breast cancer; those women with a more serious variety of this condition called hyperplasia (which is diagnosed by biopsy) face almost twice the risk.

Understanding Your Risk for Breast Cancer

The major risk factor for breast cancer is being a woman of increasing age. Seventy-five to 80 per cent of women who develop the disease do not have other typical risk factors. However, some factors are more predictive than

others. These include increasing age, a family history of breast cancer, previous breast-cancer history, radiation therapy to the chest when younger
than age thirty (e.g., to treat lymphoma), discovery of abnormal cells
during a breast biopsy, and breast density that is higher than normal.

Factors that *may* increase your risk are those related to increased exposure to reproductive hormones: early onset of menarche, later menopause,
no children, first pregnancy after age thirty, no breast-feeding.

Other factors that are implicated or are under investigation include
obesity after menopause, a high-fat diet, high alcohol consumption, HRT
use, and exposure to environmental chemicals, toxins, and estrogen in
foods. No clear evidence has surfaced to date that the use of birth-control
pills contributes to increased risk in healthy women. Other possible factors
include living in an urban area, a sedentary lifestyle, and belonging to a
higher socio-economic class. However, many questions remain unanswered regarding all of these factors.

The well-known statistic, "one in nine," is deceiving. It is based on the
fact that one of every nine women alive today will get breast cancer *at some
point in their lives*. This is more likely to happen after age seventy, since the
risk of breast cancer increases with age. Eighty per cent of breast cancers
occur after menopause. Consider, instead, your five-year risk, as shown in
this chart:[4]

Age	Five-Year Risk
30	1 in 650
35	1 in 400
40	1 in 200
45	1 in 125
50	1 in 110
60	1 in 95
70	1 in 65

Note, too, the significant finding that the risk of dying from breast cancer
is much lower than that of developing it – about one in twenty-eight by

the time a woman reaches age ninety. In 1998, breast cancer struck 178,800 American women, and 43,500 died of it.[5] In Canada, it was estimated that, in 1999, 18,700 women would develop breast cancer and 5,400 would die of it.[6]

Because more women are smoking cigarettes in both the United States and Canada, lung cancer has replaced breast cancer as the leading cause of cancer deaths among women of all ages. However, breast cancer remains the leading cause of cancer deaths among women aged forty to fifty-five. This is because breast cancers that are found at a younger age tend to be faster growing and more rapidly fatal than those found later in life. Here are some of the reasons why breast cancer has increased and why women in midlife are especially concerned about it:

- More of us are living longer.
- Improved screening techniques have meant that physicians are diagnosing more cases.
- Women today are exposed to many more menstrual cycles (due to the earlier onset of menses, fewer pregnancies, reduced time breast-feeding, and later menopause), which means our breasts are exposed to reproductive hormones longer than they were in the past.

Breast Cancer and Hormone Replacement Therapy (HRT)

There is still controversy over whether or not HRT increases one's risk for breast cancer (see Chapter 21, "Hormone Replacement Therapy: The Big Decision" for a thorough discussion). If you have concerns, consider your risk factors for breast cancer and talk with your physician about your concerns. According to current research, taking hormones to relieve menopausal symptoms for less than five years does not increase your risk. If, however, you are considering the use of HRT for longer than five years, you should carefully consider your personal risk for breast cancer.

Sometimes It Is in the Genes

There are two types of hereditary breast cancer (HBC):

- familial breast cancer, which affects 15 to 20 per cent of women with breast cancer, and
- genetic breast cancer, which affects only 5 to 10 per cent of women with breast cancer.

Familial breast cancer is the tendency for family members to develop breast cancer. This may be because of sensitivity to certain carcinogens or radiation. The most significant risk is having a first-degree relative (mother, sister, daughter) who has breast cancer. For example:

- having one first-degree relative over age 50 with breast cancer increases your risk by 9 to 11 per cent;
- having two first-degree relatives over age 50 with breast cancer increases your risk by 11 to 24 per cent;
- having a first-degree relative *under* age 50 with breast cancer greatly increases your risk.

If breast cancer is in your family, please see a physician. You may be referred to a familial breast cancer clinic (available in large cities) for genetic testing and counselling.

Women with genetic breast cancer have inherited defective genes: BRCA1 or BRCA2. Overall, about one in two hundred women inherits these genes, though Jewish women are at much higher risk (one in forty). Not all women who have the genes develop breast cancer (50 per cent by age fifty and 80 to 90 per cent by age seventy). These genes are also linked to ovarian cancer. If you have the defective BRCA1 gene, your risk of developing ovarian cancer by the age of seventy is 40 to 65 per cent. With BRCA2, your risk is 10 to 20 per cent. Ovarian cancer occurs in 1 per cent of the general population.

If you have a defective gene for breast and ovarian cancer, it is particularly important that you follow regular early-screening procedures. Talk with your physician about the use of drugs that may prevent these cancers, such as tamoxifen or raloxifene. More radical options such as preventive mastectomies and oophorectomies can be considered in consultation with genetic counsellors and your physician.[7]

Knowing you carry a gene that greatly increases your risk can cause enormous anxiety about the decisions that you make. One woman who was diagnosed as a carrier of the BRCA1 gene was advised to have a full hysterectomy and oophorectomy. When she discussed this with her family physician, she was understandably distraught. She knew that she would be in instant surgical menopause and wondered about the risks of using hormone replacement therapy. She was so frightened that she was already thinking of a preventive mastectomy. She said, "I am grieving. Everything that defines me as a female is a threat to kill me. I have small kids. I can't afford to die!"

This woman's difficult situation is all too typical of the dilemma of genetic testing. While offering hope to many, the testing poses incredibly complex and onerous decisions at the same time. Physicians are also nervous about entering this new frontier. They know they will have to educate themselves very well in order to communicate on this subject clearly and help their patients make thoughtful and informed choices.[8] There are no easy answers.

What can you do to reduce your risk for breast cancer?

- Practise a positive lifestyle (healthy eating, exercise, and reduced stress);
- Practise monthly breast self-exams;
- See a physician or nurse for regular breast exams; and
- Have regular mammograms after age fifty.

All of these are discussed in the sections that follow.

Promoting Breast Health with a Positive Lifestyle

The relationship between lifestyle and cancer prevention is complex and our knowledge is evolving. Current research strongly suggests that regular exercise, a healthy diet, not smoking, and limiting your intake of alcohol may help to reduce your risk of developing breast cancer.

Exercise

At least a dozen studies suggest a strong link between active living and lower rates of breast cancer. One Norwegian study that followed 25,000 women for nine years found that women who exercised four hours a week were 37 per cent less likely to develop breast cancer than inactive women.[9] In another study, researchers compared the exercise habits of more than 1,000 women under age forty, half of whom had been diagnosed with breast cancer. After adjusting for known risk factors, they found that exercising for a minimum of four hours per week reduced breast cancer risk by 60 per cent.[10]

Why does regular exercise reduce your risk for breast cancer? One theory is that vigorous exercise reduces a woman's production of estrogen. Another more likely explanation is that exercising four times a week burns excess calories and helps to keep you lean. In the Norwegian study, the leanest of the exercising women fared the best: they had as much as a 77-per-cent-reduced risk of developing breast cancer.

Weight Management

Extra weight after menopause appears to increase your risk for breast cancer. Researchers at the Harvard School of Public Health found that tall, overweight women had twice the risk of their thinner, shorter counterparts.[11] This may be attributed to increased estrogen production and storage in fat tissue; overweight women have higher estrogen levels in their systems.

Healthy Eating

In addition to regular exercise, both the Canadian and American cancer societies recommend a low-fat, high-fibre diet. Some researchers theorize that eating high-fat foods may increase the amount of useable estrogen in the blood and contribute to excessive weight (which also increases estrogen levels).[12] Others believe that the positive effect of a low-fat, high-fibre diet is related less to the reduction in fat and more to an increase in other nutrients, such as antioxidants and fibre. More definitive answers will come from the Diet Intervention Multicentre Study currently being undertaken with Canadian women at high risk for breast cancer. The results of this ten-year study will be available in 2005. In the meantime, it makes sense to cut back on high-fat foods and enjoy lots of vegetables, fruits, and whole grains. Studies have shown that a diet rich in these foods and others that supply fibre, beta-carotene, and vitamin C are linked to lower rates of breast cancer.[13] As already noted within the context of good prostate health for men, this kind of diet may protect you from heart disease and other health problems as well (see Chapters 8 and 20).

Other studies are examining the effects of a variety of food compounds, including a sulphur-containing element in garlic and isoflavones in soybean products. Japanese women who eat less fat and more soy foods than North American women have far lower rates of breast cancer.

Drinking milk, which is clearly associated with stronger bones, may also help prevent breast cancer. A study of 5,000 cancer-free women in Finland (where milk consumption accounts for a major portion of total dietary fat) showed that women who drank a lot of milk demonstrated a reduced risk for developing breast cancer.[14] The theory behind this finding is that milk is a good source of conjugated linoleic acid, which has been shown to suppress mammary tumours in animals and has recently been recognized as a type of anti-carcinogen.

Two other lifestyle factors increase your breast cancer risk: smoking and consuming two or more alcoholic drinks per day. Indeed, a recently published analysis of 250,000 women in the United States showed that breast-cancer mortality was 30 per cent higher in women reporting at least one drink per day, compared to non-drinkers.[15] See Chapters 5 and 9 if you want to quit smoking or cut down on the amount of alcohol you drink.

Preventing Breast Cancer with Drugs

In 1998, the National Cancer Institute in the United States announced a breakthrough in prevention research. For the first time ever, a six-year study involving more than 13,000 North American women at high risk for developing breast cancer (the Breast Cancer Prevention Trial), showed that it was possible to prevent breast cancer by taking a drug called tamoxifen. Previously the drug had been used to reduce the risk of recurrence in breast cancer. This study found an impressive 45-per-cent reduction in breast cancer among women at high risk who took a daily dose of tamoxifen, compared to those women who were given a placebo.[16]

So why aren't all women who are at high risk rushing to take tamoxifen? Because tamoxifen, like many other potent drugs, also produces some serious side-effects, including an increased risk for endometrial cancer and for lung and leg blood-clot formations. Other less severe side-effects include an increased risk of cataracts and menopausal-like symptoms such as hot flashes, vaginal dryness, nausea, and depression.[17] For women who have a high risk, whether or not to take tamoxifen is a difficult decision to make.

In addition to tamoxifen, a new drug called raloxifene (Evista) is now available. Raloxifene, a SERM (selective estrogen receptor modulator) improves bone and heart health, like estrogen, while protecting breast and uterine tissue. It was developed to prevent osteoporosis (see Chapter 17). Data presented in May 1998 suggest that it may also significantly reduce the risk of newly diagnosed breast cancer. New trials, such as STAR (Study of Tamoxifen and Raloxifene), initiated in 1999, will provide us with some clearer answers on the potential ability of these new drugs to prevent breast cancer.[18]

Detecting Breast Cancer Early

While the primary prevention of breast cancer ensures the best outcome, a second line of defence is ensuring that problems are detected early, so they can be successfully treated before it is too late. It takes ten years for a malignant cell to become a lesion or lump that can be detected, so ongoing, regular detection techniques are important in midlife and beyond. The earlier the cancer is detected (and the smaller the lump), the better one's chances for long-term survival.

Common early-detection techniques include breast self-examination, clinical breast examination, and mammography. New imaging techniques, such as ultrasound, digital mammography, and breast nuclear scanning are also in use in some places.

Breast Self-Examination

If you are over age forty, you should perform a breast self-exam once a month at approximately the same time, preferably just after your period. While the breast self-examination (BSE) is far from fail-safe, studies show that women who have good BSE techniques tend to find breast cancer at an earlier, more curable stage.

How many times have we stood in the shower or in front of a mirror, nagging ourselves to remember to do our monthly BSE, always a little worried about what we might find? Gynaecologist and holistic physician Christiane Northrup says that, when it comes to our female anatomy, we are always ready to believe that something is wrong. She articulates the conundrum for many women: "Why search meticulously each month for something you don't want to find, in an organ whose texture you don't understand?"[19] Both she and the breast-cancer expert Dr. Susan Love stress the importance of becoming very familiar with your breasts, so that you learn what is normal for you during the course of a month.

How to Do BSE Correctly

1. Stand in front of a mirror, with your arms over your head. Take a good look, then raise your arms to shoulder level, with your palms together. Look for any changes in the shape or contour, and for puckering, dimpling, rashes, red patches, or changes in the nipples (discharge, bleeding, or inversion). The best time to do this is after your period. If you no longer menstruate, pick one day of the month to check your breasts on a regular basis.

Breast Self-examination

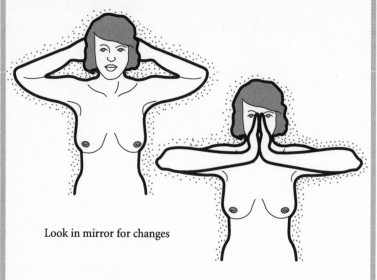

Look in mirror for changes

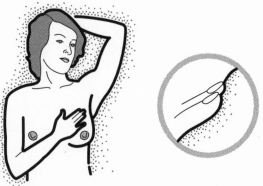

Use finger pads of 3 middle fingers to examine
your breast and underarm

2. Standing in the shower (the soap makes it easier to do) or lying down, raise one arm and place your hand behind your head. Examine the entire breast with the other hand, moving it in a circular or vertical pattern over your breast, pressing the pads of the three middle fingers firmly. Also examine your armpits.

3. Check for abnormal tenderness and for any thickening or lumps in one breast that you cannot feel in the other.

4. If you find a lump that is not familiar or discover nipple discharge or other changes in the skin or nipple, don't panic – remember that most lumps are not malignant. Make an appointment with your physician right away to check it out.

Clinical Breast Examination

A clinical breast examination (CBE) is the exam performed by a physician or nurse practitioner. All women in midlife should have a CBE done once a year. CBE is more effective at finding lumps in younger women than in older women.[20]

Mammography

Mammography is a safe, specific X-ray examination of the breast tissue that can detect lumps as small as 3 to 4 mm (0.12 to 0.16 in.) (BSE and CBE can only detect lumps as large as 10 to 20 mm (or 0.4 to 0.8 in.)). More than 90 per cent of women who find a cancerous lump before it is 10 mm in size survive and are cancer-free ten years after the diagnosis. In addition, the risk of radiation exposure is very small. This means that mammography is currently the best screening tool we have. Having said this, mammography is not foolproof – it can miss 10 to 15 per cent of breast cancers.[21]

The debate continues about the age at which women should have regular mammograms. The exception is the age group fifty to sixty-nine; studies show that regular mammograms for this group save lives. There is also no disagreement about the use of mammography when a breast abnormality is suspected, at any age. The controversy concerns whether or not to perform mammograms on healthy women with no signs of breast cancer who are younger than fifty and older than sixty-nine. In 1997, the American Cancer Society and the National Cancer Institute (U.S.) issued new guidelines recommending mammography (every one to two years) for healthy women aged forty to forty-nine.[22] The Canadian Cancer Society recommends mammography for women age fifty to sixty-nine every two years as long as results are negative.[23]

RECOMMENDATIONS FOR HEALTHY WOMEN AT NORMAL RISK FOR DEVELOPING BREAST CANCER

The American Cancer Society	*The Canadian Cancer Society*
BSE – every month	BSE – every month
CBE – once a year	CBE – once a year
Mammography	Mammography
– over age 40, once a year, as recommended by your physician	– age 50 to 69, every 2 years, as long as results are negative

---

Mammography is less accurate for younger women who have dense breasts. Why do women over age fifty (who are largely postmenopausal) benefit considerably more from mammography than women younger than fifty (who are largely premenopausal)? According to Dr. Cornelia Baines, professor in the Department of Public Health Sciences at the University of Toronto, the differences may be attributed to the menstrual cycle, which can affect the imaging achieved by mammography. Recent observations suggest that more false negative interpretations are made when a woman has a mammogram in the second half of her cycle.[24]

What Happens If You Find a Lump?
As mentioned already, if you find an unfamiliar lump in your breast, don't panic. Make an appointment to see your family physician. The following steps will then be taken to determine the nature of the lump.

- Your family physician will take a history and conduct a physical examination.
- You may be sent for a diagnostic mammogram. More views of the breast are taken in this case than in a routine screening mammogram.
- An ultrasound may be used to assess whether the lump is solid or cystic.

- If the lump is a cyst, some fluid will be removed from it with a fine needle (aspiration) and sent for analysis.
- If the lump is solid, the physician removes a small piece of tissue with a needle, guided by an ultrasound. This is called a core needle biopsy.
- If the core needle biopsy cannot be done or the service is not available in your area, the lump can be removed as a hospital out-patient procedure (called an open biopsy).

If all of these evaluations prove negative, your physician may advise one of two things:

- take no immediate action, and continue to perform BSE;
- have the benign cyst or lesion removed and biopsied, which will be done in a day hospital or out-patient clinic.

If the result of the biopsy is positive, you and your physician will need to discuss the most appropriate treatment.

THE BOTTOM LINE

Remember that most breast lumps are benign. For optimal breast health:

- Exercise regularly and avoid gaining weight.
- Eat a low-fat diet, including fruits, vegetables, whole grains, and skim milk.
- Do not smoke; drink alcohol moderately (or not at all).
- Avoid exposure to unnecessary radiation; do not use chemicals or pesticides in your home and garden.
- Practise breast self-examination monthly; have a clinical breast examination once a year and mammograms as appropriate.

Contacts and Further Information

Organizations

- American Cancer Society: contact your local unit (nationwide, U.S.): (800) ACS–2345.
- Breast Cancer Action, P.O. Box 39041, Ottawa, ON K1H 1A1. Tel.: (613) 736–5921.

- Canadian Breast Cancer Network, 207 Bank St., Suite 102, Ottawa, ON K2P 2N2. Tel.: (613) 788–3311.
- Canadian Cancer Connection Support Service: (800) 263–6750.
- Canadian Cancer Society: contact your local unit.
- Canadian Cancer Society Information Line: (toll-free) (888) 939–3333.
- Cancer Care Counselling Line (nationwide, U.S.): (800) 813–HOPE (4673).
- Cancer Information Service of the National Cancer Institute (U.S.): (800) 4–CANCER.
- National Alliance of Breast Cancer Organizations (NABCO) (U.S.), 9 East 37th St., 10th Floor, New York, NY 10016. Tel.: (212) 719–0154 (Information Services); (212) 889–0606 (office); Fax: (212) 689–1213.

Websites
- Association of Online Cancer Resources: http://www.acor.org
- Avon's Breast Cancer Awareness Crusade: http://www.avon.com
- Breast Cancer Action: http://infoweb.magi.com/^bcanet/index.htm/
- Breast Cancer Clearinghouse: http://nysernet.org/breast
- Breast Cancer Links: http://www.breastcancer.net/cgi/bcn.web.wcgi
- National Breast Cancer Coalition: http://www.natlbcc.org
- National Cancer Institute: http://rex.nc.nih.gov

Books and Booklets
- *Breast Cancer and You* (1996) and *Facts on Breast Cancer* (1998). Available from the Canadian Cancer Society Information Service. Tel.: (888) 939–3333.
- *The Complete Breast Book* by June Engel. Toronto: Key Porter, 1996.
- *Dr. Susan Love's Breast Book* by Susan Love and Karen Lindsey. 2nd ed., rev. Reading, MA: Perseus Books, 1995.
- *A Guide to Unconventional Cancer Therapies* by the Ontario Breast Cancer Information Exchange Project. Aurora, ON: R and R Bookbar, 1996.
- *Informed Decision: The Complete Book of Cancer Diagnoses, Treatment, and Recovery* by Dr. Gerald Murphy, Lois Morris, and

Diane Lange. American Cancer Society. Call (404) 320–3333 to order.
- *The Informed Woman's Guide to Breast Health* by Kerry McGinn. Palo Alto, CA: Bull Publishing, 1992.
- *What You Need to Know about Breast Cancer* (free from America's Pharmaceutical Research Companies), 1100 15th St. N.W., Washington, DC 20005. Tel.: (800) 862–4110 (U.S.).

Related Chapters in This Book
- *Chapter 5: Making Changes That Last!* provides some common-sense advice based on scientific studies on how you can make permanent lifestyle changes.
- *Chapter 7: The Active Living Solution* gives you more information on how to stay active in midlife.
- *Chapter 8: Food for Thought: Healthy Eating in Midlife* gives you more information on how a healthy diet can help prevent cancer, as well as information on how to maintain a healthy weight.
- *Chapter 9: The Boomer's Drugs of Choice* can help you quit smoking and reduce your intake of alcohol.
- *Chapter 16: Partners in Health Care* provides helpful advice on how to be an informed and assertive consumer with your physician.
- *Chapter 21: Hormone Replacement Therapy (HRT): The Big Decision* offers a decision-making guide and more information on the relationship between HRT and breast-cancer risk.

CHAPTER TWENTY

You Gotta Have Heart!

A merry heart doeth good like a medicine. – Proverbs 17:22

Fifty-two-year-old **Vincent** was a senior executive with a high-tech company. Lately, he had been under a lot of strain. When his wife finally convinced him to go in for an appointment, Vincent admitted to his doctor that he was having frequent chest pains, which got worse when he was walking the dog. He had felt the pain again during the night, and that morning while walking to the bus stop.

His doctor did a cardiogram and told Vincent that he had unstable angina, which put him at high risk for an imminent heart attack, and that he needed to go to the hospital right away. Vincent tried to persuade his doctor that he was all right. He had a big presentation that afternoon and promised to check himself in later. When his doctor insisted that he had to go right away, Vincent was furious.

The hospital confirmed the problem and kept him in overnight to stabilize his condition. Subsequently, Vincent visited a cardiologist. After a number of tests, he was booked for an angioplasty. The procedure went well and Vincent decided to enter a cardiac rehabilitation program that included supervised exercise and nutrition counselling. Vincent's initial anger at his doctor turned to gratitude as he realized how close he had come to having a major heart attack. He knew that it was time to come to terms with the way he was living. He knew that he had to quit smoking for good, relax more, and stop denying the fact that age and heredity had caught up with him.

Vincent's forty-eight-year-old wife, **June**, was also concerned about heart disease. She knew that black women are more likely than white women to have high blood pressure. Since turning forty, she had gained fifteen pounds. She was not sure what her blood-cholesterol levels were, and she had been living with a lot of stress lately, both at home and at work. Vincent's scare had been difficult and, now that he was recovering, both of them were frightened about how exertion (even the exertion of sex) might affect him.

June had helped her mother deal with a series of strokes that left her partially paralysed throughout much of her adult life. Her mother had never experienced the kind of drama that Vincent had been through. She just got weaker and more tired. Then, at age sixty-two, she had her first stroke. This was followed by several others until she died at age seventy-five. June could not bear the thought of living with the disabilities her mother had endured.

Like thousands of other North Americans in midlife, Vincent and June have good reason to be concerned. Cardiovascular disease (CVD), which consists of heart disease (including heart attack) and cerebrovascular disease (including stroke), is the leading cause of death in North America.

Vincent's and June's stories also speak to the different ways that men and women experience heart disease and stroke. While men tend to have dramatic "classic" symptoms earlier in life, women tend to experience heart disease seven to ten years later than men do, with different symptoms – and often more serious outcomes.

This chapter summarizes the differences between men and women in the ways CVD may present itself and how it is often treated. It provides a checklist to help you determine your personal risk for heart disease (or that of your partner) and gives you some helpful suggestions on how to reduce those risks. We include expanded sections on the relationship between heart health and eating, exercise, emotions, blood pressure, and blood cho-lesterol. It closes with a list of warning signs. If you suspect that you or your partner have angina pains, or signs of a heart attack or stroke, do not wait – get help immediately.

The Heart of the Matter
While four out of five deaths from heart disease occur in people over the age of sixty-five, a significant number of men and women die from or suffer

disabilities related to heart disease during midlife. Despite its reputation as an old person's disease, stroke hits thousands of North Americans in midlife each year. And it is during midlife that unhealthy living choices and high stress set the stage for a heart attack or stroke in later life.

In 1996, CVD accounted for 37 per cent of all deaths in Canada. Fifty-six per cent of these deaths were caused by ischemic heart disease (heart attacks and angina) and 19 per cent by strokes. Overall, men were slightly more likely to die of ischemic heart disease than women (22 per cent versus 19 per cent), and women were more likely to die of stroke (9 per cent versus 6 per cent).[1] Death rates due to CVD are similar in the United States; however, African Americans and Hispanics are more likely to suffer from CVD than Caucasians. African Americans between the ages of forty-five and fifty-nine are at least three times more likely to die of a stroke than white Americans in the same age group.[2]

The risk of cardiovascular disease increases with age, as the walls of the arteries become less flexible and clogged up with a fatty sludge or plaque. This condition, known as atherosclerosis, blocks the flow of oxygen-carrying blood to the heart muscle, resulting in angina (chest pain) or a myocardial infarction (heart attack). In the brain, atherosclerosis can lead to strokes; in the legs it can cause peripheral artery disease and pain in the calf muscles (called claudication) while walking. Atherosclerosis, which is part of the aging process, is exacerbated by risk factors such as smoking, sedentary living, high blood pressure, and high levels of blood cholesterol and a history of heart attacks before age fifty among close family members.

Heart disease can be prevented to a large extent by making healthy lifestyle choices. Indeed, mortality from heart disease and stroke has declined by about 2 per cent every year in North America over the last twenty years (although the rate of decline has not been as rapid in women as in men).[3] Most experts attribute this decline to dramatic reductions in smoking, increased levels of physical activity, and healthier diets (particularly a reduction in fat consumption), as well as earlier diagnoses and improved emergency treatment.

Male and Female Heart Disease: Is There a Gender Bias?

One obvious difference between men's and women's hearts is the age at which heart disease commonly strikes. In the middle decades, the rates for cardiovascular heart disease are three to four times higher for men than for women. However, the death rate from heart disease in women increases dramatically after menopause, and is significantly higher than for men by age seventy-five. Women over age seventy-five have a stroke mortality rate 26 per cent higher than men of the same age.[4] Most investigators attribute nature's bias toward younger women to the protective effects of the hormone estrogen before menopause. Estrogen has a positive effect on cholesterol levels and the walls of the arteries. It has recently become clear, however, that a human gender bias in both research and treatment may have significantly undermined women's advantages in later life.

Until recently, almost all research on heart disease was conducted on white men. This bias in research led the medical profession to assume that men's and women's experience of heart disease is the same, even though there are considerable biological differences between the sexes. Advocates for women's health suggest that knowledge about women's experience of heart disease is lacking and that women have been under-investigated, under-diagnosed, and under-treated. Others question whether men have been over-treated by the medical system.

In recent years, the medical establishment has come to realize that women's and men's experience of heart disease can differ in several ways.[5]

DIFFERENCES IN CORONARY HEART DISEASE BETWEEN WOMEN AND MEN[6, 7]

	Women	*Men*
Incidence:	By age 60, one in seven women develops CHD.	By age 60, one in five men develops CHD.
Typical age of onset:	60 to 75	40 to 50
Risk of dying of CHD:	47%	42%
Sex hormones	Estrogen decreases risk.	Testosterone increases risk.

	Women	*Men*
Risk factors:	Some factors appear to be more dangerous for women (elevated blood cholesterol and triglycerides) after menopause.	
	Some factors (diabetes) occur more often in women.	Some factors (high blood pressure) occur more often in men.
Symptoms:		
– presents as angina	47%	35%
– presents as a heart attack	29%	43%
Diagnostic tests:	Some tests may be less accurate for women.	
Treatment:		
– recurrence of heart attack	Higher in women	
– mortality in surgery	Higher in women	
– percentage receiving coronary–artery bypass surgery (1993)	15%	44%
– percentage receiving coronary-repair procedures (1993)	15%	33%
– percentage receiving treatment for heart disease	23%	70%
Outcomes:	Women are more likely to die during a first attack, to suffer a second heart attack soon after, and to die within a year of their first heart attack.	

The discovery that women's heart symptoms tend to be dramatically different from men's accounts for a great deal of the differences in the ways women and men have traditionally been treated. Physicians may not recognize that vague symptoms such as pain in the back, tingling fingers, or shortness of breath with minor exertion (such as walking up a hill) are symptoms of underlying heart disease in women. Women themselves may also dismiss these symptoms as unimportant.

In the last five to seven years, researchers have been rushing to catch up on what we know and don't know about women and heart disease. Large studies, such as the Nurses' Health Study, are looking carefully at women's experience. In addition, organizations in both Canada and the United States have set guidelines for improved diagnosis and treatment of heart disease in women.

What Is Your Risk for Coronary Heart Disease?

Whether you are male or female, your first line of defence is prevention. And prevention starts with understanding the risk factors for heart disease and what you can do about them. Some of these factors are beyond your control and others, called "modifiable risk factors," are within your control.

Check off the risk factors below that apply to you. The more boxes you check, the more likely it is that you will develop coronary heart disease.

Most important factors:
[ ] Heredity (You have a higher risk if immediate family members have or had heart disease, especially before age fifty.)
[ ] Age/postmenopausal status (You are a man over age forty or a postmenopausal woman.)
[ ] High blood pressure (hypertension)
[ ] Elevated cholesterol
[ ] Elevated blood fats (triglycerides)
[ ] Diabetes
[ ] Smoking

[ ] Obesity
[ ] Inactive lifestyle

Other important factors:
[ ] High-fat diet (More than 30 per cent of your total calories come
    from fat), especially saturated fats
[ ] High alcohol intake (You have more than two drinks a day.)
[ ] Difficulty managing stress
[ ] Hostile emotions
[ ] Work-related issues (unemployment, job insecurity, shift work)

While some risk factors have a stronger influence than others, the cumulative effect of multiple risk factors is dramatic. For example, your risk for heart disease within the next ten years is about 5 per cent if the only risk factor you have is high blood pressure. But if you have three risk factors or more, your chance of having a heart attack some time within the next ten years jumps to 39 per cent.[8]

Understanding Blood Pressure

Sheila gained eighteen pounds between the ages of forty and fifty-two. When her physician told her that her blood pressure was significantly elevated, she was determined to manage it with lifestyle changes rather than drugs. She started to exercise and to eat a moderate, healthy diet. After a fifteen-pound weight loss and an impressive improvement in her fitness level, her blood pressure returned to normal levels.

Sheila was able to manage her problem with hypertension (high blood pressure) through lifestyle changes. However, many people with high blood pressure do not even know that they have the problem. Hypertension is called "the silent killer," because there are no noticeable outward signs or symptoms. Yet inside, hypertension can quietly and insidiously damage your arteries, heart, and other organs for a decade or longer. Even though it affects 64 million Americans and some five million Canadians, including more than 30 per cent of middle-aged men, one-third of the people with hypertension are unaware they have the condition.[9] African Americans are more likely than whites to have hypertension, to develop it early, and to die from blood pressure–related problems.[10] Spanish Americans are also at high risk.

Because there are no outward signs of trouble, it is essential to have your blood pressure checked at least once a year by a health professional. Do-it-yourself blood-pressure monitors in malls and drugstores can give you a rough estimate of your blood pressure, but they are not an adequate substitute for a professional test. Blood-pressure levels vary greatly throughout the day, and can be temporarily elevated by anxiety, exercise, and caffeine. That is why your physician will want to check yours several times, especially if it is elevated.

Hypertension (generally thought of as readings higher than 140 systolic and 90 diastolic) can lead to stroke, congestive heart failure, and kidney disease. Middle-aged men with hypertension are six times more likely than men the same age with normal blood pressure to have a premature heart attack, five times more likely to die of congestive heart failure, and twelve times more likely to have a stroke. Altogether these conditions can shorten their lives by an average of ten to twenty years.[11]

KNOW YOUR NUMBERS

A blood-pressure reading measures the force with which blood pushes against the arteries, and is expressed as two numbers, such as 120/80 – the classic reading for optimal blood pressure. The upper, or systolic, number reflects the peak force when the heart is contracting and pumping blood through the arteries. The lower diastolic number measures the pressure between beats when the heart is at rest.

	Systolic	*Diastolic*
Optimal[12, 13]	less than 120	less than 80
Less than optimal	higher than 120	higher than 80

The higher your blood pressure above this optimal level, the greater your risk of heart disease, stroke, and kidney failure. Recent research suggests that damage can occur at much lower levels of elevation than was previously thought.

Heredity plays a major role in hypertension, as well as the following factors:
- age: blood pressure tends to increase with age;
- gender: at midlife, men have a higher incidence of high blood pressure than women; this difference levels off after age sixty;
- race: the ratio of hypertension between African Americans and white Americans is two to one.

Preventing and Reducing Hypertension

Preventing and reducing high blood pressure call for similar strategies:
- Control your weight and lose some pounds if you are above the healthy weight range (see Chapter 8). Excess weight is a factor in 60 per cent of cases of hypertension, and weight gain is a common factor in the number of people in middle age who have high blood pressure. Even small weight losses can lower blood pressure significantly. (See Chapter 8 for suggestions on maintaining a healthy weight.)
- Eat foods that contain potassium, magnesium, and calcium: low-fat dairy products (calcium and magnesium), whole-wheat grains (magnesium and potassium), fruits and vegetables such as potatoes, bananas, cabbage, and oranges (potassium). A recent clinical trial on the effects of diet on blood pressure found that people who ate plenty of these foods (dubbed the DASH diet – Dietary Approaches to Stop Hypertension) had lower blood-pressure levels.[14]
- Do not smoke. Nicotine raises blood pressure by constricting the blood vessels and speeding up the heart rate.
- Increase the amount of exercise that you do. Begin with moderate aerobic activities, such as brisk walking. Gradually progress to thirty minutes per day of continuous activity at a pace that suits you.
- If you drink, decrease your alcohol consumption to no more than one ounce of liquor, 24 ounces of beer, or 10 ounces of wine per day. Women and men with small physiques should aim to drink less.
- Reduce your sodium intake. Although people react to salt differently, we currently have no way to identify who is salt-sensitive and who is not. Reduce your use of table salt and restrict the amount of high-sodium foods you eat (such as potato chips and ketchup).[15]

- Avoid medication that can cause elevated blood pressure, such as ibuprofen (Advil) and oral contraceptives.

What should you do if you find you have hypertension? The first approach your physician will recommend is making the lifestyle changes suggested above. If these changes do not reduce your hypertension enough, you and your physician will need to work together to find the best possible drug-treatment regimen with the least bothersome side-effects and complications. This will take some experimenting, and it will be important that you keep your physician informed of any side-effects you notice. Once you have found a suitable medication, be sure to take it as prescribed. Do not stop taking the pills because your blood pressure appears to be under control. See your physician for regular monitoring of your condition.

Understanding Blood Fats and Cholesterol: Which One Did You Say Was the Bad One?

Cholesterol is one of several waxy-like blood fats or lipids in the blood. Lipids combine with proteins to transport fat in the blood. You have probably heard that there is "good" cholesterol (carried by high-density lipoproteins, or HDL) which carries fat away from the cells and artery walls and "bad," or "lousy," cholesterol (carried by low-density lipoproteins, or LDL), which sticks to the walls of your blood vessels, preventing blood from flowing easily to the heart. Think of LDL as the "bad" one, because "lousy" starts with "L." Smoking and high-fat eating (especially from saturated fat) increase your level of LDL.

Genetics play a fairly important role in determining whether or not you may have high blood cholesterol levels. If one or both of your parents had high cholesterol levels, you are more likely to experience the same thing, even if you are practising a healthy lifestyle. Women tend to have higher levels of HDL and lower levels of LDL than men do until they reach menopause, at which point high LDL appears to become a more serious risk to women than to men.[16]

Cholesterol-related problems have received an enormous amount of attention from the medical establishment and many clinical trials have been held both with people who have cardiovascular disease and those who do not. It is generally accepted that, for every 1-per-cent lowering of a person's blood cholesterol level, his or her risk of developing coronary heart disease is decreased by about 2 per cent.[17]

DESIRABLE CHOLESTEROL AND TRIGLYCERIDES LEVELS

Note: Canadian measures are expressed as millimoles per litre; U.S. measures are expressed as milligrams per decilitre.

Total cholesterol	LDL	HDL	Triglycerides
Can. less than 5.2	less than 3.4	more than 0.9	less than 2.3
U.S. less than 200	less than 130	more than 35	less than 200

Recent guidelines suggest that the ratio between total cholesterol and HDL levels (TC/HDL) may be as important as your total cholesterol count. Also, the more risk factors you have, the more you should aim to lower your total cholesterol level, your LDL level, and your TC/HDL ratio. They go on to suggest that other blood fats called triglycerides may play an independent role in increasing your risk for heart disease, especially if your HDL is very low.[18]

Preventing and Treating High Cholesterol

What is the best way to prevent and treat high cholesterol levels?

- When it comes to prevention, the first line of defence is a healthy lifestyle: regular physical activity, maintaining a healthy weight, little or no alcohol, no smoking, and a healthy, low-fat diet.
- Recent guidelines suggest that the treatment for elevated cholesterol should be linked to your total risk for heart disease or to already-existing problems, such as angina or as a previous heart attack. For example, if you have four or more risk factors for heart disease (e.g., smoking, high blood pressure, diabetes, and a family history of heart disease), more aggressive treatment (including lifestyle modification and medication) is called for. A person who has elevated cholesterol but has only one, or no other, risk factors may not be at risk and may not need to take medication.[19]

- The decision to use medication and what kind should be made only after all efforts have been made to control cholesterol levels with diet and other lifestyle modifications. Cholesterol-lowering drugs can have significant side-effects. Tell your physician about these as switching drugs may help. Remember, even when you find the appropriate medication, lifestyle measures such as physical activity and healthy eating still need to be followed.

In Canada, periodic testing for cholesterol is recommended for men over age forty-five and for women after menopause (who are not taking HRT) who have a number of the key risk factors for heart disease. On the other hand, the U.S. National Cholesterol Education Program suggests that "everyone should have a baseline test and know their cholesterol numbers." If your cholesterol level tests in the "desirable" range, the American and Canadian task forces on Periodic Health Examinations recommend that you then have it tested every five years. If your test results are higher, you may require more frequent testing. Keep in mind as well that what is safe and healthy can vary from person to person. Speak with your doctor about all of your risk factors and how often you require testing.

Cholesterol in food – which is found only in animal products (meats, poultry, dairy products, and eggs) – is not the same as cholesterol in the blood. Studies have shown that the best diet for maintaining low cholesterol levels is one that is low in total fat and in saturated fats in particular (as opposed to avoiding foods that contain cholesterol). Saturated fats are hard fats from animal products. Here are the most important points in reducing your blood cholesterol:

- Aim to reduce your daily intake of fat, especially saturated fat in meat, dairy, and processed foods;
- Use low-fat cooking techniques – when using fat, cook with olive or canola oil instead of butter or margarine;
- Substitute fish, beans, lentils, chickpeas, or tofu for some of the meat and poultry you eat;
- Avoid processed baked goods made with saturated fats and trans fatty acids (some margarines, shortening, french fries, pastries, cookies, crackers);
- Remember that cholesterol-free foods can be high in fat;

- Enjoy plenty of fruit, vegetables, and grains;
- Alcohol and sugars in the diet increase blood triglyceride levels, so limit your intake of these foods.

Reducing Your Risk Factors

Studies show that men aged forty-five to fifty-four are the most likely to exhibit two or three risk factors.[20] If you are in this category, it is critical that you begin to reduce or control these factors. Here is a summary of the most important things you can do to reduce your risk for heart disease. Some of these were mentioned in the previous sections on high blood pressure and cholesterol.

Quit smoking. Smokers have two to four times as high a risk for heart disease (including stroke) as non-smokers, and their heart attacks are more likely to be fatal. For women over age thirty-five, tobacco use combined with birth-control pills increases the risk by more than five times. Within five years of quitting, former smokers lower their risks by 50 to 70 per cent compared to those who continue to smoke.[21]

Active living. While sedentary living used to be seen as a secondary or less important risk factor for heart disease, a growing body of scientific evidence has recently led both the American and Canadian Heart and Stroke foundations to state that a sedentary lifestyle is now considered as potentially damaging as smoking, high blood pressure, and the other major risk factors. Studies show that inactive men have twice the risk of developing coronary heart disease as those who are physically active.[22] Increasing levels of "good" cholesterol (HDL) with aerobic exercise is particularly important for women after menopause (when reduced estrogen lowers HDL). Even small amounts of exercise can help prevent and control diabetes. See Chapter 7 for ideas on increasing your activity levels.

Eat a heart-healthy diet. Since high fat intake is linked to elevated blood cholesterol, and fibre appears to help lower blood cholesterol, aim to consume a low-fat, high-fibre diet. Maintain a healthy weight and drink alcohol conservatively, if at all. Eat plenty of plant foods that are rich in antioxidants and phytochemicals, as these have been shown to help prevent heart disease (see Chapters 4 and 8 for more information). Consider taking a vitamin E supplement (100 IU). Vitamin E is an important antioxidant, and it is almost impossible to get the amount recommended from our food in sufficient quantities to prevent heart disease. Eat fish at least once a week – the omega 3 polyunsaturated fatty acids in fish oils may have a beneficial effect on the heart.

Consider taking one Aspirin each day. Several studies, including one with 22,000 middle-aged male physicians, have shown that acetylsalicylic acid (the generic name for Aspirin) can reduce the risk of heart attack by 42 per cent.[23] As yet, the evidence is not as strong for women (since most of the studies have been done with men).

Consider the use of hormone replacement therapy (HRT) if you are menopausal and have other risk factors for heart disease. Studies have shown that HRT can reduce heart disease by 50 per cent in women at risk.[24] The decision to use long-term hormone therapy, however, must be balanced against the personal risks and side-effects (see Chapter 21 for a full explanation of how to make this decision).

Learn to cool your "hot reactions." People with high blood pressure or high lipids who also have hot reactions to situations like being held up in traffic or in a long line at the bank are at higher risk for a coronary attack or sudden death. Try to reduce the frequency and intensity of your experiences with emotions such as hostility, anger, and cynicism. These emotions increase the body's production of two major stress hormones – adrenalin and cortisol. These hormones raise blood pressure and heart rate and increase the stickiness of the platelets that form blood clots. This, in turn, increases your chances of developing a blood clot that can lead to a heart attack. Learn and practise effective stress-management techniques. Take time out to relax.

Seek help if you are depressed or experiencing panic attacks. Depression may increase your risk of a first heart attack by two to three times; panic disorder may double your risk.[25] Psychotherapy can significantly help both conditions (see Chapter 15 for more information on depression and panic disorder.)

Recognize that certain types of work (such as shift work and jobs that allow you little personal control over how you work) *are linked to a higher incidence of heart disease.*[26] Unemployment and job insecurity, which have become an alarming fact of life for many middle-aged men and women in the 1990s, are also linked to the early development of heart disease. If you find yourself in this situation, it becomes especially important to pay attention to the other risk factors that you can control, such as smoking, diet, stress management, and physical activity.

If you have diabetes, manage it carefully and follow your doctor's advice. Diabetes increases both men's and women's mortality from heart disease. However, it is a more serious risk factor for women. Diabetic women are three times more likely than non-diabetic women to suffer heart disease.[27] Many people with Type II diabetes are overweight, have high blood pressure and elevated blood lipids. Once again, losing weight helps control all of these conditions and reduces your overall risk for life-threatening heart disease.

Some studies have shown that *elevated levels of homocysteine* in the blood may be an important risk factor for CVD. Homocysteine is a byproduct of methionine, an essential amino acid found mainly in animal proteins. The more homocysteine you have, the higher your risk. It is estimated that about 10 to 20 per cent of North Americans may have elevated homocysteine levels. Adding folic acid, B12, and B6 to your diet may help lower your homocysteine level.[28, 29]

Warning Signs: Get Help Fast!

Immediate treatment of a heart attack or stroke is critical to recovery. If you or a friend or family member experiences the symptoms of a heart attack or stroke, you must act quickly. Call 911 or an emergency ambulance service immediately and tell the dispatcher you suspect you or another person is having a heart attack or stroke. Since most heart attacks and strokes occur in the home, make sure your family members know how to deal with these medical emergencies and how to administer CPR (cardiopulmonary resuscitation).

Warning Signs of a Heart Attack

- persistent, vague chest pain, sometimes radiating to the arms (more common in men);
- vague discomfort in the chest, neck, jaw, shoulder, or arm (typical signs of angina – more common in women), and not relieved by nitroglycerin;
- tightness or squeezing feeling in the chest, shoulder, arm, neck, or jaw;
- nausea, vomiting, or indigestion;
- pale skin, shortness of breath, sweating;
- severe anxiety or denial – refusal to believe that anything serious is wrong.

Warning Signs of a Stroke

Studies show that the immediate treatment with clot-busting drugs called streptokinase and TPA (tissue plasminogen activator) can make a substantial difference in the progress of the damage. Here are the classic signs of stroke in both men and women:

- sudden weakness, numbness, or tingling of the face, arm, or leg;
- difficulty speaking or understanding simple sentences, sudden confusion;
- sudden loss of vision, particularly in one eye, or double vision;
- sudden, severe headaches of unknown cause;
- sudden dizziness, loss of balance or co-ordination, especially accompanied by any of the above signs.

Heart and the Emotions

In his book *Love and Survival*, Dean Ornish says, "When the emotional heart and the spiritual heart begin to open, the physical heart often follows."[30]

The heart is more than a well-designed pump, and affairs of the heart are more than cholesterol levels and lipids. We've always known that people die of broken hearts, that love makes the world go round, and that you've gotta have heart to survive and thrive. As with many topics in this book, once we know and understand the medical information, it is matters of the psyche and soul that capture our interest.

Numerous studies have shown that both depression and hostility are significantly linked to a higher incidence of heart disease and heart attacks. In a study of 1,200 white males, who were followed every five years from 1948 to 1995, depressed men were twice as likely as non-depressed men to develop CHD, suffer a myocardial infarction, or succumb to a sudden cardiac death.[31] In addition, patients who suffer a major depression while in hospital recovering from a heart attack are more likely to die in the six months after their myocardial infarction than their non-depressed cohorts.[32]

Research has also shown that hostility and cynicism have a very deleterious effect on the heart. Redford Williams of Duke University studied the hostility component of the Type-A behaviour profile and found it to be a stronger predictor of heart disease than the full Type A pattern. Williams went on to do a long-term study on levels of hostility in male physicians. He and his collaborators found that those physicians who had high hostility scores on a test taken twenty-five years earlier in medical school were dying at a rate six and a half times greater than those with low hostility ratings.[33]

The suppression of emotional expression also seems to have negative effects, as seen in measures of hypertension. Some studies suggest that high blood pressure may be linked to both extremes of emotional behaviour – suppression and explosiveness.[34] While women have been largely neglected in long-term heart studies, current research indicates that inappropriate expression of anger is also a cardiac risk factor for women. Studies say that women tend not to be as explosive as men, but are more likely to ruminate on their anger in a repetitive, obsessive way. It has been suggested that pre-menopausal women who don't deal effectively with their anger appear to lose the cardioprotective effects of estrogen. The Framingham Heart Study showed that women who "hold in" their anger are also at significantly increased risk for CHD.[35]

Many respected researchers, including Joan Borysenko, formerly of Harvard Medical School, and Jon Kabat-Zinn, of the University of Massachusetts Medical School, have cautiously put forth the premise that, if negative emotions can harm the heart, then perhaps positive emotions can protect it.

Borysenko, in her book, *Minding the Body, Mending the Mind*, points to the Roseto Study as an example of this. The town of Roseto, Pennsylvania, was extensively studied, because of its very low death rates from CHD. While the townspeople turned out to have numerous high-risk medical factors, they seemed to be protected by the close, supportive nature of their social network. People knew each other for a long time, seldom moved away, and took care of each other in simple, everyday ways. Borysenko writes, "Social support, the great stress buffer, turned out to be more important than health habits in predicting heart disease."[36]

Dean Ornish cites a number of studies that indicate that being in a loving relationship protects against heart disease. He describes a particularly fascinating study of male Harvard students, started in the 1950s. The students were asked to describe their relationships to their mothers and fathers on a scale from "very close" to "strained and cold." Thirty-five years later, their current medical records were obtained and detailed histories taken. The results were unequivocal. Ninety-one per cent of the participants who did not see themselves having a close relationship with their mothers had seriously diagnosed diseases in midlife (such as CHD and high blood pressure), compared to 45 per cent who perceived their relationships with their mothers as warm. This was independent of family histories of illness, smoking, and current emotional stress. Ornish quotes the researchers: "The perception of love itself . . . may turn out to be a core biopsychosocial–spiritual buffer, reducing the negative impact of stressors and pathogens and promoting immune function and healing."[37]

How serendipitous to discover that doing what we love to do, enjoying ourselves and spending time with people for whom we have great affection are not only fine ways to spend time, but are also very good for our health!

THE BOTTOM LINE

Your chance of developing heart disease depends on the number of risk factors you have. Since we can't control heredity, we must reduce or eliminate those risk factors we can control through a healthy lifestyle. Close personal relationships and community involvement are beneficial to the heart. So take time to relax and laugh with your family and friends.

Contacts and Further Information

Organizations
- American Heart Association: Contact your local organization.
- Heart and Stroke Foundation of Canada: Contact your local organization (check the phone book).

Websites
- American Heart Association: http://www.amhrt.org
- Heart to Heart Volunteers: http://www.csusm.edu/public/guests/
- Heart and Stroke Foundation of Canada: http://www.hsf.ca
- National Institutes of Health and the National Heart, Lung and Blood Institute: http://www.nhlbi.nih.gov/nhlbi/nhlbi.htm
- National Stroke Association (U.S.): http://www.stroke.org

Books
- *Anatomy of an Illness: As Perceived by the Patient* by Norman Cousins. New York: Bantam Books, 1979.
- *The Canadian Family Guide to Stroke: Prevention, Treatment, Recovery* by the Heart and Stroke Foundation of Canada and the American Heart and Stroke Foundation. Toronto: Random House, 1996.
- *A Change of Heart* by Brian Baker and Paul Dorian. Toronto: Random House with the Heart and Stroke Foundation of Canada, 1998.
- *Healing Hypertension: Uncovering the Secret Power of Your Hidden Emotions* by Samuel Mann. New York: John Wiley, 1999.
- *Heart and Soul: A Psychological and Spiritual Guide to Preventing and Healing Heart Disease* by Bruno Cortis. New York: Pocket Books, 1995.
- *Love and Survival: Eight Pathways to Intimacy and Health* by Dean Ornish. New York: HarperPerennial, 1998.
- *Natural Medicine for Heart Disease: The Best Alternative Methods for Prevention and Treatment* by Glen Rothfield and Suzanne LeVert. Philadelphia, PA: Rodale Press, 1996.

Related Chapters in This Book

- *Chapter 4: The Search for the Fountain of Youth* provides more information on the role of antioxidants and physical activity in the prevention of heart disease.
- *Chapter 7: The Active Living Solution.* Look here for information and practical advice on how to start and stay active.
- *Chapter 8: Food for Thought: Healthy Eating in Midlife.* Here you will find more information on heart-healthy eating and advice on how to maintain a healthy weight.
- *Chapter 9: The Boomer's Drugs of Choice.* Look here for solid advice to help you quit smoking and reduce your alcohol intake.
- *Chapter 13: Stress-Proofing in Midlife* provides ideas on managing stress in midlife.
- *Chapter 21: Hormone Replacement Therapy (HRT): The Big Decision.* This chapter reviews the evidence on HRT and heart health, and provides a simple guide to help you make the choices about HRT that are right for you.
- *Chapter 23: Body, Mind, and Soul* further explores the role of spiritual well-being in prevention and healing.

Hormone Replacement Therapy (HRT): The Big Decision

> Risks that apply to the general population may or may not apply to an individual woman. No two women are alike. Each woman has to make the difficult choice.
>
> – Janine O'Leary Cobb[1]

The decision to take hormones or not is both complex and unique to each individual woman. Each of us needs to be well informed about what we can and cannot expect from hormone replacement therapy (HRT). This chapter discusses the benefits and risks of HRT and provides a straightforward guide to help you make your personal decision.

HRT is not used to replicate premenopausal hormone levels or to suppress normal hormone production, as is the case with the birth-control pill. The intent of HRT is to provide the lowest levels of estrogen and progesterone required to manage symptoms and protect the bones and heart.

Throughout this chapter (and in the rest of the book) we use the phrase "hormone replacement therapy" or HRT, even though we are uncomfortable with what it implies. "Hormone replacement therapy" assumes that menopause is a deficiency problem and that the "replacement" of missing hormones is required. After a long discussion, however, we decided to stick with this term (and to refer as well to simply "hormone therapy"), since these are the terms you are most likely to hear or read in other sources. We have rewritten this chapter many times to include new information as it became available. We very much want to present an open and balanced picture of the pros and cons of HRT to encourage women to make informed decisions that feel right for them.

In our seminars, after we have gone through a detailed explanation of why each woman must make a decision based on her own beliefs, health, and family history, it is not unusual to have women come up at the end of a presentation and ask, "So, do you think I should take it?"

This question reflects the confusion and need for support that many women feel when it comes to HRT. Even physicians are confused by the conflicting scientific studies that seem to hit the media almost weekly. For example, the results of two studies on HRT and the risk of breast cancer were released in June and July of 1995. One study claimed there was no increased risk for breast cancer with HRT; the other claimed a 40-per-cent increased risk with HRT. While many women are confused about the results of these scientific studies, the lack of rigorous research on alternative therapies is just as troubling. Given all this confusion on so many fronts, no wonder we still want someone to tell us what to do!

This chapter gives you the information you need to discuss the use of HRT with your physician confidently. He or she, in turn, should be prepared to discuss your individual risk factors, medical history (family and personal), and preferences. We encourage you to keep up to date with the results of studies as they are released and to re-evaluate your own position on HRT use in consultation with your doctor every six to twelve months.

Each Woman Is Unique

Consider the situations of the following six women, each with a significantly different experience of menopause:

Sara underwent a hysterectomy (removal of the uterus) and oophorectomy (removal of the ovaries) at age forty and has been taking estrogen to relieve severe menopausal symptoms after her surgery. She took comfort knowing that HRT would also help protect her against bone loss that can lead to osteoporosis. Now, at age forty-eight, she is wondering how long it is safe to continue to take hormones and whether or not she should talk with her doctor about adding testosterone to help with her diminished sexual drive. Ever since the surgery, she has had little interest in sex.

Barb started a regimen of estrogen and progesterone to help her handle the hot flashes and night sweats that were keeping her awake and making her life a misery. Almost immediately, the night sweats disappeared and the number of daytime hot flashes was greatly reduced. It was only after she started to sleep well again that Barb realized how much her joints and muscles had ached and how tired she had been. She was also relieved that she no longer had to get up in the night to urinate. She assumed that her use of hormones would be short term – until the hot flashes, night sweats, and troubled sleeping associated with the earlier phases of menopause have passed.

Martha had no intention of trying HRT. She was disturbed by the conflicting studies reported in the press and had always been an avid user of alternative therapies. She was well versed in nutrition and had done her research on the benefits of eating soy and flax products that contain phytoestrogens. She took calcium, vitamin D, and other mineral and vitamin supplements. Martha enjoyed walking and had recently started to work out with light weights. Her family physician supported this regimen, and she was happy to be in control of her symptoms.

Sandy sailed through the menopausal period with only minor complaints and never suspected that she might be at high risk for osteoporosis. Sandy is an avid walker and swimmer, and eats well. She is small and thin and has chosen not to have children. Her mother was diagnosed with osteoporosis when she fell and broke her hip at age sixty-five, but Sandy thought it was because she smoked and never took good care of herself. Sandy was in shock when her doctor sent her for a bone-density test and told her that she had low bone mass.

Because of her concern about breast cancer, her physician advised Sandy to consider the use of one of the new "designer" estrogens called SERMs (selective estrogen receptor modulators). She decided to do some research on her own and a few months later, after consultation with a specialist, Sandy decided to go ahead and try the SERMs.

Linda was faced with a difficult decision. She was really suffering with menopausal complaints: hot flashes, fatigue, and upsetting mood swings. Yet she was not prepared to take hormones. Her mother had died of breast cancer, and her sister was a breast-cancer survivor. Even though she knew from all she was reading that the link between hormone therapy and breast cancer was inconclusive, she was too uncomfortable with the idea to take the chance. When she explained how she felt, her physician made a number of other suggestions, including some fundamental changes in her lifestyle. She suggested that Linda exercise regularly and include soy products such as tofu and soy protein shakes in her daily diet. She also advised Linda to increase her intake of calcium and to eat lots of fruits and vegetables.

Over time, Linda began to eat better and to work out on a stationary bicycle every other evening. She researched the use of alternative remedies and began to take vitamin E, in addition eating a high soy diet to help control her hot flashes.

Coping with the psychological turmoil of midlife was every bit as hard as changing her physical behaviours. But gradually, with the help of psychotherapy, she began to make changes: to work less and to take more time for herself. Over the next twelve months, Linda began to feel better, not only about her health but also about her accomplishments. Menopause had forced her into some fundamental changes that she knew were right for her and her family.

Maureen had a very stressful job as lawyer in a large firm. Despite her general assertiveness, when the flashes started she was suddenly not "in charge" of her emotions. She hated her heavy periods and the very little time she had between them. Maureen told her doctor how badly she wanted hormones: "I can't stand it. I either have PMS or my period. I can't deal with the aging. I want my skin to stay young and my bones to stay strong. I want to get rid of this midlife acne. I've had enough!" After a thorough assessment and discussion of her options with her physician, Maureen decided to take a low-dose oral contraceptive to bridge the difficult perimenopausal period.

The experiences of Sara, Barb, Martha, Sandy, Linda, and Maureen mirror some common situations for women in the menopausal period. Indeed, as mentioned earlier, "Should I take hormones?" is the most common question we hear in our seminars.

Women like Maureen who are fed up with distressing symptoms and are looking for immediate relief are more likely to view the use of HRT favourably than those who prefer to view menopause as a natural process that all women go through.[2] Some of the women we see in our clinic decide to manage their minor menopausal complaints with healthy lifestyle choices. They see little reason to consider HRT, especially if they are not at risk for heart disease or osteoporosis. One said, "I'd like to think I can just accept some inconveniences and get on with my life." Others decide to use HRT while remaining prepared to reconsider how to proceed as new research becomes available.

Whatever your situation, it is important to remember that taking HRT or not taking HRT is not a once-in-a-lifetime decision. You can always change your approach to menopause.

The decision to use HRT for short-term symptom control is a relatively easy one. The short-term use of HRT is considered effective and safe for most women, except for a small number who have contraindications to taking it. Many other women find relief from menopausal symptoms through the use of alternative therapies and diet changes, such as increasing their intake of phytoestrogen-rich foods.

The difficulty comes when you must make a decision on the long-term use of HRT as a way of preventing or treating disease. While we have learned a lot about the role of HRT in these areas, there are still many questions about both the benefits and risks of long-term use.

An Introduction to Hormones and Hormone Replacement Therapy (HRT)
There are two female sex hormones: estrogen and progesterone. Most of the estrogen in the body is produced by converting cholesterol into estrogen in the ovaries and body fat cells. Progesterone is secreted by the corpus luteum in the ovary during the second half of the menstrual cycle. Women also produce small amounts of the male sex hormone, testosterone. Sometimes, testosterone is converted into estrogen at various sites throughout the body, including the brain. Hormone production decreases dramatically during menopause, leading to menopausal discomforts and other age-related changes in the body.

Main Reasons for Using HRT
For now, there are three main reasons for considering the use of HRT:
- to relieve menopausal discomforts;
- to prevent osteoporosis and heart disease;
- to treat existing osteoporosis.

1. *Using HRT to relieve menopausal discomforts is the number-one reason that healthy women choose to take hormones.*[3] As one woman told us, "When my hormones dropped, so did my energy, interests, and sense of humour." HRT can eliminate or relieve menstrual-flow disturbances, hot flashes, sleep disturbances, fatigue, mood changes, a dry vagina, and urinary incontinence. Barb chose HRT for this reason and she is right in believing that her use of hormones will be fairly short term (less than five years). She and her physician will continue to monitor her bone and heart health to see if she should consider taking hormones for disease-prevention purposes later. Sara is taking hormones to deal with an early menopause that was surgically induced, causing immediate, severe symptoms and an increased risk for osteoporosis and heart disease. Eight years later, when she would naturally be coming into menopause, she is correct in thinking that it will be time to re-evaluate her position. Different hormone dosages and regimens can have quite different effects.

2. *The second reason to take hormones is to prevent osteoporosis and heart disease.* Sandy is healthy and relatively free of menopausal complaints. She is taking SERMs to prevent osteoporosis, because she is at high risk for developing this crippling disease. This therapy also has a protective effect on the heart.

    For women with no risk for breast cancer or osteoporosis, the use of traditional HRT has been shown to be effective in preventing heart disease by as much as 50 per cent. Preventing heart disease and osteoporosis (whether you have a surgically induced or natural menopause) requires you to take hormones for a longer period of time (ten to fifteen years), with re-evaluations on a regular basis.

3. *The third reason to take hormones is to treat osteoporosis.* Women who have been diagnosed with osteoporosis may derive the greatest benefit from SERMs or traditional hormone therapies.

Results of Some Recent Studies
Until recently, many studies looking at the effect of HRT on heart disease showed significantly less hardening of the arteries among women who took estrogen and some benefits for women with heart disease who took estrogen combined with progesterone. This indication dramatically changed with

the release of the Heart and Estrogen–Progestin Replacement Study (HERS) – a randomized, double-blind trial – in August 1998. This study followed 2,763 randomly selected women with documented heart disease between the ages of fifty-four and seventy-nine. The women were divided into two groups and received either a placebo or a combined hormone regimen (.625 mg estrogen and 2.5 mg progesterone on a continuing basis). After four years, there was a slightly higher incidence of heart attacks and death in the HRT group, especially during the first year. Women in the HRT group also had a higher incidence of complications such as gall-bladder disease and phlebitis (inflammation of a vein, often accompanied by formation of a blood clot).[4]

The results of this study were an enormous surprise, since many previously published observational studies had shown the opposite. Many questions remain. Was it the type of estrogen and progesterone used, or was it the dosage? Obviously, more prospective trials are needed before estrogen and progesterone are used routinely as a therapy for the treatment of heart disease.

At the same time there is still a large body of evidence supporting the use of HRT for preventing heart disease in women at high risk. Hence there are additional questions and confusion about its use. Female baby boomers find themselves once again part of a living research experiment, this time on the benefits and risks of various hormone therapies. Fortunately, large ongoing studies are now under way that will give us and our daughters much clearer direction in the future. These include:

- Soy Estrogen Alternative Study (SEA), 1996–1999
  A randomized, double-blind trial of 240 perimenopausal women aged forty-five to fifty-five. The goal is to study the effects of phytoestrogens in soy products on menopausal symptoms, plasma lipids, thickness of the lining of the carotid artery, bone density, and mood.
- Women's International Study of Long-Duration Oestrogen after Menopause (WISDOM), 1997–2017
  A randomized, double-blind, placebo-controlled study of 18,000 postmenopausal women aged fifty to sixty-four. The goal is to evaluate the relationship of hormone therapy to heart disease, stroke, and fractures resulting from osteoporosis.

- Women's Health Initiative (WHI), 1991–2006
  A randomized, double-blind, placebo-controlled trial involving forty clinical sites and 68,000 postmenopausal women aged fifty to seventy-nine. The goal is to study the effects of hormone therapy and diet on coronary heart disease, cerebrovascular events, breast and colorectal cancer, and fractures because of osteoporosis.

Until results are available from these comprehensive studies, there is no reason to advise all healthy women to routinely take HRT to prevent heart disease and osteoporosis. If you are *not* at risk and your health is monitored regularly, there is little evidence that adding HRT will significantly prolong your life or prevent bone fractures.[5] There is, however, sufficient research to indicate that women at high risk for developing either heart disease or osteoporosis may benefit greatly from hormone or SERMs treatment. Each woman needs to carefully analyse her own situation and discuss with her doctor the potential benefits and risks in her own case. The charts presented later in this chapter will help you do just that.

The Advantages of HRT

Prescribing estrogen for the treatment of menopausal symptoms became popular in the early sixties. Ten years later, physicians realized that women taking estrogen without the addition of progesterone had a much higher incidence of endometrial (uterine) cancer. Since then, progesterone – which actually protects the uterus from endometrial cancer – has been added. Indeed, studies have shown that women taking a combination of estrogen and progesterone have a lower risk of developing endometrial cancer than women taking no hormones.

In addition to relieving the discomforts of menopausal symptoms, and reducing risk for osteoporosis and heart disease among women at high risk, hormone therapy has been shown in reliable studies to have other significant health benefits for some women.

- Hormone therapy helps prevent urinary incontinence (the involuntary loss of urine) and sexual problems by strengthening the vaginal and urethral walls.
- Hormone therapy may have a positive effect on mood disturbances.

Studies show that estrogen withdrawal may be linked to depression and that HRT can improve these conditions.[6]

- Hormone therapy may have a beneficial effect on memory and concentration. As one woman said to us, "When I started taking hormones, I felt like someone had taken an oil can to my rusty brain." Several studies have linked estrogen deficiency to Alzheimer disease, but the clinical trials have varied in their methodology. A growing body of evidence suggests that estrogen may help prevent or delay the onset of Alzheimer disease. One five-year study by a team at Columbia University showed that, among 1,124 women aged seventy and older, just under 3 per cent of women taking estrogen developed the degenerative brain disease compared to 8 per cent of women who took no hormones. Women on HRT long-term had the lowest incidence. Researchers suggested that estrogen may slow down the development of Alzheimer disease by protecting nerve cells in the brain or by improving blood flow to the brain.[7] Be cautious in interpreting these results, however. These are positive findings but not absolute proof that estrogen reduces the risk. More studies are needed on the relationship between hormones and Alzheimer disease; the Women's Health Initiative, which is studying more than 5,000 women in this connection, will report on this in 2006.[8]

- Other emerging benefits for HRT include a possibility that it alleviates the symptoms of rheumatoid arthritis[9] and Parkinson disease,[10] prevents cancer of the colon,[11] maintains the collagen content and thickness of the skin,[12] prevents a receding jaw line (oral bone loss is strongly correlated with osteoporosis and tooth loss is reduced in women who use estrogen), and prevents gingivitis (gum disease).[13] All of these claims require more rigorous scientific inquiry.

HRT Is Not for Everyone

In light of all these emerging claims, why aren't all women beating down their doctors' doors to get on HRT? Indeed, in Canada only 15 per cent of postmenopausal women start HRT and less than half of those women continue to use it after one year. Most women take HRT for short-term symptom control, and 20 per cent stop taking hormones before the end of nine months.[14]

There are several reasons why women reject hormone therapy:

- fear of breast cancer
- negative side-effects such as the return of their periods and PMS symptoms
- the belief that menopause is a natural phenomenon that does not require medical treatment
- resentment of the medical community's tendency to prescribe without involving women in their own health-care decisions

Studies show that, when it is a woman's own choice to use hormone therapy, her compliance with use is 89 per cent over a twelve-month period.[15] Other reasons women we interviewed gave for not using HRT include mistrust of conflicting medical studies, a concern that we may not know all of the long-term effects and concerns about weight gain. Women who do not have drug plans may find the monthly prescription costs prohibitive.

So HRT is not for everyone. Nor is it a once-in-a-lifetime decision. The passage through midlife is a journey that requires constant re-evaluation. A healthy woman with an active, positive lifestyle, few uncomfortable symptoms of menopause, and no risk for heart disease or osteoporosis will likely decide against using hormones. She can re-evaluate that decision later, if she sees symptoms or changes in her health (such as a loss of bone density beyond the average). Similarly, a woman who takes HRT for menopausal discomforts should continue to re-evaluate this decision in consultation with her physician.

Some women should avoid hormone therapy because of the following absolute contraindications:

- personal history of breast cancer*
- vaginal bleeding of unknown cause
- active liver disease
- active vascular thrombosis (blood clots in legs or lungs)

Women with any of the following conditions should carefully consider the risks and benefits of HRT and agree to be monitored by their physicians:

- gall-bladder disease

---

* Some women who have been free of breast cancer for two to five years and are suffering from heart disease or osteoporosis may take hormones under close supervision. This is further discussed later in this chapter.

- uterine fibroids
- early, treated stages of uterine cancer
- endometriosis
- migraine headaches
- familial hypertriglyceridaemia (high lipids)
- chronic liver disease
- history of blood clots in the legs or lungs (personal or family members)

Guidelines for the use of hormone therapy with these conditions have changed dramatically over the last few years. Fibroids and endometriosis used to be considered absolute contraindications to HRT, but recent studies have shown that hormone therapy does not stimulate their growth and can be used when closely monitored. Women with fibroids, however, should be aware that the return of their periods may mean heavy bleeding such as they experienced before menopause. Some women with migraines may find their headaches worsen with hormone therapy; others may find that hormones alleviate their headaches. Recently, the use of a low-dose estrogen patch with oral progesterone has been shown to help some women who suffer more from these headaches.[16] This treatment can help reduce migraine severity and frequency.

On the other hand, some women have negative side-effects using hormones. They may decide that it is not worth compromising their quality of life to continue with them. Negative side-effects that resemble premenstrual syndrome (PMS) are linked largely to the progesterone component of the therapy. Women with a history of PMS are more likely to suffer these side-effects than women who never had PMS. While some women encounter none of these, the side-effects of HRT can include:

- return of periods
- water retention
- nausea
- migraine, recurrence of PMS headaches
- leg cramps, breast tenderness, limb pain
- eye irritations
- increased vaginal secretion
- fatigue, negative moods, mood swings
- cravings (for chocolate, sugar, alcohol)

Many of these side-effects can be eliminated with changes in the hormone regimen or in the type of product. For example, women tolerate a newer form of progesterone (Prometrium) much better than the synthetic versions. You can use this product if you tend toward PMS-type complaints. (Other therapy options and product choices are discussed later in this chapter.)

HRT and Breast Cancer

While the relationship between estrogen replacement and endometrial cancer (and the protective effect of progesterone) is well known, the evidence and understanding of the association between HRT and breast cancer are much less conclusive. (See Chapter 19.)

Studies to date have generated equivocal results in the debate about hormone therapy and breast cancer. In 1995, the Nurses' Health Study of more than 120,000 women revealed a 32-per-cent higher risk for developing breast cancer in those using estrogen and a 41-per-cent higher risk in those women using estrogen and progesterone.[17] Simultaneously, a prospective study showed that the risk for estrogen use was 0 per cent and 20 per cent for estrogen and progesterone.[18] One month after the release of the data from the Nurses' Study, in the *Journal of the American Medical Association*, Stanford and colleagues reported no link between hormone use and breast cancer.[19, 20]

Coming to any conclusion about hormone use and breast cancer is further complicated because the amount or dosage of estrogen has been drastically reduced over the years. Earlier studies were based on estrogen only, rather than the estrogen-progesterone combination commonly prescribed today. In addition, most studies rely on patients' recall about the dosage and the length of time they used hormones. "Ever-users" can include women who used hormones for a short time or a long time. Sometimes lifestyle factors such as smoking and diet are not taken into account. Fortunately, several studies are under way that will shed more light on the relationship between HRT use and breast-cancer risk.

Epidemiologists (scientists who study the health of populations as opposed to individuals) also point out that heart disease, not breast cancer, kills the large majority of women. Breast cancer is a frightening and significant disease – although lung cancer caused by increased smoking by women has now surpassed breast cancer as the number-one cause of cancer death among women. The familiar "one-out-of-nine" statistic, how-ever, is often misunderstood. Most breast cancers develop after age seventy; it is only after age eighty that a woman's risk for breast cancer rises to one in nine. At age forty or fifty, her risk for breast cancer is dramatically lower than one in nine. (See Chapter 19.)

PUTTING THE RISKS OF HRT AND BREAST CANCER INTO PERSPECTIVE

As this table shows, other factors in your lifestyle may increase your risk of breast cancer far more than the use of HRT.

Factor	Effect on Breast Cancer
HRT	2.3% increased risk per year of use
Late menopause	2.8% increased risk per year of delay
Body Mass Index	3.1% increased risk for every additional kg/m^2
Alcohol consumption	60% increased risk if alcohol consumption exceeds 2 drinks per day
Lack of regular exercise	60% increased risk

Source: Adapted from "HRT: An Update," *Journal of the Society of Obstetricians and Gynecologists of Canada* 20 (1998): 490–96.

In 1993, 46,000 women in the United States died of breast cancer, compared to 350,000 who died from heart disease.[21] In Canada in 1998, 5,300 women died of breast cancer, while 39 per cent of all female deaths were from heart disease.[22] Since hormone therapy could potentially reduce heart disease significantly in women at risk, some researchers argue that the benefits of hormone therapy outweigh the risks associated with breast cancer.

Many women object to this reasoning, because of their experience watching friends and family members suffer with breast cancer. Assertions that "the risk is not significant" or "even if you get it you won't die from it" are just not enough. Another factor often overlooked is that, while heart disease is definitely more common than breast cancer, it is primarily a disease of older age (average age at diagnosis is seventy-four).

Studies show that the risk may be almost negligible if you take hormones for a short time.[23] If, however, you are at high risk for osteoporosis or heart disease and may need to take hormones for more than five years, you should carefully consider your risk for breast cancer.

Clear risks include:

- increasing age (most breast cancer occurs in women over age seventy);
- family history of breast cancer;
- previous diagnosis of cancer of the breast;
- radiation therapy to the chest when younger than age thirty;
- discovery of abnormal cell during a breast biopsy;
- dense breasts.

Factors that *may* increase your risk include:

- early onset of menstruation and/or late onset of menopause;
- delayed child-bearing or no pregnancies;
- regular alcohol consumption;
- high-fat diet;
- excessive exposure to environmental chemicals and toxins.
- sedentary lifestyle;
- postmenopausal obesity.

A Question of Risks and Benefits

Hormone therapy will give a fifty-year-old woman who is at risk for heart disease or osteoporosis about 1.5 extra years of life; however, the more important factor may be the age at which she is diagnosed with osteoporosis or heart disease, and the quality of her life during the time that she is ill. Living with a chronic, painful disease, such as a hip or spinal fracture, is very hard. If hormone therapy can delay the onset and progression of the disease, it becomes an important factor to consider.

The other problem with performing a risk-benefit analysis is the lack of comparisons in the medical literature on how effectively lifestyle changes and alternative medicines can reduce your risk when compared to HRT.

Active, healthy living, for example, may do as much as HRT to both reduce menopausal complaints and prevent disease. At the moment, we lack the long-term studies we need to evaluate how successfully lifestyle changes compare to HRT.

How to Use the HRT Decision-Making Guide

The HRT Decision-Making Guide that follows will help you decide whether you should consider the use of hormone therapy. The results are based on the intensity of your symptoms and how they respond to changes you make to the way you live and an assessment of your risks for osteoporosis, heart disease, and breast cancer. You can work through the chart yourself or take it with you to discuss with your physician.

1. Check to be sure that you do not have any contraindications (Checklist 1).
2. Review Checklist 2 to see if you have any of the conditions that may increase your risk for problems with hormone therapy. Weigh any of these conditions carefully and talk with your physician about them.
3. Review Checklists 3 and 4 to see if you are at risk for osteoporosis and/or heart disease.
4. Choose the column that applies to you (bothered by menopausal discomforts, high risk of osteoporosis, or high risk of heart disease) and work through the steps that follow.

Checklist 1: ABSOLUTE CONTRAINDICATIONS TO HORMONE REPLACEMENT THERAPY

[ ] Personal history of breast cancer*
[ ] Vaginal bleeding of unknown cause
[ ] Active liver disease
[ ] Active blood clots in the legs or lungs

* Some women who have been free of breast cancer for 2 to 5 years may take hormones under the close supervision of their physicians.

Checklist 2: RELATIVE CONTRAINDICATIONS OR CONDITIONS THAT REQUIRE CAREFUL CONSIDERATION AND CLOSE MONITORING IF HRT IS USED

[ ] Gall-bladder disease
[ ] Fibroids
[ ] Endometriosis
[ ] Migraine headaches
[ ] Personal or family history of blood clots in the legs or lungs
[ ] Family history of hypertriglyceridaemia (high blood fats)
[ ] Chronic liver disease
[ ] Two or more risk factors for breast cancer (see previous section)
[ ] Previous history of uterine cancer (later stages)

Checklist 3: ARE YOU AT RISK FOR OSTEOPOROSIS?

Check off the risk factors that apply to you. The more boxes you check, the more likely you are to develop osteoporosis.
[ ] Family history of osteoporosis
[ ] Postmenopausal state
[ ] Prolonged use of certain medications (cortisone, prednisone, thyroid hormone, anticonvulsants, aluminum-containing antacids)
[ ] Ovaries surgically removed or early menopause (before age 45)
[ ] History of little or no regular exercise; or over-exercise (to the point of losing periods – amenorrhea)
[ ] History of anorexia or bulimia
[ ] Thin with small bones
[ ] White or Asian
[ ] Smoker (or ex-smoker) or heavy alcohol user
[ ] Low intake of calcium throughout life

Checklist 4: ARE YOU AT RISK FOR HEART DISEASE?

Check off the risk factors that apply to you. The more boxes you check, the more likely you are to develop heart disease.

[ ] Hypertension (high blood pressure)
[ ] Hyperlipidemia (elevated cholesterol or blood fats)
[ ] Diabetes
[ ] Smoking
[ ] Obesity, especially around the waist
[ ] Inactive lifestyle
[ ] High-fat diet
[ ] Premature menopause (surgical or natural)
[ ] Difficulties dealing with stress

More Choices: How Should I Take HRT?

Estrogen and progesterone come in a number of forms and doses. Some women prefer to use estrogen that is derived from plants rather than that from the urine of pregnant horses. Many women prefer a natural-source progesterone (such as Prometrium) because it causes fewer PMS-like side-effects than synthetic products. Most women take their hormones before going to bed, because progesterone naturally causes sleepiness and estrogen can ease troublesome night sweats.

You and your physician should base your decision as to which form of HRT to take according to your needs and personal preferences. He or she will guide you by looking at your lipid profile, your tendencies regarding blood clotting, and whether you have gall-bladder disease and/or low bone mass. One advantage of taking pills is that this form of HRT has been studied the most.

There are several advantages to using a patch over taking pills. It releases comparatively low doses of estrogen, which are absorbed slowly and steadily through the skin into the bloodstream. Because estrogen bypasses the liver, the patch may be cautiously used by women who have mild liver or gall-bladder disease. Women with digestive problems,

A GUIDE TO DECISION-MAKING ABOUT HORMONE REPLACEMENT THERAPY (HRT)

Menopausal woman with no contraindications (Checklists 1 and 2)

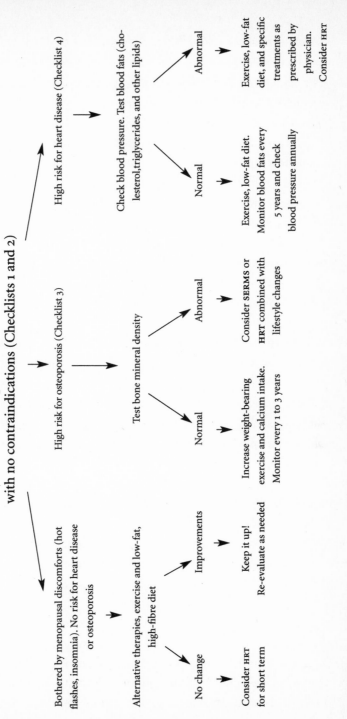

Bothered by menopausal discomforts (hot flashes, insomnia). No risk for heart disease or osteoporosis

Alternative therapies, exercise and low-fat, high-fibre diet

No change → Consider HRT for short term

Improvements → Keep it up! Re-evaluate as needed

High risk for osteoporosis (Checklist 3)

Test bone mineral density

Normal → Increase weight-bearing exercise and calcium intake. Monitor every 1 to 3 years

Abnormal → Consider SERMS or HRT combined with lifestyle changes

High risk for heart disease (Checklist 4)

Check blood pressure. Test blood fats (cholesterol, triglycerides, and other lipids)

Normal → Exercise, low-fat diet. Monitor blood fats every 5 years and check blood pressure annually

Abnormal → Exercise, low-fat diet, and specific treatments as prescribed by physician. Consider HRT

Remember: Re-evaluate annually or when you notice any changes in your health.

smokers, women with migraines, and those with high triglycerides may do better with the patch than a pill. The patch also has its disadvantages. Some women become allergic to the glue and end up with itchy red marks on their buttocks. Others have told us embarrassing stories about losing their patches in bathtubs while staying with friends, or waking in the morning to find their patches stuck to their partners' leg or chest hairs! Fortunately, new less-allergenic and better-sticking patches are now available.

Another new option is Estrogel – the first estrogen available in gel form. You apply the gel to the skin in a particular area of your abdomen, arms, and inner thigh once a day. It is absorbed within two minutes, there is no sticky residue, and women who react to the patch tolerate this form of the hormone well.

You may need to try several different doses and forms until you find the regimen that works best for you. Your physician should be willing to help you try different options and to discuss fully the pros and cons of each one. Here are some of your options:

- *Estrogen without progesterone* is commonly prescribed for women without a uterus who therefore have no danger of developing cancer of the endometrium (uterine lining).

- *Cyclical estrogen and progesterone.* This common form of HRT involves the cyclical use of estrogen and progesterone, by mouth or through a skin patch. For example, you might take estrogen on days 1 to 25, add progesterone on days 14 to 25, and take no hormones for the last three to five days of the month. Another option for women with very troubling menopausal symptoms during the week they are not taking hormones is to take estrogen every day and progesterone on a cyclical basis. A withdrawal bleed will begin during or immediately after you take the progesterone. This return to periods has prompted many women to switch to another option: a combination of continuous estrogen and progesterone.

- *Continuous combined estrogen and progesterone each day of the month.* Women who have stopped menstruating naturally and use this approach find that, after a time, the monthly bleeding brought on by hormones gradually disappears. In addition, because progestin doses are very low, there are fewer PMS-like side-effects, including headaches.

- **Progesterone only.** Used continuously or cyclically, progesterone alone can provide relief from hot flashes, help prevent vaginal atrophy (including dryness), and promote bone strength. If taken cyclically, progesterone produces a withdrawal bleed. This option is important for women with estrogen contraindications, including a high risk for breast cancer.

- **Estrogen-androgen and cyclic progestin.** Adding androgen (the male hormone testosterone) to the mix is a growing trend in HRT. While women produce a fairly small amount of androgen compared to men, they lose at least 50 per cent of that production at menopause. This depletion has been implicated in decreased libido, loss of sensation in the clitoris and nipples, thinning of pubic hair, skin dryness, loss of energy, overwhelming fatigue, and mild depression.

  Testosterone supplementation may be especially indicated for women who have had their ovaries removed. Studies confirm that these women are very likely to have a reduced sexual drive and lubrication and to have less pleasure from sex than women who have their ovaries intact.

  Some studies show that an androgen-estrogen-progestin mixture, given as pills or an injection, makes some women feel more energetic and interested in sex.[24] Other studies show that testosterone has no effect on libido in menopausal women with normal testosterone levels and helps only women with testosterone levels below the normal range.[25] Androgen also promotes bone formation and inhibits bone resorption.[26] Drawbacks include the lowering of HDL cholesterol (the good one), masculinizing effects such as increased chin hair, deepening of the voice, and weight gain. In addition, testosterone has been shown to stimulate breast-cancer cell division in the laboratory.[27] However, a study of 4,000 women found no increase in breast cancer among the women taking testosterone.[28]

- **Vaginal estrogen creams and tablets.** If vaginal dryness is your main complaint, a cream containing estrogen (about one-quarter of the amount taken orally) is normally prescribed. You apply the cream to the vulva and vaginal area once a week. Vaginal tablets may also be used.

- *Estradiol vaginal ring (Estring).* A vaginal ring that releases low doses of hormones on a continuous basis is now available. It is inserted high in the vagina and worn continuously for ninety days. The ring is soft and you and your partner will not feel it during intercourse.
- *Low-dose birth-control pill.* Historically, physicians have advised against the use of oral contraceptives after age thirty-five, but recent studies have produced new guidelines on the use of the Pill for women in their later reproductive years. For healthy, non-smoking women with no direct contraindications (breast cancer, thrombosis, liver dysfunction), low-dose oral contraceptives provide a safe, effective method of birth control. This can be a bonus for perimenopausal women who experience menopausal symptoms while they are still menstruating. The low-dose pill offers relief from heavy bleeding and bleeding irregularities, hot flashes, and atrophy of the genital urinary tract, while serving as an effective way to prevent pregnancy at the same time. Oral contraceptives can reduce profuse bleeding in as many as 20 per cent to 50 per cent of the women taking it.[29]

Emerging Trends

Lower Doses

Today we are seeing a trend toward a dramatic lowering of the dosage that is commonly prescribed. In late 1998, in a debate organized by the North American Menopause Society, one of the participants stated, "The results of the HERS study indicate the need to change the way we prescribe HRT for older women.[30] Some researchers agree that using lower-dose estrogens and smaller doses of natural progesterone may prove to be more appropriate.

SERMS

Another exciting trend is the development of selective estrogen receptor modulators (SERMs), discussed in Chapter 17. These have a protective estrogenic effect on the bones and heart but work as an anti-estrogen in the uterus and breast. This opens up another important choice for women who are at risk for breast cancer and have osteoporosis or low bone mass. Raloxifene (sold as Evista) is available in the United States and Canada. It has been shown to decrease bone loss, increase bone density, and decrease fractures by 52 per cent. It has a protective effect on the heart by lowering blood fats and has been shown to reduce the incidence of newly diagnosed cases of breast cancer. It does not stimulate the lining of the uterus; therefore your periods do not return. Raloxifene, however, will not help hot flashes and may aggravate them. It provides no relief for bladder problems or dry vagina. It may also cause cramps and blood clots in the legs.[31]

Alternatives to Hormones

Despite the hype surrounding HRT, there is no evidence that all healthy postmenopausal women need hormone therapy. Some prefer using alternatives to deal with the complaints of menopause and one and one-half million breast-cancer survivors in North America cannot use HRT. Here are some of the alternatives to hormones that may help you manage irritating menopausal complaints and increase your chances for a healthy old age, free of both heart disease and osteoporosis. (See Chapter 2 for more information on these.)

- Consider alternative therapies such as vitamins, herbs, acupuncture, and biofeedback, in consultation with a trained naturopath, nutrition therapist, and other practitioners (Chapters 2 and 22).
- Exercise regularly, including sexual activity (Chapters 7 and 11).
- Kegel. Kegel. Kegel. (See Chapter 2 for explanations of how to do these exercises.)
- Maintain a healthy weight (Chapters 7 and 8).
- Enjoy healthy eating, including foods that fight hot flashes (Chapter 8). Cut back on alcohol and coffee; drink more water; avoid hot spices.
- Don't smoke or misuse alcohol.
- Modify your environment. Lower the thermostat, dress in layers, and make sure your bedroom promotes sound sleeping.
- Join a menopause support group or pursue individual counselling to help you deal with the turmoil of midlife.

DID YOU KNOW?

HORMONES ARE BIG BUSINESS[32]

In the late seventies, reports of increased incidences of endometrial cancer from estrogen use led to a major decline in prescriptions. In the eighties, use was revived again when it was discovered that estrogen protects against heart disease and osteoporosis and that the addition of progesterone actually reduces a woman's risk for endometrial cancer. In 1992, some 35-million prescriptions for menopausal hormones were dispensed in the United States. Today it is the most widely prescribed drug. By 2013, there will be more than 50 million women over age fifty in North America. Their attitudes toward HRT will prove a highly significant commercial force!

THE BOTTOM LINE

To use or not to use HRT is a complex decision, unique to each of us. Be informed of the pros and cons and of current research. Take your time and discuss the matter thoroughly with your family physician or gynaecologist. You will then be in a good position to make a sound, sensible, and reasoned choice for yourself. Remember that trying it does not commit you to a lifetime of use. You can change your mind at any time. Be sure to look at lifestyle changes and alternatives as well.

Contacts and Further Information

Organizations

- American Menopause Foundation Inc., 350 Fifth Ave., Suite 2822, New York, NY 10118. Tel.: (212) 714–2398.
- The Canadian Continence Foundation, P.O Box 66524, Cavendish Mall, Côté St. Luc, QC H4W 3J6. Tel.: (514) 932–3535; (800) 265–9575 (Canada); Fax: (514) 932–3533.
- National Action Forum for Midlife and Older Women (NAFOW), P.O. Box 816, Stony Brook, NY 11790. A clearinghouse of information for women at midlife and beyond; newsletter called *Hot Flash*.
- North American Menopause Society (NAMS), c/o Department of OB/GYN, University Hospitals of Cleveland, 11100 Euclid Ave., Cleveland, OH 44106. Tel.: (216) 844–8748; Fax: (216) 844–8708; E-mail: nams@atk.et

Websites

- A Friend Indeed Website (sponsored by the Manitoba Women's Health Centre): http://www.afriendindeed.ca (Can also be contacted at: Main Floor, 419 Graham Ave., Winnipeg, MB. R3C 0M3, or, in the U.S., at P.O. Box 260, Pembina, ND 58271-0260. E-mail is afi@panagea.ca)
- *Menopause* (journal of the North American Menopause Society): http://www.menopause.org/journal.htm
- National Kidney and Urologic Diseases Information Clearinghouse (information on urinary incontinence): http://www.niddk.nig.gov/uibcw/index.htm
- Newsletter on complementary approaches: http://www.aimnet.com/~hyperion/meno/menotimes.index.html
- North American Menopause Society: http://www.menopause.org
- Obgyn.net (The Universe of Women's Health by David Ashley Hill, MD, and various sponsors): http://www.obgyn.net/woman.htm
- Wide-ranging discussions about all aspects of perimenopause and menopause: http://alt.support.menopause

Books, Kits, and Booklets

- *Dr. Susan Love's Hormone Book* by Dr. Susan Love and Karen Lindsey. New York: Random House, 1998.
- *Making Choices: Hormones after Menopause: A Decision Aid for Women*. Available from the Ottawa Health Decision Centre, University of Ottawa.
- *Making Hormones and Women's Health*, a booklet from the National Women's Health Network (U.S.), 514 10th St., N.W., Suite 400, Washington, DC 20004. Cost is $7.50 plus $1.00 handling fee.
- *What Every Woman Needs to Know about Estrogen: Natural and Traditional Therapies for a Longer, Healthier Life* by Karen Anne Hutchinson and Judith Sachs. New York: Plume Books, 1997.

Please see Chapter 2 for additional recommended books.

Related Chapters in This Book

- *Chapter 1: The Midlife Journey* situates menopause within the larger journey of midlife.
- *Chapter 2: Understanding the Female Menopause* provides an overview on the short- and long-term consequences of menopause, as well as some practical ideas for handling common menopausal complaints.
- *Chapter 7: The Active Living Solution* provides more information and some practical advice on improving your motivation to get active.
- *Chapter 8: Food for Thought: Healthy Eating in Midlife* gives you more information on foods and estrogen and healthy eating during menopause.
- *Chapter 16: Partners in Health Care* provides some tips on how to be a well-informed and assertive consumer with your health care provider.
- *Chapter 17: Keep Your Bones Strong* explains osteoporosis further and explores the role of HRT in preventing and managing the disease.
- *Chapter 19: Breast Health* provides more information on how to assess your risk for breast cancer.
- *Chapter 20: You Gotta Have Heart!* gives you the facts about female heart disease and how you can take steps to prevent it.
- *Chapter 22: Complementary and Alternative Medicine Is Coming on Strong* provides more information on alternative therapies.

Complementary and Alternative Medicine Is Coming on Strong

Human nature is such that we are frequently prevented from seeing that what is taken for today's unorthodox is probably tomorrow's convention.

– Charles, Prince of Wales, speaking as honorary president of the British Medical Association[1]

Herbal medicine has formed the basis for healing throughout recorded history. The ancient practices of yoga and Chinese and Ayurvedic medicine are sophisticated systems geared to returning the ill person to wholeness, balance, and harmony.

While the advances of Western medicine have been of incalculable value, they sometimes came at the cost of ignoring and discrediting many of the older systems. In the last half of the twentieth century, disillusionment with the high-tech direction and confusing studies of Western medicine has led to tremendous interest in natural healing and traditional practices. Only recently has a welcome new direction emerged, whereby Western and Eastern or alternative approaches are beginning to work together to promote good health.

Complementary and alternative medicine (CAM) covers a broad range of healing philosophies, treatments, and therapies. Sometimes these are used alone (often referred to as "alternative"), in combination with other alternative therapies, or in conjunction with conventional Western therapies (sometimes referred to as "complementary").

This chapter begins with a discussion about why interest in CAM is increasing with both the general public and the medical community. It provides some guidelines on how to safely and effectively choose complementary and alternative therapies, and then reviews some of the specific options and techniques available to you.

The Growing Popularity of Complementary and Alternative Medicine (CAM)

In 1994, a national survey showed that 15 per cent of Canadians had used CAM in the previous year.

A study by D. M. Eisenberg and colleagues, published in the influential *New England Journal of Medicine*, found that one in three adults used CAM in some form in the United States in 1990; 72 per cent did not tell their physicians, and 47 per cent did not consult either a medical or alternative practitioner about the use of such medicines. The same study reported that consumers were willing to spend $13.7 billion (U.S.) in 1990 for these services – more than the $12.8 billion (U.S.) spent on hospitalization during the same period.[2] The Canadian market for herbal medicines alone was estimated at $150 million in 1995.[3]

Who are the people most likely to use CAM and why aren't they telling their family physicians? A national study in Canada showed that use was most common among midlife women, aged forty-five to sixty-four, and by people in higher-income groups. CAM practitioners report that, depending on their orientation and expertise, the range of problems brought to them include musculoskeletal disorders (such as chronic back pain), headaches, chronic fatigue, anxiety, and cancer.[4]

Until recently, many physicians in Canada and the United States were both uneasy and uninformed about the potential value of alternative therapies. Only now are they beginning to consider CAM as a complement to conventional medical practice. Many therapies can be used in conjunction with medical care and vice versa. For example, chiropractic treatments may be combined with prescription pain relievers to relieve low-back pain; medical treatment for migraine headaches may be complemented with massage therapy, biofeedback, and acupuncture.

Popular interest has prompted the U.S. National Institutes of Health to establish a National Center for Complementary and Alternative Medicine to evaluate the safety and effectiveness of a number of alternative therapies and see how they might augment conventional treatments. This group has developed an excellent website (see the end of this chapter), which should be the first stop for consumers who are considering the use of alternative therapies. In Canada at the time of writing, the federal Minister of Health had just announced the development of a national strategy on CAM and a variety of medical groups have created websites and published papers and special supplements on the subject.

The increased interest has also resulted in some medical schools in Canada and the United States adding the study of CAM to their curriculae. In the United States, some insurance companies now cover selected complementary therapies. In Canada, medical insurance coverage varies across the country and, again at the time of writing, was generally limited to a specific number of select treatments, including massage therapy, chiropractic treatments, and acupuncture.

Why Are People Attracted to CAM?

People turn to complementary and alternative medicine for many reasons. Some like the focus on prevention in CAM. Others prefer the style of complementary and alternative practitioners, who focus on treating the individual as a whole person. Some people turn to CAM when they feel that Western medicine has let them down. For example, people often use complementary and alternative therapies when they have multiple complaints or illnesses such as chronic fatigue or cancer that are not addressed or cured by conventional medicine.

The basic principle behind most complementary and alternative therapies is that illness represents a lack of harmony in the way the body, mind, and spirit work together. Treatment primarily aims at mobilizing the body's own healing mechanisms to restore balance and health in the whole system. This holistic philosophy sees sickness as a combination of physical illness, emotional disharmony, and environmental stress which negatively affects the immune system and makes us vulnerable to more disease.

Certain complementary and alternative therapies, such as naturopathy and homeopathy involve a very detailed look at all aspects of a person's life, from nutrition and sleep patterns to the amount of self-awareness and social support one has. Because CAM works on the basis of a healing partnership between clients and practitioners, clients usually feel that they are taking charge of their illness, often for the first time.

Research indicates that having a sense of control and playing an active role in one's own health care promotes healing. In a world in which we often feel that so much is out of our control, it is empowering to feel in charge of our own health and to be able to do something about a problem that often cannot be solved by modern medicine.

At the same time that consumers are seeking out complementary and alternative practitioners, they are also looking for alternative pills and elixirs that can ease their pains and cure various conditions. In today's highly stressful and exhausting environment, what middle-aged man or woman has not been tempted to look for an easy fix, if not by prescription, then in the local pharmacy or health-food store? Every day the media headlines tell of another "natural" way to feel better – St. John's wort for the blues, ginseng for fatigue, echinacea to ward off the common cold. The demand for information about CAM is front-page news in many popular magazines. In 1997, *Good Housekeeping*, *Psychology Today*, the *Town and Country Monthly*, *Canadian Living*, and *Time* all featured articles on alternative medicine. Medical journals are publishing frequent articles on complementary and alternative therapies.[5]

It is not surprising that the boomers are the most frequent users of CAM. Unlike our parents, who tended to see the onset of chronic illnesses such as arthritis or back pain as part of aging, we refuse to believe that aging must be associated with a decline in our health. One man said to us, "It's not fair! How can I possibly have heart disease? I always ate well, exercised, meditated, took vitamins and garlic. How can I possibly need bypass surgery?"

Women in menopause who are concerned about the potentially negative effects of hormone replacement therapy are looking for alternatives that will relieve hot flashes and other discomforts in the short term, and protect them from osteoporosis and heart disease in the long term. The 1997 Menopause Survey carried out by the North American Menopause Society found that, among 750 menopausal women, 25 per cent were using yoga or relaxation techniques, 3 per cent used acupuncture, and 25 per cent were using herbal remedies or other "natural" products to control menopausal complaints.[6] Similarly, middle-aged men who are unwilling to put up with the symptoms of an enlarged prostate or who want to prevent prostate problems in the future are looking to alternative medicines for help.

Western Medicine Has Concerns

Mainstream medicine has three basic concerns about CAM. One is a lack of hard scientific data to confirm the effectiveness of such remedies. Most physicians are unwilling to recommend therapies without this objective evidence. However, an increasing number of clinical trials and published results are appearing in the medical journals. The results of these studies will dramatically affect whether or not Western physicians will accept and recommend complementary and alternative therapies to their patients.

Second, health professionals worry that people with new symptoms who choose alternative therapies without also seeing a physician may delay an important diagnosis for an illness that should have been treated immediately with conventional medicine.

The third concern – which largely centres around the use of herbal medicines – is more immediate. Because herbal remedies do not come under the strict safety regulations that govern conventional medicines, it is always a case of buyer beware. Does the bottle really contain what it says it does? In addition, the side-effects of herbs and their interaction with regular medicines have not been well documented or studied.

In the United States, herbal medicines and other alternative drugs are sold as "dietary supplements," which removes them from Food and Drug Administration (FDA) control. This means that manufacturers can say almost anything in their ads and on their packages, although, in theory, they cannot make medical claims. In Canada, regulations concerning herbal products are currently consideration by Health Canada.

While most herbs are relatively safe in small doses, some have side-effects and some can become toxic if they accumulate in your body. Their long-term effects are generally not known, and in some cases mixing herbal preparations with conventional medicines can be counterproductive or dangerous. This is why it is essential to tell both your physician and your alternative practitioner what you are taking – prescribed, over-the-counter pharmaceuticals, and herbal or homeopathic remedies. In fact, it is a good idea to bring all of your medicines with you, so that your health care provider can check both the type of medication and the ingredients in it.

Before You Use a Complementary or Alternative Therapy

In the same way that it is important to be a savvy consumer with conventional medicine and Western physicians, it is important to check out both the complementary or alternative therapy and the practitioner that you plan to visit. Here is a checklist you can use:

[ ] Get a referral from a reliable source (a physician or a recognized organization that is accountable for professional practice).

[ ] Assess the safety and effectiveness of the therapy. Ask the practitioner if there have been any controlled scientific trials on the effectiveness of a given therapy. Be an informed consumer – seek out information from credible sources in libraries, on-line, or from professional organizations and universities (see the end of this chapter).

[ ] Find out about a practitioner's education and credentials: Does he or she belong to a recognized organization that oversees that profession?

[ ] Question anyone who suggests a fast solution to a complicated problem.

[ ] Make sure your alternative practitioner will contact your family physician if you have been in treatment for a particular concern – and vice versa. This is especially important if your condition is not improving. Alternative and Western medicines should be complementary, not contradictory.

[ ] Consider the costs. Find out what other practitioners charge for the same or similar service or consult a professional association for this information. Find out which (if any) treatments are covered by insurance.

Before You Use Herbal or Other Complementary and Alternative Medicines
Before trying herbal or other complementary and alternative medicines, consider the following DON'Ts of being a good consumer:

[ ] Do not collect or grow medicinal herbs unless you are very knowledgeable about plants.

[ ] Do not buy herbs through mail order or the Internet unless the supplier is personally recommended by a physician or alternative practitioner.

[ ] Buy herbal preparations from a credible source. Make sure the ingredients, instructions for use, contraindications, and side-effects are listed on the bottle.

[ ] Do not use herbal remedies for longer than six months without re-evaluating their effectiveness.

[ ] Do not mix herbs with conventional medicines unless you discuss it with your physician and alternative practitioner.

Complementary and Alternative Therapies: Some of Your Options

While it does not provide an exhaustive list, the following section gives some helpful information about some of the most common CAM approaches. They are classified thematically under four headings: holistic healing therapies, hands-on physical therapies, mind-body therapies, and herbal medicine. It is impossible to do justice to the complexity and history of these approaches in one chapter. Please refer to the Contacts and Further Information at the end of the chapter if you would like to learn more about any of these therapies. See the National Center for Complementary and Alternative Medicine website for a useful and expanded classification of alternative and complementary therapies and techniques.

Holistic Healing Therapies

Naturopathic Medicine is based on the premise that the body has the ability to heal itself. Illness is the result of a weakening of an individual's vital force by viruses, bacteria, allergens, stress, environmental pollution, and unhealthy lifestyle choices. Naturopaths help you restore your inner harmony, or homeostasis, by combining traditional natural therapies (including botanical medicine, homeopathy, acupuncture, clinical nutrition, and others) with modern diagnostics and standards of care. In North America, naturopaths must be licensed.

Homeopathic Medicine is practised world-wide and is very popular in Europe: in Britain, 42 per cent of physicians refer their patients to homeopaths; 32 per cent of family doctors in France and 20 per cent of doctors in Germany are using some form of homeopathic therapies in combination with Western medicine.[7] There are more than 1,300 homeopathic remedies created from a range of plants, animals, and minerals; many are available without prescription in local pharmacies. Homeopathic remedies are highly diluted medicines. Recent clinical trials suggest that homeopathic remedies have a positive effect on allergic rhinitis, fibrositis, and influenza.[8]

Traditional Oriental Medicine strives to help people maintain balance in their bodies, minds, spirits, and environments. A sense of harmony and the disruptions that affect it are described in terms of two complementary forces, yin and yang. Yin is hot and masculine, while yang is cold and feminine. Qi (pronounced chee) is the vital, nourishing energy we receive in the womb and later in food. It constantly flows between the yin and yang forces. Traditional oriental medicine includes a sophisticated set of techniques, including acupuncture, acupressure, oriental massage, qi gong (breath and movement meditation to stimulate energy), and herbal remedies, to restore balance and harmony.

Acupuncture involves direct stimulation with needles on specific points of "energy meridians." It is one of the most thoroughly researched and documented alternative practices. Studies have shown its efficacy in treating a variety of conditions, including arthritis, chemotherapy-induced nausea, asthma, back pain, painful menstrual cycles, bladder instability, and migraines, as well as in the management of chronic pain and drug addiction.[9]

Environmental Medicine is based on the premise that similar symptoms in two different people will require very different treatments based on the unique environment to which each person is exposed. Our surroundings are filled with chemicals, pollen, and other allergens in food and the environment. When a person can no longer cope with his or her total allergic load, he or she suffers illness and environmental hypersensitivities. Treatment involves assessing and changing the diet and surrounding environment.

Ayurvedic Medicine is a method of holistic healing practised in India since ancient times. As with oriental medicine, the principle behind this approach is balancing one's energies. Here, the five elements are represented by different parts of the body: water (body fluids), earth (bones), fire (digestion), air (nervous system), and ether (blood vessels and other channels). Treatment includes lifestyle intervention, meditative techniques, and herbal therapies. Published studies have documented reductions in cardiovascular disease risk factors, including high blood pressure, high cholesterol, and stress for those who practise Ayurvedic methods.[10]

Hands-On Physical Therapies
Chiropractic medicine focuses mainly on musculoskeletal disorders such as

spinal problems, neck and head pain, disc problems, posture abnormalities, sports injuries, and muscle sprains. Chiropractors use manual procedures and interventions, not surgical or chemotherapeutic treatments.

Osteopathic Medicine – the science of body mechanics – employs a holistic approach that focuses on your mental and emotional state of being, as well as your physical health. Typically, osteopaths work manually on conditions such as back pain, sports injuries, and arthritis. Through gentle, delicate manipulation, the practitioner works to bring the tissues back to their normal functioning. An extensive body of scientific work supports the use of osteopathic techniques for musculoskeletal problems.[11]

Craniosacral Therapy operates on the theory that strain in the symmetrical rhythm of the cerebrospinal fluid can cause physical and emotional disorders. Craniosacral therapy is most often used for headaches, fatigue, anxiety, and postviral syndromes.

Therapeutic Massage, including traditional Swedish massage, concentrates on the muscles rather than the joints (as in manipulation). Massage therapies are often used in spas and sports-medicine clinics to relieve tension, stress, and aches and pains. Therapeutic massage is practised by a registered massage therapist and is sometimes combined with aromatherapy and other techniques.

Other forms of massage include:
- *Shiatsu therapy* is a combination of massage, acupressure, and components of physiotherapy. It is most often used for stress-related conditions such as headaches, migraine, tension, anxiety, fatigue, insomnia, back pain, sprains, and injuries.
- *Therapeutic touch* is based on the belief that all human beings are energy fields and part of a universal life force. Ill health results from an imbalance of this energy flow, which the practitioner tries to rebalance. At least 30,000 American nurses practise therapeutic touch in hospitals – usually with palliative-care patients and people with anxiety and stress-related conditions.

- *Rolfing* compares the body to a child's tower of blocks. If any of the blocks is out of alignment, the whole structure becomes unstable. The aim of rolfing is to relieve pain through deep massage and manipulation. This is not a soothing massage; it is uncomfortable, even painful, at times.
- *Aromatherapy* uses medicinal oils to enhance well-being, relieve stress, and rejuvenate the body. The oils are absorbed through the skin during a massage or in the bath or inhaled through the nose. For example, peppermint oil is used to soothe an irritable bowel, and lavender oil is used for healing wounds.
- *Reflexology* consists of an examination of the feet and then thumb pressure applied to particular points on the feet that correspond to various organs and other body parts. Evidence of the use of foot massage dates back to ancient Egypt. It is easy to learn and simple to perform; indeed, it may be a new and pleasurable way for midlife couples to relax and enjoy each other.

Mind-Body Therapies

Meditation can decrease blood pressure and slow your heart rate and breathing rate. To achieve the state of relaxed awareness that meditation brings, you need the following: a quiet environment, a comfortable position, an object of attention to focus on, such as a mantra, and an attitude of passive awareness.

Yoga, which is Sanskrit for "union," has been practised in India for more than six thousand years. As well as gentle stretching, strengthening exercises and breath control, many yoga practices include spiritual and mental exercises intended to lead one to mystical harmony with a higher consciousness. Yoga exercises are excellent for developing flexibility and preventing many of the aches and pains associated with aging.

Tai chi, sometimes called "meditation in motion," is a series of slow, graceful movements developed by the eleventh-century Chinese philosopher Chang San Feng. Tai chi is best practised in the open air, which is why it is often performed in parks in Chinese communities. Like yoga, tai chi is an excellent way to relieve stress and build flexibility.

Biofeedback uses monitoring instruments to measure changes in the body (such as muscle tension, body temperature, heart rate, and blood pressure) in response to stress or anxiety. Learning when these changes occur and how your body reacts in certain situations can help you learn to consciously control stress reactions and may relieve or prevent conditions such as migraines and anxiety.

The Feldenkrais method, which was developed by a Russian physicist in the 1940s, helps people develop an ease of movement with minimum effort and maximum efficiency. Students learn to be aware of their body posture and tension and respond by re-organizing their movements. Feldenkrais is used for general fitness, recovering movement after a stroke, and for the treatment of chronic pain and scoliosis.

Alexander technique, which was developed by an Australian actor and dancer in the late nineteenth century, teaches you to improve your posture, so you can stand and move efficiently and gracefully without straining your body.

Pilates technique was developed by a dancer in Germany thirty to forty years ago to heal himself from an injury. It combines controlled breathing with precise movements in a carefully designed sequence performed on a mat. The emphasis is on stretching, posture, and breathing, to increase strength and flexibility.

Dance, music, and art therapy are employed in a variety of settings to foster self-awareness and to reduce anxiety, stress reactions, and emotional conflicts.

Herbal Medicine

More than 13,000 plant species are used for medicinal purposes. It would be impossible to do justice to the range and complexity of herbal medicines in this section. As much as possible, we have tried to include information on herbal therapies throughout the book. This chart summarizes where you can find additional information in other chapters:

INFORMATION ON HERBAL REMEDIES

To find information on	*See*
Female herbal remedies: black cohosh, chaste tree berry, don quai, wild yam root, motherworth, evening primrose oil	Chapter 2: Understanding the Female Menopause
Male herbal therapies: saw palmetto, pygeum bark	Chapter 18: Prostate Health
Anti-aging herbs: ginseng, gingko biloba, bee pollen	Chapter 4: The Search for the Fountain of Youth
Aphrodisiacs: ginseng, yohimbine, and others	Chapter 11: Enjoying Sex in Midlife
Herbs for depression and sleep problems: St. John's wort, valerian, kava-kava	Chapter 15: When Times Are Tough: Depression, Anxiety, and Insomnia

The section that follows presents an overview of some additional popular herbal medicines often used in midlife.

NATURE'S PHARMACY: SOME POPULAR HERBAL REMEDIES

Devil's Claw	Promoted for the treatment of arthritis. Appears to reduce inflammation; however, little is known about its long-term toxicity and interactions with other anti-inflammatory drugs. Talk with your physician before you use this remedy.
Echinacea	Used to boost the immune system and prevent infections. Not recommended for use for longer

than two weeks, since you develop a tolerance. There is no evidence that its use prevents colds; in some studies it shortened the duration of colds and lessened cold and flu symptoms.[12] Not recommended for children.

Fenugreek	An ancient herb which may help to minimize menopausal symptoms, lower cholesterol, and help control Type II diabetes. In American folk medicine it was used as a "menstruation promoter"; in the nineteenth century it was patented as America's medicine for "female weakness." Recent studies show it may also be helpful in reducing the formation of kidney stones. Used as a powder or a medicinal tea.[13]
Feverfew	Proven effective in controlled trials to reduce the frequency of migraines by 25 per cent and approved for treatment in Canada and the United States. Can upset stomach and cause mouth ulcers in some people. Should not be taken by people with hay fever or allergies to ragweed.[14]
Ginger Root	A digestive spice. Useful to counteract nausea caused by drugs, such as antidepressants and chemotherapy. May help prevent morning sickness and nausea related to flu; relieves gas and indigestion.
Glucosamine and Chondroitin Sulphates (shark cartilage)	Shown to lead to a gradual reduction in inflammation and pain associated with arthritis.[15] They appear to be safe, but long-term studies are needed. Talk with your physician about using them.
Licorice Root	A protective agent that increases stomach mucus; useful for indigestion and heartburn.

Milk Thistle	Contains silymarin, an antioxidant that protects the liver; sometimes used to treat hepatitis and cirrhosis of the liver caused by excessive alcohol or chemical toxins. No studies show that it will prevent liver illness that results from excessive drinking.
Tea tree oil	Use mainly for anti-microbial effect without irritating sensitive tissue. It can be applied to cuts, stings, acne, and burns.[16]
Mahonia Aquifolium	A remedy for psoriasis used by North American native peoples for centuries. It is made from the bark of a bush found on the west coast of North America and in Central Europe.[17]
Witch Hazel	A native medicine with astringent properties, popular for soothing irritated skin, healing minor skin wounds, and for hemorrhoid therapy.[18]

DID YOU KNOW?

Cranberry juice has an antibacterial effect. One glass per day lowers urine acidity, which prevents infections and reduces odour from bladder leakage.

THE BOTTOM LINE

Complementary and alternative medicine offers a holistic, preventive approach to good health, which involves a healing partnership between practitioner and client. CAM is best used in conjunction with, not in place of, Western medicine. Develop a trusting relationship with both your alternative practitioner and your family physician so they can communicate with each other about your health care, if necessary. Make sure they both know all the medications and supplements you are taking. Remember that herbs are strong medicines; treat them with respect.

Contacts and Further Information

Organizations

- American Academy of Environmental Medicine, Box CN 1001–8001, New Hope, PA 18938. Tel.: (215) 862–4544.
- American Academy of Medical Acupuncture, 500–5820 Wiltshire Blvd., Los Angeles, CA 90036. Tel.: (213) 937–5514; Web: http://www.medicalacupuncture.org
- American Academy of Osteopathy, 3500 DePauw Blvd., Suite 1080, Indianapolis, IN 46268. Tel.: (317) 879–1881; Web: http://www.aao.medguide.net
- American Association of Naturopathic Physicians, 601 Valley, Suite 105, Seattle, WA 98109. Tel.: (206) 298–0126; Web: http://www.naturopathic.org
- American Chiropractic Association, 1701 Clarendon Blvd., Suite 200, Arlington, VA 22209. Tel.: (703) 276–8800; Web: http://www.amerchiro.org
- American Herbalists Guild, P.O. Box 1683, Soquel, CA 95073. Tel.: (408) 469–4372; Web: http://www.healthy.net/herbalist
- American Massage Therapy Association, 820 Davis St., Suite 100, Evanston, IL 60201. Tel.: (847) 864–0123; Web: http://www.amtamassage.org
- Ayurvedic Institute, P.O. Box 23445, Albuquerque, NM 87192. Tel.: (505) 291–9698.
- Canadian Association of Ayurvedic Medicine, P.O. Box 749, Station B, Ottawa, ON K1P 5P8. Tel.: (613) 837–5737.
- Canadian Chiropractic Association, 1396 Eglinton Ave. W., Toronto, ON M6C 2E4. Tel.: (416) 781–5656; Fax: (416) 781–7344; Web: http://www.ccachiro.org
- Canadian Medical Acupuncture Society/World Natural Medicine Foundation, 9904–106 St. N.W., Edmonton, AB T5K 1C4. Tel.: (403) 462–2760; Fax: (403) 426–5650; Web: http://www.acupuncture.com/referrals/can.htrr
- Canadian Naturopathic Association, 304–4174 Dundas St. W., Etobicoke, ON M8X 1X3. Tel.: (416) 233–1043.

- Homeopathic College of Canada, 280 Eglinton Ave. E., Toronto, ON M4P 1L4. Tel.: (416) 481–8816.
- National Center for Complementary and Alternative Medicine (U.S.), sponsored by the National Institutes of Health: OAM Clearinghouse, P.O. Box 8218, Silver Spring, MD 20907. Tel.: (888) 644–6226; Web: http://altmed.od.nih.gov
- National Center for Homeopathy, 801 N. Fairfax St., Suite 306, Alexander, VA 22314. Tel.: (703) 548–7790; Web: http://www.homeopathic.org

Websites

In addition to the websites listed with the Organizations above:
- Alternative Medicine Resources (sponsored by McMaster University): http://www.-hsl.mcmaster.ca/tomflem/altmed.html
- Sympatico Health Directory for Alternative Medicine: http://www.bc.sympatico.ca/contents/health/directory
- Tzu Chi Institute for Complementary and Alternative Medicine (sponsored by the Vancouver Hospital Health Sciences Centre and the Buddhist Tzu Chi Foundation): http://wwwicam.healthcare.ubc.ca/TCICAM.htm
- University of Pittsburgh alternative-medicine home page: http://www.pitt.edu/~cbw/altm.htm
- Quackwatch: Your Guide to Health Fraud, Quackery, and Intelligent Decisions (sponsored by a panel of 127 physician specialists, pharmacists, and academics): http://www.quackwatch.com

Books
- *Alternative Health Care: The Canadian Directory* by Bonnie and Craig Harden. Toronto: Nobel Ages Publishing, 1997.
- *Complete Illustrated Holistic Herbal* by David Hoffmann. New York: Barnes & Noble, 1996.
- *Encyclopedia of Natural Medicine* by Michael Murray and Joseph Pizzorno. London, U.K.: Little, Brown, 1990.
- *Herbs of Choice: The Therapeutic Use of Phytochemicals* by Tyler Varro. Binghamton, NY: Haworth Press, 1993.

- *The Honest Herbal: A Sensible Guide to the Use of Herbs and Related Remedies* (3rd ed.) by Tyler Varro. New York: Pharmaceutical Products Press, 1993.

Related Chapters in This Book
- *Chapter 2: Understanding the Female Menopause* describes some alternative regimens for dealing with menopausal complaints.
- *Chapter 4: The Search for the Fountain of Youth* describes alternative therapies and medicines related to aging.
- *Chapter 11: Enjoying Sex in Midlife* lists some popular aphrodisiacs and herbs associated with sexual potency.
- *Chapter 15: When Times Are Tough: Depression, Anxiety, and Insomnia* describes some herbs and alternative therapies used for depression and sleep problems.
- *Chapter 16: Partners in Health Care* gives you some more information on understanding research and using the Internet to find reliable information.
- *Chapter 18: Prostate Health* describes several male herbal therapies.
- *Chapter 23: Body, Mind, and Soul* talks about the power of prayer for healing.

PART FOUR

Looking Ahead . . .

CHAPTER TWENTY-THREE

Body, Mind, and Soul

You ought not to attempt to cure the body without the soul . . .
for the part will never be well unless the whole is well.

— Plato

In previous generations, religious faith was a major support for people entering the midlife transition. But many baby boomers – perhaps more than previous generations – have rejected organized religion during their adolescence and young adulthood. Now, as they face the challenges of midlife, the desire and need to experience greater meaning in life begin to take precedence over their striving for day-to-day material success. Evidence of this spiritual quest fills bookstore shelves, newsstands, and prime-time television slots.

The enormous sales of books about the soul and new-age theories, the renewed interest in angels, and the incredible popularity of writers such as Marianne Williamson, Thomas Moore, and Jack Canfield are the outward signs of a burgeoning movement. Some boomers have returned to their childhood faiths; others are working to reshape traditional religions to increase their relevance. Still others are finding ways – outside the church, mosque, temple, or synagogue – to be spiritual people.

In our interviews with midlife men and women, we met people who are deeply spiritual and who believe that spiritual well-being is every bit as important as physical and psychosocial health. We went back to some of these people to help us write this chapter by asking them more about their experiences with spirituality in midlife.

This chapter relies on their collective wisdom and experience. It also draws on the work of a number of writers who have explored the importance of spirituality in midlife. Lastly, this chapter looks to a growing body of scientific evidence that links spirituality, health, and healing.

We hope that this chapter will inspire you to reflect on your own spirituality and how it fits within your midlife journey. Maybe you will decide to discuss it with your partner or a good friend. As we have stated many times in this book, no two people will follow exactly the same midlife journey the same way. Undoubtedly, midlife is a time of upheaval, re-assessment, and growth. We can no longer deny that roughly half of our lives is over and that death is a reality we all must face. This realization can make midlife an entranceway to the soul and bring us to a richer experience of ourselves.

Spirituality and the Boomers

In the questionnaires we first used to collect information on the experience of midlife, we often received a note at the bottom, asking why we hadn't included questions about spirituality. We began to realize that spiritual considerations were a matter of great concern to both the people we interviewed and to us.

When we thought back to our youths, we realized that the sixties culture of experimentation and rebellion had moved many of us away from the dutiful religious observances of our parents' generation in search of a more direct experience of something "spiritual." Timothy Leary and Richard Alpert (Baba Ram Dass) – the psychedelic gurus of the time – promoted the notion of direct experience, telling us to "turn on, tune in, and drop out." Researchers such as Czech psychiatrist Stanislav Grof conducted experiments that showed the importance and impact of direct experience. He did controlled, double-blind studies with clergy, some given LSD and some not. It was soon evident who had received the LSD, as they immediately reported profound spiritual experiences.[1] Then, the Beatles went to meditate at the feet of Maharishi Mahesh Yogi in India and shared what they learned with a generation who grew up listening to their music.

The boomers were "turned on" by these leaders, not just to drugs but to some direct experience of the divine which many found sadly lacking in the traditional forms of worship with which they had grown up. One fifty-three-year-old told us, "We used to go to church because it was good for us, our duty, our responsibility, not because it was invigorating and restorative. Today, spirituality has to have a more immediate sense to it to be appealing."

Another person told us, "I remember growing up in a Protestant congregation in the fifties that felt like a social club more than a place of worship. The contact with the music, drugs, and Eastern mysticism of the sixties opened my mind and heart, like nothing before had done. While I became disillusioned with that lifestyle over time, the feelings stay with me still. It is largely how I know that something exists that is greater than the individual."

Other boomers experimented with alternative forms of psychotherapy, such as primal-scream and encounter groups. The line between psychological growth and spiritual development blurred for many people as their involvement with these and other therapy techniques became an extension of their spiritual search.

Along with a growing interest in Eastern traditions such as Buddhism and Hinduism, many boomers developed an interest in native American traditions and in the feminine experience of divinity. Some women who felt marginalized by the patriarchal orientation of the Judeo-Christian faiths embraced the ancient goddess traditions, which gave a feminine face to God and made spiritual pursuits more accessible and meaningful to women. As one fifty-year-old woman said with a smile, "The Great Mother rocks! She provides me with a kind of comfort, nurturing, and juiciness, a means of connecting with the divine that I never had growing up as a Catholic girl. Many people think this is 'fringey' and touches on the occult. It doesn't. It is just a different face for what we call God."

Returning in middle age to things rejected in adolescence is not unique to the boomers. The search for the spiritual self is characteristic of all generations. Carl Jung said that we seek to define ourselves and succeed as individuals in the first half of life; in the second half of life we reach for psychospiritual wholeness. To do this, we need to develop the parts of ourselves that have been neglected or rejected. We need to honour what has been hidden in our souls.[2]

Winifred Gallagher, in her book *Working on God*, writes about a dinner party of successful midlife professionals who all described a sense of something lacking – and that something seemed to be spirituality or religion. Gallagher said, "Maybe that's the thread running through human experience, that reminds our species of what's most important and real, yet so easily forgotten."[3] She writes of the boomer "neoagnostics," who require direct experience of spiritual matters, and quotes sociologist Wade

Clark Roof, a researcher into the religious lives of the baby boomers. He puts it this way: "People are in a 'searching' rather than commitment mode. They have enormous interest in religion, but in the form of exploring and checking out and mixing things together that may or may not lead to an old-style faith."[4]

The "seekers" are looking in many different directions, so that you may find Jews who practise Buddhist meditation and Christians who say Friday-night Shabbat blessings and women who combine the ancient goddess traditions with a reverence for Mary that is shared by Roman Catholics. Many of us have lost the sense of continuity and belonging that comes from actively being part of a religious community to which our parents and grandparents belonged. At the same time we have gained a sense of adventure and a belief that we can find a form of spiritual expression that works for us. As with other areas of our lives, spirituality is largely a matter of personal choice – of picking and choosing what feels right and makes sense for us.

Peter Emberley, author of a forthcoming book on the spiritual search of Canada's baby boomers, says that there are two main themes in their search. One is the belief that spirituality is primarily a turning inward to a wisdom that lives deep within oneself. The other is a deep cynicism about the established religious institutions of society. He adds that, with all the difficulties in modern-day life, "many of the boomers are simply looking for a little grace and an opportunity to express indebtedness, fidelity, and reverence."[5]

For many boomers, "looking for a little grace" involves forging a new path or redefining an old one that can bring them closer to a source of inspiration. At the end of this century and the beginning of the next, it will be hard to ignore the Big Generation's search for spiritual meaning and the revitalized forms of worship that bear its mark.

What Is Spirituality?
Defining and understanding spirituality is a complex question which has occupied scholars and mystics for countless centuries. We do not pretend to be experts, but will try to present some of what we believe the boomers are thinking about in this area. Quite often, the question "What is spirituality?" is more easily answered in the negative. As mentioned earlier, for some, it is not found in organized religions, especially not in the ones in which they

grew up. As one man told us, spirituality is not what you find in pop culture. He found spiritual renewal through a return to the ancient religion of his childhood, in a revitalized form, in which he and other laypeople play a vital part. "The spiritual awakening is real," he says. "For me, it is about connection, responsibility, awe, and inheritance. When I wear my talus, I am connected through joy and suffering to a thousand years of Jewish civilization."

For some people, the direct experience of spirituality is most immediate in nature. One woman told us, "Increasingly, I feel that a grove of redwoods or a mountaintop is the holiest place I can be. I feel my whole being slow and calm, and I simply know that there is a power much greater than me at work."

Other people talked about the links among spirituality, social action, and community. "It is hard to be spiritual outside community," one man said. "When we enter the arena as Christians, we do not face the lions alone."

Facing the lions alone is a pervasive concern in midlife, when we long for a sense of meaning and relief from the loneliness of being human. As people move into midlife and encounter in a very personal way the inevitability of dying, the search for meaning, the "What's it all about, Alfie?" questions loom large. Because we live in a culture that supports an almost manic denial of death, it is only as our bodies begin to slow down and as we witness the deaths of parents and friends that these questions can no longer be pushed aside.

One woman we spoke with said that, as she approached her fiftieth birthday, she had moments of "a chilling reality," knowing her life was very likely more than half over. "Suddenly," she said, "an intellectual knowing (that I would die one day) collided with a visceral awareness (that I *will* die one day), and I felt scared. Of course, that's when we turn to spiritual matters. We do not have a clue about how to die!"

This reckoning with mortality causes many of us to re-assess what we have achieved, where we are now, and what is important in the time ahead of us. In Chapter 1, we wrote about the midlife journey as the loss of a certain way of knowing ourselves that plunges us into "the dark night of the soul." From the necessary descent into this turbulent place, we re-emerge with a more integrated and re-focused sense of self. For many people, this renewed sense of self incorporates a spiritual dimension.

Several of the people we interviewed linked spirituality with reaching out and connecting with others in the forms of altruism, friendship, and social action. In modern times, no one has exemplified selflessness more than the tiny Albanian nun, Mother Teresa of Calcutta, whose life of devotion struck a chord in the collective conscience of the "me" generation. Daniel Osmond, a University of Toronto professor who writes about questions of meaning and purpose in life, suggests that Mother Teresa's tireless efforts to heal the world's most vulnerable people showed that "there is a moral force that cares about the poor and the suffering."[6] Robert Choquette, a member of the University of Ottawa's religious studies department, called her an international symbol of the kind of Christianity that people in the twentieth century trust and want to demonstrate. Yet Mother Teresa never tried to convert those who came to her. In India she used to say, "I hope that you will be a better Hindu having met me, just as I will try to be a better Christian having met you."[7]

Spirituality Is Good for Your Health

Through most of recorded history, spiritual practices have been an integral part of physical healing. Shamans were called to drive the evil spirits from the sick; prayers were said and incantations recited in all early religions. With the advent of the scientific study of the body, the practice of medicine became increasingly divorced from the care for the soul. As philosopher Ken Wilber points out in his book, *The Marriage of Sense and Soul: Integrating Science and Religion*, both science and religion are guilty of dismissing and undermining the other. Now, at the end of the twentieth century and beginning of the twenty-first, Wilber sees working toward a union of the two as the "greatest challenge of our time."[8] Fortunately, we now have evidence of science and religion tentatively reaching out toward each other.

For example, in May 1998, *New York* magazine featured a visit by His Holiness the Dalai Lama to a meeting of fifty neuroscientists and biologists at Beth Israel Medical Center. The scientists hoped to "hook him up" while in a meditative state to lend further "scientific" credence to the power of meditation. One neurologist called it the most unusual intellectual discussion in his twenty-five years of medical training. At the same meeting, cardiothoracic surgeon Mehmet Oz was quoted as saying, "The fundamental argument I have always made is that, to a certain extent, we can augment our own ability to heal."[9]

Some mainstream medical schools now offer brief courses on shamanic healing and other alternative therapies to their students and continuing education credits on the power of faith and prayer in healing. Books such as Bernie Siegel's *Love, Medicine, and Miracles*, Larry Dossey's *Prayer Is Good Medicine*, and Dean Ornish's *Love and Survival* are all best-sellers.

Mind-body disciplines such as tai chi, yoga, and meditation are increasingly an accepted part of heart-disease rehabilitation programs. Who would have believed a few years ago that part of the preparation for bypass surgery would be individual sessions in hypnosis and meditation?

Larry Dossey, an internationally known expert on the healing aspects of prayer and spirituality, says that prayer is "the desire to contact the Absolute, however it may be conceived." More than 120 studies have documented the healing power of prayer, regardless of a person's religious affiliations or beliefs.[10] In his book *Healing Words*, Dossey describes one study at the San Francisco General Hospital. Over a period of ten months, home prayer groups prayed for one group of patients who were compared to a control group who were not remembered in prayer. No one knew which group the patients were in. The prayed-for patients were two and one-half times less likely to suffer congestive heart failure, less likely to suffer cardiac arrest, and five times less likely than the unremembered group to require antibiotics. Dossey suggests that the feelings of care, warmth, and love that accompany prayer are a significant part of the healing power. "Prayer is a reminder of our unbounded nature, of the part of us that is infinite in space and time," says Dossey. "It is an affirmation that we are not alone."[11]

Practising Spirituality in Day-to-Day Life

There is a Zen teaching that says: "Before enlightenment, chop wood and carry water. After enlightenment, chop wood and carry water." This points, in true Zen fashion, to the importance of how we live our everyday lives. All world religions acknowledge the need for a special time in the day and/or week for spiritual practice; it can take many forms.

We asked the people we interviewed to tell us how they practised spirituality in their daily lives, and who or what helps them the most. Their answers were as varied as their ways of worship. Here are some of the ideas we heard:

- Commune with nature. One forty-year-old West Coast woman told us, "I realize that I have to be in touch with the ocean and the mountains every day. It's not a conscious practice for me at all. But it is my spiritual grounding."
- Read stories about and by the great teachers – Buddha, Jesus, Ramana Maharshi, the Dalai Lama, and others. Read the Bible, the Torah, or the teachings of Taoism, Hinduism, and the Eagle Clan. These "teaching" stories help us gain wisdom and reflect on our purpose in life.
- Meditate. Meditation can foster a direct experience of the divine that can be calming and centring. Periodical silent, spiritual retreats can enhance your meditation practice.
- Explore poetry, both spiritual and secular. Read aloud from Rumi, Kabir, Leonard Cohen, Mary Oliver, William Butler Yeats, Robert Bly, and others.
- Sing and listen to spiritual music. One woman told us, "Sometimes, when I sing 'O Lamb of God' I feel as if my sins really have been taken away."
- Join a faith community. This is a central aspect of all spiritual traditions. In Buddhism, there are three main components: the Buddha, the dharma, and the sanga. These are the embodiment of the divine, the teachings about the divine, and the community in which to practise. A Jewish man told us, "Since I returned to the synagogue, I feel connected, like I live in a small village inside a large city."
- Find a spiritual teacher and cultivate role models: a Sufi master, an advocate for social justice, a teacher of meditation and prayer, a clergy member you admire.
- Reach out and support others: be a mentor, a community activist, a caring neighbour, aunt, uncle, or grandparent.
- Be here now. Take time to stop and savour the sunset, hug your partner, and find special moments with your children and grandchildren.
- Create rituals that are meaningful for you and your family – such as a moment of thanks before eating.

THE BOTTOM LINE

The quest for meaning and purpose is central to who we are. In midlife, this search is highlighted as we struggle to understand and accept the inevitable losses that occur. Take time to learn what nurtures your soul and awakens a sense of the sacred. As Thomas Moore puts it, "caring for the soul means making all life sacred, and then appreciating that sacredness everywhere."[12]

Contacts and Further Information

Organizations

- Contact a local place of worship or local college or university about their religious-studies courses.

Books

- *The Blooming of a Lotus: Guided Meditation Exercises for Healing and Transformation* by Thich Nhat Hanh. Boston: Beacon Press, 1993.
- *Care of the Soul: A Guide for Cultivating Depth and Sacredness in Everyday Life* by Thomas Moore. New York: HarperPerennial, 1992.
- *The Faith Factor: Proof of the Healing Power of Prayer* by D. Matthews and C. Clark. New York: Viking, 1998.
- *The Heart of the Goddess: Art, Myth, and Meditations of the World's Sacred Feminine* by Hallie Inglehart Austen. Berkeley, CA: Wingbow Press, 1990.
- *A History of God: The 4,000-Year Quest of Judaism, Christianity, and Islam* by Karen Armstrong. New York: Ballantine Books, 1993.
- *Prayer Is Good Medicine* by Larry Dossey. New York: HarperCollins, 1996.
- *Spiritual Passages* by Dean Leder. New York: Jeremy P. Tarcher/Putnam, 1997.
- *Working on God* by Winifred Gallagher. New York: Random House, 1999.
- *A Year to Live: How to Live This Year as if It Were Your Last* by Stephen Levine. New York: Belltower, 1997.

Related Chapters in This Book

- *Chapter 1: The Midlife Journey* describes the psychological journey of midlife that is intimately related to the spiritual journey.
- *Chapter 10: Growing Apart and Together: Relationships in Midlife* discusses in more detail the value of social connections to health.
- *Chapter 13: Stress-Proofing in Midlife* describes some of the mind-body techniques mentioned in this chapter.
- *Chapter 20: You Gotta Have Heart!* explores the relationship between heart health and the emotions.

Conclusion: The Time of Your Life

This book contains a lot of information about physical health. But like the seminars we give, we find that once this information has been provided, a discussion of midlife health always turns to questions of psychosocial, and then spiritual, well-being. In developing this book, we began in Chapter 1 with a description of the midlife journey. It seems fitting to end with a poem we often use at the close of our seminars. It is particularly meaningful to us and to our seminar participants. The poem is called "Warning," by Jenny Joseph:*

When I am an old woman I shall wear purple
With a red hat that doesn't go, and doesn't suit me.
And I shall spend my pension on brandy and summer gloves
And satin sandals, and say we've no money for butter.
I shall sit down on the pavement when I am tired
And gobble up samples in shops and press alarm bells
And run my stick along public railings
And make up for the sobriety of my youth.
I shall go out in my slippers in the rain
And pick the flowers in other people's gardens
And learn to spit.

You can wear terrible shirts and grow more fat
And eat three pounds of sausages at a go
Or only bread and pickles for a week
And hoard pens and pencils and beer mats and things in boxes.

---

* Copyright © Jenny Joseph, reprinted with premission.

But now we must have clothes that keep us dry
And pay our rent and not swear in the street
And set a good example for the children.
We must have friends for dinner and read the papers.

But maybe I ought to practise a little now?
So people who know me are not too shocked and surprised
When suddenly I am old, and start to wear purple.[1]

Joseph's poem is funny and outrageous. We love it because it reminds us in a teasing way to dare to become our unique true selves now, instead of waiting for some far-off time. Finding an increased comfort with ourselves is a theme that we heard repeatedly from women and men who have moved through the midlife years. One fifty-eight-year-old woman told us, "I feel so much more accepting of myself now than I did in my thirties and forties. I know my strengths and my limitations, and I can say what I want. I feel surprisingly at ease with myself." Similarly, a man in his late fifties said, "I've been through a lot and life is not always smooth sailing. But I know who I am and I feel okay about that."

In one of the Hasidic teaching stories, Rabbi Zusya, who was dying, surveyed the meaning of his life. He said, "In the coming world, they will not ask me, 'Why were you not Moses?' They will ask me, 'Why were you not Zusya?' God does not ask us to be someone else, but only to be our truly unique selves."[2]

Since midlife reminds us that our personal existence is finite, it challenges us to finish with the intense self-preoccupation that has so defined our generation. Midlife experiences encourage us to move on, to recognize that we are but a small part of something much greater than ourselves.

So maybe – just maybe – as we embrace the midlife journey, we had better practise a little of our true selves now.

A Final Word

Advances in research happen so quickly these days that, by the time you read this book, some of the information will already need updating. Yet our basic premise remains the same. Our well-being in midlife depends on not only caring for our physical health, but also for the emotional, spiritual, and social aspects of life. It depends on caring for each other as well as ourselves.

We would be happy to receive your comments and to hear about your experiences in midlife. Please contact us at:

The Toronto Midlife Health Institute*
90 Eglinton Avenue East, Suite 402
Toronto, Ontario
M4P 2Y3
Canada
Web: www.healthyboomer.com

* formerly The Mature Women's Clinic

Notes

Abbreviations

A Friend Indeed – A Friend Indeed: For Women in the Prime of Life by Jeanine O'Leary Cobb

CMAJ – *Canadian Medical Association Journal*

DSM-IV – *Diagnostic and Statistical Manual of Mental Disorders,* 4th edition

Health After 50 – Johns Hopkins Medical Letter: Health After 50

JAMA – *Journal of the American Medical Association*

Journal SOGC – Journal of the Society of Obstetricians and Gynaecologists of Canada

JSOG – *Journal of the Society of Obstetricians and Gynaecologists*

Menopause Management – Menopause Management: The NAMS Publication for Health Professionals

NAMS – The North American Menopause Society

NIH – National Institutes of Health (U.S.)

UC at Berkeley Wellness Letter – University of California at Berkeley Wellness Letter

Chapter 1: The Midlife Journey

1. Hollis, J., *The Middle Passage: From Misery to Meaning in Midlife* (Toronto: Inner City Books, 1993), p. 94.

2. Maltas, C., "Trouble in Paradise: Marital Crises of Midlife," *Psychiatry* 55 (May 1992): 122–31.

3. Gray, J., *Men Are from Mars, Women Are from Venus* (New York: HarperCollins, 1994).

4. U.S. Census Bureau (http://www.census.gov), and Foot, D. with Stoffman, D., *Boom, Bust and Echo* (Toronto: Macfarlane, Walter & Ross, 1996).

5. Official Website of the Boston Athletic Center and the Boston Marathon: http://www.bostonmarathon.org

6. Barry, D., *Dave Barry Turns 40* (New York: Crown Publishers, 1990), p. 76.

7. Organization for Economic Cooperation and Development, "OECD Health Data 1996" (CD-ROM), cited in Statistics Canada, "Deaths 1996," *The Daily*, April 16, 1998. Note: Life expectancy is slightly higher in Canada than in the United States.

8. Taylor, D.; and Sumrall, A. C. (eds.), *Women of the 14th Moon* (Freedom, CA: Crossing Press, 1991), p. 151.

9. Bly, R., *The Sibling Society* (New York: Addison Wesley, 1996), p. 35.

10. Hollis, J., *The Middle Passage*.

11. Erikson, E., "Generativity and Ego Integrity," in *Middle Age and Aging*, ed. B. L. Neugarten (Chicago: University of Chicago Press, 1968), p. 86.

12. Le Guin, U., "The Space Crone," in Taylor, D.; and Sumrall, A. C. (eds.), *Women of the 14th Moon*, p. 6.

Chapter 2: Understanding the Female Menopause

1. Greer, G., *The Change: Women, Aging, and the Menopause* (New York: Alfred A. Knopf, 1992), p. 31.

2. McKinlay, S.; Brambilla, D.; Posner, J., "The Normal Menopause Transition," *Maturitas* 14 (1992): 103.

3. McKinlay, S.; Bigano, N.; and McKinlay, J., "Smoking and Age at Menopause," *Annals of Internal Medicine* 103 (1985): 350.

4. McKinlay, S.; and McKinlay, J., "The Impact of Menopause and Social Factors on Health," in Hammond, C.; Maseltine, F.; and Schiff, I. (eds.), *Menopause: Evaluation, Treatment and Health Concerns* (New York: Allan R. Riss, 1989), pp. 137–61.

5. NAMS, *The NAMS 1997 Menopause Survey*, released at the Eighth Annual Conference of NAMS. Boston, 1997. On-line.

6. Editors, "Clinical Practice Guidelines for Diagnosis and Management of Osteoporosis," *CMAJ* 155, no. 8 (October 15, 1996): 1,118.

7. Fleming, L. A., "Osteoporosis: Clinical Features, Prevention and Treatment," *Journal of General Internal Medicine* 7 (1992): 554–61.

8. Castelli, W., "Cardiovascular Disease in Women," *American Journal of Obstetrics and Gynaecology* 158 (1988): 1,553.

9. Wenger, N.; Speroff, L.; and Packard, B., "Cardiovascular Health and Disease in Women," *New England Journal of Medicine* 329 (1993): 247.

10. Heart and Stroke Foundation of Canada (CHSF), *Cardiovascular Disease in Canada*. Ottawa, 1993.

11. Semmens, J.; and Wagner, G., "Effects of Estrogen Therapy on Vaginal Physiology During Menopause," *American Journal of Obstetrics and Gynaecology* 66 (1985): 15.

12. Farrell, S., "A Triage Approach to the Investigation and Management of Urinary Incontinence in Women," *Journal SOGC* 20, no. 17 (October 2, 1998): 1,153–62.

13. Bobinski, B., "Add Progesterone to Curb Obesity," *Family Medicine* (November 15, 1997).

14. Kronenberg, F., "Hot Flashes: Epidemiology and Physiology," *Annals of New York Academy of Sciences* 592 (1990): 56–86, 123–33.

15. Landau, C.; Cyr, M. G.; and Moulton, A., *The Complete Book of Menopause* (New York: Grosset/Putnam, 1994).

16. Lock, M., "Medicine and Culture: Contested Meanings of the Menopause," *The Lancet* 337 (1991): 1,270–72.

17. Ravnikar, V. A., "Physiology and Treatment of Hot Flashes," *Obstetrics and Gynaecology* 75 (1990): 35–85.

18. Starr, B. D.; and Weiner, M. B., *The Starr-Weiner Report on Sex and Sexuality in the Mature Years* (New York: McGraw-Hill, 1981), cited in "The Menopause: Psychosexual Context," *Journal SOGC* (special supplement) (May 1994): 1,653–54.

19. Kaplan, H., "Sex, Intimacy and the Aging Process," *Journal of the American Academy of Psychoanalysis* 18, no. 2 (1990): 185–205, cited in "The Menopause: Psychosexual Context," *Journal SOGC* (special supplement) (May 1994): 1,653–54.

20. Sarrell, P., "Sexuality and Menopause," *American Journal of Obstetrics and Gynaecology* 75, no. 4 (1990), cited in "The Menopause: Psychosexual Context," *Journal SOGC* (special supplement) (May 1994): 1,653–54.

21. Kaplan, H., *Disorders of Sexual Desire* (New York: Brunner Mazel, 1979), cited in "The Menopause: Psychosexual Context," *Journal SOGC* (special supplement) (May 1994): 1,653–54.

22. Zussman, L.; Zussman, S.; Sunley, R.; and Bjornson, E., "Sexual Response After Hysterectomy and Oophorectomy: Recent Studies and Reconsideration of Psychogenesis," *American Journal of Obstetrics and Gynaecology* 140 (1981): 725–29, cited in "The Menopause: Psychosexual Context," *Journal SOGC* (special supplement) (May 1994): 1,653–54.

23. NAMS, "The NAMS 1997 Menopause Survey," released in Boston at the Eighth Annual Meeting of NAMS, September 1997. On-line.

24. Kronenberg, F.; O'Leary Cobb, J.; and McMahon, D., "Women and Alternatives: Prevention Magazine Menopause Survey," presented at the Eighth Annual Meeting of NAMS, September 1997.

25. DerMarderosian, A. (ed.), *Facts and Comparisons: The Review of Natural Products* (St. Louis, MO: Facts and Comparisons, 1997).

26. Editors, "Menopause: Complementary Approaches," The Canadian Consensus Conference on Menopause and Osteoporosis. *Journal SOGC* (December 1998): 1,375–80.

27. Jary, H.; Harnischfeger, G.; and Duker, E., "Studies on the Endocrine Effect of the Contents of Cimufuss Racemosa 2: Invitro Binding of Components to Estrogen Receptors," *Planta Medica* 4 (1983): 316–19.

28. Etinger, B.; Mirata S.; Swiersal, L.; et al., "Clinical Trial of Don Quai for Menopausal Symptoms," presented at the Eighth Annual Meeting of NAMS, Boston, September 4 to 6, 1997.

29. Lindgreen, R.; Mattsson, L.; and Moir, W., "Effect of Ginseng on Quality of Life in Postmenopausal Women," presented at the Eighth Annual Meeting of NAMS, September 1997. On-line.

30. Chenoy, R.; Hussain, S.; Tayob, Y.; et al., "Effect of Oral Gamma-Linoleic Acid from EPO on Menopausal Flushing," *British Medical Journal* 308 (1994): 501–3.

31. Delaney, J.; Lupton, M. J.; and Toth, E., *The Curse: A Cultural History of Menstruation* (Chicago: University of Illinois Press, 1998), p. 216.

32. Freud, S., cited by Silberman, I., in "A Contribution to the Psychology of Menstruation," *International Journal of Psycho-Analysis* 31 (1950): 266.

33. Wilson, R. A., *Feminine Forever* (New York: M. Evans, 1966).

34. Gifford-Jones, H., *The Modern Woman's Guide to Gynaecology*, 1971. Out of print.

35. Evans, B., *Life Change: A Guide to the Menopause, Its Effects and Treatment*, 4th ed. (London: Pan Books, 1980), p. 11, cited in Greer, G., *The Change: Women, Aging, and the Menopause.*

36. Griffen, J., "A Cross-Cultural Investigation of Behavioural Changes at Menopause," *Social Science Journal* 14, no. 2 (1977): 52, cited in Barbach, L., *The Pause: Positive Approaches to Menopause* (New York: Dutton/Penguin Books, 1995), p. 198.

37. Shinoda Bolen, J., *Wise Woman Archetype: Menopause as Initiation* (audiotape) (Boulder, CO: Sounds True Recordings, 1991).

38. NAMS, *The NAMS 1997 Menopause Survey.*

39. Evans, Marie, and Shakeshaft, Ann, *The Noisy Passage* (Bridgeport, CT: Hysteria Publications, 1996).

40. Heilbrun, Carolyn, "Naming a New Rite of Passage," *Smith Alumnae Quarterly* (Summer 1991): 28.

Chapter 3: Is There a Male Menopause?

1. Goethe (On-line): http://www.annabene.net/topics/age.html

2. Skolnick, A., "Is Male Menopause Real or Is It Just an Excuse?" *JAMA* 18 (November 11, 1992): 2,486.

3. Valpy, M., "Man, Oh Man!" *Globe and Mail*, sec. D (August 22, 1998): 1–3.

4. Carruthers, M., quoted in the *Daily Telegraph*, from an article by Victoria MacDonald, in the *Ottawa Citizen* (January 7, 1996).

5. Sheehy, G., quoted in "Mind Over Manliness," by Sharon Doyle Driedger, *Maclean's* (June 8, 1998): 21.

6. Van Han, E.; Verdel, M.; and Van der Veldun, J., "Perimenopausal Complaints in Women and Men: A Comparative Study," *Journal of Women's Health* 3 (1994): 45–49.

7. Nichols, M., "When the Male Equipment Fails," *Maclean's* 112, no. 8 (February 22, 1998): 33.

8. Hynes, R.; and Grantmyre, J., "Current Opinions on Andropause. Part One – The Pathophysiology," *Mature Medicine Canada* 1, no. 5 (September/October 1998): 15–17.

9. McKinlay, J. B.; and Feldman, H. A., "Changes in Sexual Activity and Interest in the Normally Aging Male: Results from the Massachusetts Male Aging Study," in

Chapter 1, "Epidemiology of Impotence," in Bennett, A. (ed.), *Impotence: Diagnosis and Management of Erectile Dysfunction* (Philadelphia: Saunders, 1992).

10. McKinlay and Feldman, "Changes on Sexual Activity and Interest."

11. Tenover, J., "Effects of Testosterone Supplementation in the Aging Male," *Journal of Clinical Endocrinology and Metabolism* 75 (1992): 1,092–98.

12. Weksler, M., "Hormone Replacement Therapy for Men: Has the Time Come?" *Geriatrics* 50, no. 10 (October 1995): 52–55.

13. Tremblay, R.; and Morales, A., "Canadian Practice Recommendations for Screening, Monitoring, and Treating Men Affected by Andropause or Partial Androgen Deficiency," *The Aging Male – The Official Journal of the International Society of the Aging Male* I, no. 3 (July 1998): 213–18.

14. Editor, "Should You Take Testosterone?" *Health After 50* 8, no. 6 (August 1996): 3.

15. O'Leary Cobb, J., "Male Menopause," *A Friend Indeed* 11, no. 4 (1994): 1–2.

16. U.S. Bureau of the Census, "Population Projections of the United States by Age, Sex, Race and Hispanic Origin: 1993 to 2050," *Current Population Reports* 1996: 38–39.

17. Quoted in an article by Howard, J.; and Wagenheim, J., "Men on Midlife," *New Age Journal* (July/August 1993).

18. Ibid.

19. Diamond, J., *Male Menopause* (Napierville, IL: Sourcebooks Inc., 1997), p. 9.

Chapter 4: The Search for the Fountain of Youth

1. Moore, E. (ed.), *Collins Gem Quotations* (Glasgow: HarperCollins, 1997), p. 9.

2. Statistics Canada, Health Statistics Division, *Health Indicators*. Ottawa, 1994.

3. National Cancer Institute of Canada (NCIC), *Canadian Cancer Statistics, 1998*. Toronto, 1998.

4. Begley, S.; Hagar, M.; and Murr, A., "The Search for the Fountain of Youth," *Newsweek* (March 5, 1990).

5. "DHEA – The Promise of Youth and Health," *UC at Berkeley Wellness Letter* 12, no. 4 (January 1996): 1–2.

6. Dyner, T.; Lang, W.; and Geaga, J., "An Open Label Dose Escalation Trial of Oral DHEA Tolerance and Pharmacokinetics on Patients with HIV Disease," *Journal of Acquired Immune Deficiency Syndrome* 6 (1993): 459–65.

7. Brzezinski, A., "Melatonin in Humans," *New England Journal of Medicine* 349 (1997): 186–95.

8. Charbonneau, L. (ed.), "Melatonin: Miracle or Myth?" *Medical Post* 7 (November 1995).

9. Pierpaoli, W.; and Regelson, W., *The Melatonin Miracle: Nature's Age-Reversing, Disease-Fighting, Sex-Enhancing Hormone* (New York: Simon and Schuster, 1995).

10. Rudman, D.; Fellor, A.; et al., "Effects of Human Growth Hormone in Men Over 60 Years Old," *New England Journal of Medicine* 323, no. 1 (July 5, 1990): 323.

11. Editors, "Creatine and Androstenedione–Two Dietary Supplements," *Medical Letter on Drugs and Therapeutics* 40, no. 1,039 (November 6, 1998).

12. DerMarderosian, A. (ed.), *Facts and Comparisons: The Review of Natural Products* (St. Louis, MO: Facts and Comparisons, 1997).

13. Cadario, B., "Replace Misinformation with Facts about Herbal Medicine," *Patient Care Canada* 9, no. 1 (January 1998): 64–89.

14. Pearson, D.; and Shaw, S., *Life Extension: A Practical, Scientific Approach* and *The Life Extension Companion* (New York: Warner Books, 1982).

15. Greenburg, D., "Can Aging Be Stopped?" *Men's Journal* (February 1996).

16. Statistics Canada, "Life Expectancy Statistics, 1996" (reported in the *Ottawa Citizen*, April 24, 1998), pp. 1–2.

17. Barry, D., *Dave Barry Turns 40* (New York: Crown, 1990), p. 19.

18. Bonner, J.; and Harris, W., *Healthy Aging* (Claremont, CA: Hunter House, 1988).

19. Stavric, B.; Alabaster, O.; Blumberg, J.; and Stampfer, M., "Do Antioxidants Really Prevent Disease?" *Patient Care Canada* 7, no. 4 (April 1996).

20. Ames, B.; Shigenaga, M.; and Hagen, T., "Oxidants, Antioxidants, and the Degenerative Diseases of Aging," *Proceedings of the National Academy of Science USA* 90, no. 17 (September 1993): 7,915–22.

21. Brewer, S., *The Complete Book of Men's Health* (Glasgow: HarperCollins, 1995), p. 358.

22. Alpha-Tocopherol, Beta Carotene Cancer Prevention Study Group (Finland), "The Effect of Vitamin E and Beta Carotene on the Incidence of Lung Cancer and Other Cancers in Male Smokers," *New England Journal of Medicine* 330 (1994): 1,029–35.

23. Rimm, E. B.; Stampfer, M. T.; and Ascheriol, A., "Vitamin E Consumption and Risk of Coronary Heart Disease in Men," *New England Journal of Medicine* 328, no. 20 (May 20, 1993): 1,451.

24. Liebman, B., "The Selenium Surprise," *Nutritional Action Health Letter* (January/February 1997): 8–9.

25. Editor, "Beta Carotene Pills: Should You Take Them?" *UC at Berkeley Wellness Letter* 12, no. 7 (April 1996).

26. McGeer, E. G.; and McGeer, P. L., "Aging, Neurodegenerative Disease, and the Brain," *Canadian Journal of Aging* 16 (1997): 218–36.

27. Editor, *Active Living* (January 1984), reporting on an article published in *Medicine and Science in Sports and Exercise* (May 1994).

28. Kushi, L.; Fee, R.; Folsom, A.; et al., "Physical Activity and Mortality in Post-menopausal Women," *JAMA* 277, no. 16 (April 1997): 1,287–92.

29. Shephard, R.; and Thomas, S., *Fit after Fifty* (Vancouver and Washington, DC: Self-Counsel Press, 1989).

30. Blair, S.; Kohl, H.; Paffenbarger, R.; et al., "Physical Fitness and All-Cause Mortality: A Prospective Study of Healthy Men and Women," *JAMA* 262 (1989): 2,395–401.

31. Warga, C., *Menopause and the Mind* (New York: The Free Press, 1999).

32. *British Medical Journal* 315, no. 7,123 (1997): 164–45 (cited in World Health Network, Website for the American Academy of Anti-Aging Medicine).

33. Ross, G., "Report from the National Institute on Aging" (cited in World Health Network, Website for the American Academy of Anti-Aging Medicine).

34. Speroff, L.; Glass, R.; and Kase, N., Chapter 18, "Menopause and Postmenopausal Hormone Therapy," in *Clinical Gynaecologic Endocrinology and Infertility*, fifth ed. (Montreal: Upjohn Canada), p. 586.

35. Marmot, M.; and Mustard, J., "Heart Disease from a Population Perspective," in Evans, R.; Barer, M.; and Marmor, T. (eds.), *Why Are Some People Healthy and Others Not?* (New York: Aldine de Gruyter, 1994).

36. Stroebe, M.; and Stroebe, W., "Who Suffers More?: Sex Differences in Health Risks of the Widowed," *Psychological Bulletin* 93, no. 2 (1983): 279.

37. Hawkes, K. "Nature's Food Furnishing Granny Factor," *Proceedings of the National Academy of Science* 95 1995: 1,336.

38. Rinzler, C., *Why Eve Doesn't Have an Adam's Apple: A Dictionary of Sex Differences* (New York: Facts on File, 1996), quoting "New Twist to Marriage and Mortality," *Science News* (October 27, 1990): 93.

39. Cayol, T., "Frenchwoman, 122, Known as Oldest Person," *Globe and Mail*, August 5, 1997, pp. A1, A15.

Chapter 5: Making Changes That Last!

1. Kettering, C., quoted in McWilliams, J.-R.; and McWilliams, P., *Life 101* (Los Angeles: Prelude Press, 1991), p. 224.

2. Health and Welfare Canada, *Achieving Health for All: A Framework for Health Promotion* (Ottawa, 1986).

3. Ornstein, R.; Sobel, D., *Healthy Pleasures* (New York: Addison Wesley, 1989).

4. Leonard, G., *Mastery: The Keys to Success and Long-Term Fulfillment* (New York: Plume Books, 1992).

5. Prochaska, J.; Norcross, J.; Diclemente, C., *Changing for Good* (New York: Avon Books, 1995).

Chapter 6: Wrinkles, Chin Hairs, and Baldness

1. Shephard, R.; and Thomas, S., *Fit after Fifty* (Vancouver and Washington, DC: Self-Counsel Press, 1989).

2. Northrop, C., *Women's Bodies, Women's Wisdom* (New York: Bantam Books, 1994).

3. Editors, University of Toronto Faculty of Medicine, "New Help for Wrinkles," *Health News* 13, no. 5 (October 1995): 6–7.

4. National Cancer Institute of Canada (NCIC) and Statistics Canada, *Canadian Cancer Statistics, 1997*. Toronto, 1997.

5. Statistics Canada, *National Population Health Survey, 1996–97* (special tabulations).

6. Editors, "Deadly Sunspots," *American Health* (January/February 1996): 13.

7. Statistics Canada, *Sun Exposure Survey*, 1996, Ottawa: Statistics Canada, 1996 (special tabulations).

8. Adamson, P.; and Pollack, S., "Help for Aging Skin," *Patient Care Canada* 6, no. 7, (September 1995).

9. Groot, D.; and Johnston, P., *Young as You Look: Medical and Natural Alternatives to Improve Your Appearance* (Edmonton, AB: InForum, 1993).

10. Wigod, R., "Fit to Be Old: How to Stay Young and Vibrant as You Age," *Ottawa Citizen* (October 26, 1996).

11. Kuster, W.; and Happle, R., "The Inheritance of Common Baldness: Two B or Not Two B," *Journal of the American Academy of Dermatology* 11 (1984): 921–26.

12. Roberts, M., "Finasteride Study Presents New Hope for Balding Men," *Family Practice* 10, no. 9 (April 6, 1998).

13. Editors, "Hair Loss: Does Anything Really Help?" *Consumer Reports* 61, no. 8 (August 1996): 62.

14. Brewer, S., *The Complete Book of Men's Health* (Glasgow: HarperCollins, 1995), p. 231.

15. Cobb, K., *Men's Fitness Magazine's Complete Guide to Health and Well-Being* (New York: HarperCollins, 1996), p. 134.

16. Rinzler, C., *Why Eve Doesn't Have an Adam's Apple: A Dictionary of Sex Differences* (New York: Facts on File, 1996), p. 4.

17. Melamed, E., *Mirror, Mirror: The Terror of Not Being Young* (New York: Linden Press/Simon & Schuster, 1983).

18. Heilbrun, C., "Naming a New Rite of Passage," *Smith Alumnae Quarterly* (summer 1991): 27.

19. Greer, G., *The Change: Women, Aging, and the Menopause* (Toronto, New York: Knopf Canada, Knopf, 1991), p. 378.

Chapter 7: The Active Living Solution

1. Orban, W., "Active Living for Older Adults: A Model for Optimal Active Living," in Quinney, A.; Gauvin, L.; and Wall, T. (eds.), *Toward Active Living: Proceedings of the International Conference on Physical Activity, Fitness and Health* (Champaign, IL: Human Kinetics, 1994).

2. Blair, S.; Brill, P.; Barlow, C., "Physical Activity and Disease Prevention," in Quinney, A.; Gauvin, L.; and Wall, T. (eds.), *Toward Active Living*.

3. Fiatarone, M.; Marks, E.; Ryan, N.; et al., "High Intensity Strength Training in Nonagenarians," *JAMA* 263 (1990): 3,029–34.

4. Bouchard, C.; Shephard, R.; and Stephens, T. (eds.), *Physical Activity, Fitness and Health-Consensus Statement* (Windsor, ON: Human Kinetics, 1993).

5. Melpomene Institute for Women's Health Research, *The Bodywise Woman* (Champaign, IL: Prentice-Hall, 1993).

6. McCauley, E., "Enhancing Psychological Health Through Physical Activity," in Quinney, A.; Gauvin, L.; and Wall, T. (eds.), *Toward Active Living.*

7. Libby, R., "Love Muscles," *Prime Health and Fitness* (summer 1997): 63–67.

8. Wells, C., "Physical Activity and Women's Health" (President's Council on Physical Fitness and Sports), *Physical Activity and Fitness Research Digest* 2, no. 5 (March 1996): 1–2.

9. Federal, Provincial, and Territorial Advisory Committee on Population Health, Chapter 52, "Exercise," *Report on the Health of Canadians* (Toronto: Health Canada, 1996), pp. 218–21.

10. Bombeck, E., cited in John-Roger and McWilliams, P., *Life 101* (Los Angeles: Prelude Press, 1991), p. 272.

11. Centers for Disease Control and Prevention, *Surgeon General's Report on Physical Activity and Health* (Washington, DC: U.S. Department of Health and Human Services and the President's Council on Physical Fitness and Sports, 1996).

12. Barbara Drinkwater, "Physical Activity and Health Outcomes in Women," in Quinney, A.; Gauvin, L.; and Wall, T. (eds.), *Toward Active Living.*

13. Bailey, C., *The New Fit or Fat* (Boston: Houghton Mifflin, 1991).

14. Nelson, M., *Strong Women Stay Young* (New York: Bantam Books, 1997).

15. Ibid.

16. Califano, J., "Just Look at Us Now!" *American Health* (May 1997): 46–49.

Chapter 8: Food for Thought: Healthy Eating in Midlife

1. In Fuchs, R. D., *You Said a Mouthful: Wise and Witty Quotations about Food* (New York: St. Martin's Press, 1996).

2. Canadian Foundation for Dietetic Research, Dietitians of Canada, and Kraft Canada, *Speaking of Food and Eating: A Consumer's Perspective* (Toronto: Canadian Foundation for Dietetic Research, 1997).

3. Federal, Provincial, and Territorial Advisory Committee on Population Health, *Report on the Health of Canadians* (Toronto: Health Canada, 1996), p. 283.

4. Centers for Disease Control and Prevention, National Center for Health Statistics (U.S.), *National Health and Nutrition Examination Survey, 1991.* http://www.cdc.gov/nchswww

5. World Cancer Research Fund, American Institute for Cancer Research, *Food, Nutrition and the Prevention of Cancer: A Global Perspective* (Washington, DC: American Institute for Cancer Research, 1998). See www.aicr.org for more information on this 670-page report.

6. National Cancer Institute website: cancernet.nci.nih\gov

7. U.S. Department of Agriculture, Agricultural Research Service, *Pyramid Services Data: Results from USDA's 1995 and 1996 Continuing Survey of Food Intakes by Individuals,* 1997. On-line.

8. Health Canada, *Nutrition for a Healthy Pregnancy: National Guidelines for the Childbearing Years* (Ottawa: Minister of Public Works and Government Services Canada, 1997).

9. NygÅrd, O.; et al., "Plasma Homocysteine Levels and Mortality in Patients with Coronary Artery Disease," *New England Journal of Medicine* 337 (1997): 230–36.

10. Rimm, E. B.; Willett, W. C.; Hu, F. B.; et al., "Folate and Vitamin B6 from Diet and Supplements in Relation to Risk of CHD among Women," *JAMA* 279 (1998): 359–92.

11. Stampfer, M.; Hennekensch, C.; Manson, S.; et al., "Vitamin E Consumption and the Risk of CHD in Women," *New England Journal of Medicine* 328, no. 20 (May 20, 1993): 1,444–49.

12. Ibid.

13. Liebman, B., "Vitamins and Minerals," *Nutrition Action* 25, no. 4 (May 1998): 6.

14. Morris, M., "Healthy Eating During Perimenopause," *Canadian Journal of Diagnosis* (1998): 47–60.

15. National Institute of Nutrition, "Antioxidant Vitamins and Health," *NIN Review* 25 (winter 1996): 1–6.

16. Ibid.

17. Ibid.

18. Blake, J., "Phytoestrogens: The Food of the Menopause?" *JSOG* 20, no. 5 (May 1998): 451–60.

19. Ibid.

20. Skelly, A., "The Garden of Estrogen," *Nutrition Post* 5, no. 2 (summer 1998), pp. 8–9.

21. Anderson, J.; Johnstone, B.; and Cook-Newell, M., "Meta-analysis of the Effects of Soy Protein Intake on Serum Lipids," *New England Journal of Medicine* 333, no. 5 (August 1995): 276–82.

22. Schwartz, R., "Soy Your Patients Want to Eat Healthier?" *Family Practice* 10, no. 9 (April 6, 1998): 22.

23. Wing, R.; Matthews, K.; Kuller, L.; et al., "Weight Gain at the Time of Menopause," *Archives of Internal Medicine* 151 (1991): 97–102.

24. Espeland, M.; et al. "Effect of Postmenopausal HRT in Body Weight and Waist and Hip Girth," *Journal of Clinical Endocrinology and Metabolism* 82 (1997): 82.

25. Kahn, H.; Calle, E.; Thun, M. J.; et al., "Stable Behaviours Associated with Adult's Ten Year Change in Body Mass Index and Likelihood of Gain at the Waist," *American Journal of Public Health* 87 (1997): 747–54.

26. Health and Welfare Canada, *Canadian Guidelines for Healthy Weights.* (Booklet.) Ottawa, 1988.

27. Health and Welfare Canada, *Promoting Healthy Weights: A Discussion Paper.* (Booklet.) Ottawa, 1988.

28. National Heart, Lung and Blood Institute Obesity Education Initiative Expert Panel in co-operation with the National Institute of Diabetes and Digestive and

Kidney Diseases, *Clinical Guidelines on the Identification, Evaluation and Treatment of Obesity in Adults*. See *Obesity Research* 6, no. 2 (1998).

Additional General References

- Barr, S., "Food for Thought: Nutrition after 50," *Canadian Journal of Continuing Medical Education* (November 1996): 89–100.
- Mestel, R., "Soy Wonder," *Health* (January/February 1998): 83–86.
- Morris, M., "Healthy Eating During Menopause," *Canadian Journal of Diagnosis* (January 1998): 27–47.
- Nutrition Promotion Program, *Nutrition Matters*, newsletter produced by Toronto Public Health Department and Regions of York and Peel, summer/fall 1997 and winter 1998 issues.

Chapter 9: The Boomer's Drugs of Choice

1. Fitzgerald, F. Scott, in *Collins Gem Quotations* (Glasgow: HarperCollins, 1997).
2. Federal, Provincial, and Territorial Advisory Committee on Population Health, "Cigarette Smoking," *Report on the Health of Canadians* (Toronto: Health Canada, 1996), pp. 184–90. Note: Statistics in the United States are similar.
3. Editors, "Alcohol: Weighing the Benefits and Risks for You," *UC at Berkeley Wellness Letter* 13, no. 11 (August 1997): 4.
4. Federal, Provincial, and Territorial Advisory Committee on Population Health, "Alcohol and Drug Use," *Report on the Health of Canadians*, pp. 193–202.
5. Editors, University of Toronto Faculty of Medicine, "Is Moderate Drinking Good for You?" *Health News* 13, no. 12 (April 1995): 2.
6. Addiction Research Foundation of Ontario, Canadian Centre on Substance Abuse, "Moderate Drinking and Health: A Joint Policy Statement Based on the International Symposium on Moderate Drinking and Health (1993)," *CMAJ* 151, no. 6 (1994): 821–24.
7. CrownLife and ParticipACTION, *Quality of Life* newsletter, fall 1997.
8. Editors, *Executive Health's Good Health Report* 32, no. 11 (August 1996): 6.
9. Ashley, M. J.; and the Tobacco Research Unit, University of Toronto, *The Health Effects of Tobacco Use* (Ottawa: National Clearinghouse on Tobacco and Health, March 1995).
10. Editors, "Smoking Your Sex Life Away?" *American Health*, reporting on a study published in the *Journal of Urology* (December 1991): 11.
11. Editors, "Fearing Impotence?" *Smoking or Health Update*, reporting on a study in *Quit Newsletter*, 1994, and *La Presse* (Montreal), October 23, 1994. Canadian Council on Smoking and Health 22, no. 1 (spring 1995): 11.
12. Editors, *UC at Berkeley Wellness Letter*, reporting on a study published in *The Lancet* (December 1996); 13, no. 6 (March 1997): 8.

13. Ashley, M. J.; and the Tobacco Research Unit, University of Toronto, *The Health Effects of Tobacco Use*.

14. Rinzler, C. A., *Mayo Clinic Health Letter* (April 1987), quoted in Rinzler, C., *Why Eve Doesn't Have an Adam's Apple* (New York: Facts on File, 1996).

15. Ashley, M. J.; and the Tobacco Research Unit, University of Toronto, *The Health Effects of Tobacco Use*.

16. Adapted from a story told in Prochaska, J.; Norcross, J.; and Diclemente, C., *Changing for Good* (New York: Avon Books, 1995).

17. Marcus, B.; Emmons, K.; Simkin, L.; et al., "Women and Smoking Cessation: Current Strategies and Future Directions," *Medicine, Exercise, Nutrition and Health* 3 (1994): 17–31.

18. Editors, Canada Health Monitor, *Survey #14* (May/June 1996): 11.

Chapter 10: Growing Apart and Together: Relationships in Midlife

1. Gibran, K., *The Prophet* (New York: Alfred A. Knopf, 1923), p. 19.

2. Swenson, C.; Eskew, R.; and Kohlhepp, K., "Stages of Family Life Cycle: Ego Development and the Marriage Relationship," *Journal of Marriage and the Family* 49 (1987): 751–60; cited in Maltas, C., "Trouble in Paradise: Marital Crises of Midlife," *Psychiatry* 55 (May 1992): 122–31.

3. MacArthur Foundation Research Network, "Study on Successful Midlife Development," described in Goode, E., "The Best Years of Our Lives," *Globe and Mail* (February 27, 1998): D5.

4. Jamuma, D.; and Ramamurti, P., "Age, Adjustment and Husband-Wife Communication of Middle-Aged and Older Women," *Journal of Psychological Research* 28 (1984): 145–57; cited in Maltas, C., "Trouble in Paradise," pp. 122–31.

5. Bly, R., Orillia Conference on Healing Relationships, Orillia, Ontario, May 1989.

6. Strachey, J. (ed.), *The Standard Edition of the Complete Psychological Works of Sigmund Freud*, Vol. XII (London: The Hogarth Press and the Institute of Psycho-Analysis, 1933), p. 106.

7. Scarf, M., *Intimate Partners: Patterns of Love and Marriage* (New York: Random House, 1987).

8. Maltas, C., "Trouble in Paradise," 122–31.

9. Tannen, D., *You Just Don't Understand* (New York: Ballantine Books, 1990), p. 298.

10. Gottman, J.; and Silver, N., *The Seven Principles for Making Marriage Work* (New York: Crown Publishers, 1999), pp. 19–21.

11. Asbell, B.; and Wynn, K., *The Book of You* (New York: Ballantine Books, 1991), p. 202.

12. Kumpusalo, E., *Social Support and Care*, National Agency for Welfare and Health: Sundsvall Conference on Healthy Environments, 1991.

Chapter 11: Enjoying Sex in Midlife

1. Friedan, B., *The Fountain of Age* (New York: Simon & Schuster, 1993), p. 59.
2. Lamont, J., "Sexuality Today: Counselling Older Patients, First the Facts," *Patient Care Canada* 7, no. 10 (November/December 1996): 95–98.
3. Kaye, M., "Sex Is Forever," *Canadian Living* (October 1991): 146.
4. Lamont, J., "Sex and the Older Woman," *Journal SOGC* 20, no. 5 (May 1990): 461–66.
5. Winn, R.; and Newton, N., "Sexuality and Aging: A Study of 106 Cultures," *Archives of Sexual Behaviour* 11, no. 4 (1982): 283–98.
6. American Medical Association, "Sexual Functioning at Midlife," *Guide to Health and Well-Being after Fifty* (New York: Random House, 1984), pp. 126–45.
7. Skalka, P.; and the American Medical Association, *The AMA Guide to Health and Well-Being After 50*.
8. Landers, A., "Men Found to Prefer 'The Act' over Cuddling," *Toronto Star* (November 26, 1995): E3.
9. Levinson, D., *The Seasons of a Woman's Life* (New York: Ballantine Books, 1996), pp. 172–79.
10. Zilbergeld, B., "Tips to Keep the Sexual Spark Alive," *Executive Health's Good Health Report* 29, no. 8 (May 1993): 1, 4, 5.
11. Lamont, J., "Sexuality Today: Counselling Older Patients, First the Facts."
12. Mitchell, D., *Nature's Aphrodisiacs: Safe, Holistic Approaches to Intensified Sexual Responses and Enjoyment* (New York: Dell Publishing, 1999).
13. Michael, E.; and Reid, R., "Non-Contraceptive Benefits of Oral Contraceptives in the Perimenopausal Woman," *SOGC* (supplement) (May 1994): 1–7.
14. Goldstein, M., "No-scalpel Vasectomy: A Kinder, Gentler Approach," *Patient Care Canada* 6, no. 5 (June 1995): 29ff.
15. Hendry, W., "Vasectomy and Vasectomy Reversal," *British Journal of Urology* 73 (1994): 337–44.
16. Giovannucci, E.; Ascherio, A.; Rimm, E.; et al., "A Prospective Cohort Study of Vasectomy and Prostate Cancer in U.S. Men," *JAMA* 269 (1984): 128–32.
17. National Center for Health Statistics, Centers for Disease Control (U.S.) [On-line]. http://www.cdc.gov/nchwww/default.htm
18. World Health Organization (WHO), *Global AIDS Surveillance: Weekly Epidemiological Record, 26 June, 1998.* Geneva, 1998.
19. Health Canada, Laboratory Centre for Disease Control, *Epi update, 1998*.
20. "Practical Guidelines for Obstetrical and Gynaecological Care of Women Living with HIV," *Journal SOGC* (supplement) (May 1994).

Chapter 12: Dealing with Impotence

1. Johansen, S., quoted in Chidley, J., "Viagra Fever," *Maclean's* (June 8, 1998): 16.

2. Sabbath, L., "The High Cost of Organic Impotence," *Family Practice* (July 18, 1994): 17–21.

3. Feldman, H. A.; Goldstein, I.; Hatzichristou, D.; et al., "Impotence and Its Psychosocial Correlates: Results of the Massachusetts Male Aging Study," *Journal of Urology* 151 (1994): 54–61.

4. Sheehy, G., *Understanding Men's Passages* (New York: Random House, 1998), p. 184.

5. Wysong, P., "Most Men Don't Seek Treatment for Impotence," *Medical Post* 33, no. 44 (Apr. 8, 1997): 46.

6. Casey, R., "Male Aging and Sexual Dysfunction," *Mature Medicine Canada* 9, no. 1 (January/February 1998): 16–17.

7. Sheehy, G., *Understanding Men's Passages*, p. 198.

8. Schneider, S., "Update on Impotence: More Treatment Options than Ever," *Executive Health's Good Health Report* 28, no. 10 (1992): 1, 4.

9. Grantmyre, J.; and Keresteci, A., "Impotence: Treating Erectile Dysfunction," *Patient Care Canada* 6, no. 7 (September 1995): 38–47.

10. Goldstein, I.; and Hatzichristou, D., Chapter 1, "Epidemiology of Impotence," in ed. Bennett, A., *Impotence: Diagnosis and Management of Erectile Dysfunction* (Philadelphia: W. B. Saunders, 1994).

11. Ibid.

12. Bain, J., "Erectile Insufficiency: Not Just 'His' Problem," *Canadian Journal of Diagnosis* 13, no. 6 (June 1996): 53–60.

13. Goldstein, I.; Luc, T.; Padma-Nathan, H.; et al., "Oral Sildenafil in the Treatment of Erectile Dysfunction," *New England Journal of Medicine* 338, no. 20 (May 14, 1998): 1,397–404.

14. Brock, G., "A Potent Pill: News for Erectile Dysfunction," *Parkhurst Exchange* (April 1997): 64–66.

15. Carani, C.; Zini, D.; Baldina, A.; et al., "Effect of Androgen Therapy in Impotent Men with Normal and Low Levels of Free Testosterone," *Archives of Sexual Behaviour* 19, no. 3 (1990): 223–34.

16. Korenman, S.; and Lue, F., *Erectile Dysfunction* (Kalamazoo, MI: Upjohn, 1994).

17. Witherington, R., "Mechanical Devices for the Treatment of Erectile Dysfunction," *American Family Physician* 43 (1991): 1,611–20.

18. Ibid.

Chapter 13: Stress-Proofing in Midlife

1. Selye, H., *The Stress of Life* (New York: McGraw-Hill, 1956), p. xv.

2. Kobasa, S.; Maddi, S. R.; and Kahn, S., "Hardiness and Health: A Prospective Study," *Journal of Personality and Social Psychology* 42 (1982): 168–77, cited in Benson, H.; and Stuart, E., *The Wellness Book* (New York: Fireside Books, 1992), pp. 178–79.

3. Selye, H., *The Stress of Life*, p. 11.

4. Ibid., p. 78.

5. Kabat-Zinn, J., *Full Catastrophe Living: Using the Wisdom of Your Body and Mind to Face Stress, Pain, and Illness* (New York: Delta Books, 1990), p. 236.

6. Barrett, J. A., *Yoga Journal for Health and Conscious Living* (February 1998): 38. (series of articles on stress)

7. Kabat-Zinn, J., *Full Catastrophe Living*, p. 174.

8. Editors, "Stress: How Big a Heart Attack Risk?" *Health After 50* 8, no. 10 (December 1996): 1, 2.

9. Ornish, D., *Love and Survival: Eight Pathways to Intimacy and Health* (New York: HarperCollins, 1998).

10. Bly, R., *The Sibling Society* (New York: Addison Wesley, 1996).

11. Paulson, B., "A Nation Out of Balance," *Health* (December 1994): 45–48.

12. Shenk, D., *Data Smog: Surviving the Information Glut* (New York: HarperEdge, 1997), p. 36.

13. Jeffrey, S., "On-the-Job Stress More Common than Injuries," *Medical Post* 34, no. 15 (April 21, 1998): 6.

14. Freudenberger, H., *Burnout: The High Cost of High Achievement* (Garden City, NY: Anchor Press, 1980), p. 16.

15. Marshall, V.; and Clarke, P., "Facilitating the Transition from Employment to Retirement," in *Determinants of Health: Adults and Seniors: National Forum on Health* (Montréal: Éditions Multi Mondes, 1998).

16. Benson, H., *The Relaxation Response* (New York: William Morrow, 1975).

17. Ibid.

18. Cassileth, B., *The Alternative Medicine Handbook: The Complete Reference and Guide to Alternative and Complementary Therapies* (New York: W. W. Norton, 1998).

19. Kabat-Zinn, J., *Full Catastrophe Living*, p. 45.

20. Hanh, Thich Nhat, *The Miracle of Mindfulness: A Manual on Meditation* (Boston: Beacon Press, 1976), p. 60.

21. Carlson, R., and Bailey, J., *Don't Sweat the Small Stuff . . . and It's All Small Stuff* (New York: Hyperion, 1997), p.45.

22. Ornish, D., *Love and Survival*, p. 13.

23. Ibid.

24. Frankl, V., *Man's Search for Meaning* (Boston: Beacon Press, 1963).

25. Kobasa, S.; Maddi, S. R.; and Kahn, S., "Hardiness and Health: A Prospective Study," *Journal of Personality and Social Psychology* 42 (1982): 168–77, cited in Benson, H.; and Stuart E., *The Wellness Book*, pp. 178–79.

26. Posen, D. B., *Staying Afloat When the Water Gets Rough: How to Live in a Rapidly Changing World* (Toronto: Key Porter, 1998).

Chapter 14: Now Where Did I Put Those Glasses?

1. Richler, M., *Barney's Version* (Toronto: Knopf Canada, 1997), p. 11.

2. Cottin Pogrebin, L., *Getting Over Getting Older* (New York: Berkeley Books, 1997), p. 99.

3. Cowley, G.; and Underwood, A., "Memory," *Newsweek* 131, no. 24 (June 15, 1998): 39–44.

4. Cottin Pogrebin, L., *Getting Over Getting Older*, p. 98.

5. Cowley and Underwood, "Memory," *Newsweek*, pp. 39–44.

6. Ibid., pp. 39–44.

7. McClearn, G. E., "Substantial Genetic Influence on Cognitive Abilities in Twins 80 or More Years," *Science* 276 (1997): 1,560–63, cited in Hister, A., *Midlife Man* (Vancouver: Greystone Books, 1998).

8. Plouffe, L.; and Schulkin, J., "The Clinical Relevance of Estrogen in Cognition, Memory and Mood," *Journal SOGC* 20, no. 10 (September 1998): 929–41.

9. Shank, D., *Data Smog: Surviving the Information Glut* (New York: HarperEdge, 1997), p. 42.

10. Sherwin, B.; and Carlson, L., "Estrogen and Memory in Women," in *Journal SOGC* (supplement) (1997): 7–13.

11. Warga, C., *Menopause and the Mind* (New York: The Free Press, 1999).

12. Love, S., with Lindsey, K., *Dr. Susan Love's Hormone Book: Making Informed Choices about Menopause* (New York: Times Books, 1998), p. 53.

13. Josse, R., "The Evolving Concept of SERMS" (presented at the conference on Postmenopausal Health, Toronto, May 1999).

14. Coffey, C.; et al., "Sex Differences in Brain Aging: A Quantitative Magnetic Resonance Imaging Study," *Archives of Neurology* 55 (1998): 169–79.

15. Simpkins, J.; Green, P.; Gridley, K.; and Shi, J., "Estrogens and Memory Protection," *Journal SOGC* (supplement) (1997): 14–20.

16. Hamilton, J., "Estrogen, Memory, and Alzheimer's Disease," *CMAJ* 151, no. 10 (November 15, 1994).

17. Lebars, P. L.; Katz, M. N.; Berman, N.; Itil, T. M.; et al., "A Placebo-Controlled, Double-Blind, Randomized Trial of an Extract of Ginkgo Biloba for Dementia," *JAMA* 278 (1997): 1,327–32.

18. Alzheimer Society of Canada, "Is It Alzheimer Disease?: 10 Warning Signs," *Canadian Alzheimer Disease Review* 1, no. 2 (March 1998): 13.

19. Landsberg Warga, C., "Estrogen and the Brain."

Chapter 15: When Times Are Tough: Depression, Anxiety, and Insomnia

1. Longfellow, H. W., quoted in Maggio, M., *Quotations for a Man's Soul* (Paramus, N. J.: Prentice Hall, 1998).

2. Cagnacci, A.; Volpe, A.; Arangino, S.; et al., "Depression and Anxiety in Climacteric Women: Role of HRT," *Menopause, Journal of NAMS* 4, no. 4 (1997): 206–11.

3. University of Toronto Faculty of Medicine, *Health News* 16, no. 2 (April 1998): 1.

4. American Psychiatric Association, *Diagnostic and Statistical Manual of Mental*

Disorders, 4th ed. (*DSM-IV*) (Washington, DC: American Psychiatric Association, 1994), p. 345.

5. Ibid., p. 3.

6. Lesperance, F.; and Frasure-Smith, N., "Depression Following Myocardial Infarction: Impact on Six-Month Survival," *JAMA* 270, no. 15 (October 20, 1993): 1,819–24.

7. Styron, W., *Darkness Visible: A Memoir of Madness* (New York: Vintage Books, 1992), pp. 33, 50.

8. Statistics Canada, Health Statistics Division, *Health Indicators, 1997*. Statistics Canada Catalogue 82–221–XDE.

9. Health Canada, *Suicide in Canada: Update of the Report of the Task Force on Suicide in Canada* (Ottawa: Ministry of Supply and Services Canada, 1994).

10. Levitan, R., "An Overview of Seasonal Affective Disorder," *Psychiatry Rounds* (Dept. of Psychiatry, University of Toronto, Centre for Addiction and Mental Health, Toronto, Canada), 2, no. 7 (October, 1998): 3, 4.

11. *DSM-IV*, p. 363.

12. Real, T., *I Don't Want to Talk About It!: Overcoming the Secret Legacy of Male Depression* (New York: Scribner, 1997), p. 24.

13. Statistics Canada, *Mental Health Statistics, 1990–91*. Statistics Canada Catalogue 83: (1991): 45.

14. Cagnacci, A.; Volpe, A.; Arangino, S.; et al., "Depression and Anxiety in Climacteric Women: Role of HRT."

15. *DSM-IV*, p. 397.

16. Shaila, M., "Anxiety Disorder and Menopause," *Journal SOGC* 20, no. 4 (March 1998): 251–57.

17. Kinzler, E.; et al., in *Arzneimittleforschung* 41, no. 6 (1991): pp. 584–88.

18. Matthews, J.; et al., *Med. J. Australia* 148, no. 11 (1988): 548–55.

19. Coren, S., *Sleep Thieves: An Eye-Opening Exploration into the Science and Mysteries of Sleep* (New York: Free Press Paperbacks, 1996), p. 39.

20. Cadario, B., "Replace Misinformation with Facts about Herbal Medicine," *Patient Care Canada* 9, no. 1 (January 1998): 64–88.

21. Brezinski, A., "Melatonin in Humans," *New England Journal of Medicine* 336, no. 3 (January 6, 1997): 186–95.

22. Lipman, D., "Snore No More," *Prime Health and Fitness* (summer 1997): 72–74.

Chapter 16: Partners in Health Care

1. Northrup, C., *Women's Bodies, Women's Wisdom* (New York: Bantam Books, 1994), p. 544.

2. Editors, "How Is Your Physician Treating You?" *Consumer Reports* (February 1995): 81–88.

3. Ibid.

4. Ibid.

5. Editors, University of Toronto Faculty of Medicine. *Health News* 16, no. 4 (October/November 1998): 10.

6. Matis, M., "Genetics: Managing the Benefits to Outweigh Potential Harm," *Family Practice* 11, no. 5 (March 3, 1999) 1–2.

7. Jussim, D., "The Check-Up Challenge," *American Health* (April 1998): 110–13.

8. Buchan, L., "Networking: Searching for Health Information On-Line," *Canadian Women's Health Network* 1, no. 4 (fall 1998): 10–11.

Chapter 17: Keep Your Bones Strong

1. Osteoporosis Society of Canada (OSC), *Osteoporosis: Let's Talk about It!* (booklet) (Toronto: OSC and the Society of Obstetricians and Gynaecologists of Canada, 1997), p. 1.

2. Scientific Advisory Board, Osteoporosis Society of Canada, "Clinical Practice Guidelines for the Diagnosis and Management of Osteoporosis," *CMAJ* 155, no. 8 (October 15, 1996): 1,113–33.

3. National Osteoporosis Foundation (U.S.), "Fast Facts on Osteoporosis," fact sheet, 1996.

4. Harvard Medical School and Harvard Health Letter, *Osteoporosis: A Special Report* (Boston: Harvard Medical School Health Publications Group, 1991).

5. Editor, "What Men Don't Know about Their Bones," *Executive Health's Good Health Report* 33, no. 10 (July 1997): 2–3.

6. Osteoporosis Society of Canada, "Men and Osteoporosis," Fact Sheet Series No. 6. Toronto 1997.

7. Ibid.

8. Riggs, B.; and Melton, L., "The Worldwide Problem of Osteoporosis: Insights Afforded by Epidemiology," *Bone* 17, no. 5 (supplement) (November 1995): 5,055–115.

9. Peck, W.; et al., "Conference Report: Consensus Development Conference: Diagnosis, Prophylaxis, and Treatment of Osteoporosis," *American Journal of Medicine* 94 (June 1993): 646–50.

10. Osteoporosis Society of Canada, "How Strong Are Your Bones?: Assessing Your Risk and Testing for Bone Loss," Fact Sheet Series No. 4. Toronto, 1998.

11. Osteoporosis Society of Canada, "Calcium: An Essential Element for Bone Health," Fact Sheet Series No. 3. Toronto, 1998.

12. Yendt, E., "Vitamin D and Osteoporosis," *Osteoporosis Bulletin for Physicians* 2, no. 4 (May 1994). Toronto: OSC.

13. Osteoporosis Society of Canada, "Calcium: An Essential Element for Bone Health."

14. Osteoporosis Society of Canada, "Calcium Supplementation: When You Can't Get Enough from Food," Fact Sheet Series No. 5, 1998.

15. Scientific Advisory Board, Osteoporosis Society of Canada, "Clinical Practice Guidelines for the Diagnosis and Management of Osteoporosis."

16. Chow, R., "Exercise, Osteoporosis, and the Prevention of Bone Loss," *Osteoporosis Bulletin for Physicians* 2, no. 6 (March 1995): 1–4.

17. Barrett-Connor, E., "Risks and Benefits of Replacement Estrogen," *Annual Review of Medicine* 43 (1992): 239–51.

18. Schneider, D. L.; Barrett-Connor, E. L.; and Morton, D. J., "Timing of Post-menopausal Estrogen for Optimal Bone Mineral Density," The Rancho Bernardo Study. *JAMA* 277 (1997): 543–47.

19. Genant, H. K.; Lucas, J.; et al., "Low Dose Esterified Estrogen Therapy: Effect on Bone, Plasma, Estradiol Concentration, Endometrium, and Lipid Levels," *Archives of Internal Medicine* 157 (1997): 2,609–15.

20. Editors, "Canadian Consensus Conference on Menopause and Osteoporosis," *Journal SOGC* 20, no. 13 (November 1998).

21. Hoskin, D.; Chilvers, C.; et al., "Prevention of Bone Loss with Alendronate in Postmenopausal Women under Sixty Years of Age," *New England Journal of Medicine* 338 (1998): 485–92.

22. MacLusky, N., "New Concepts in Hormone Management: Selective Estrogen Receptor Modulators (SERMs)," *Journal SOGC* (supplement) (November 1997): 1–56.

Chapter 18: Prostate Health

1. Wickens, B., "Middle-age Suffering: New Hope for Prostate Problems," *Maclean's* (March 16, 1992): 45.

2. Ibid.

3. Birkhoff, J., "Natural History of Benign Prostatic Hypertrophy," in *Benign Prostatic Hypertrophy*, ed. Hinman, F. (New York: Springer Verlag, 1983): 5.

4. World Health Organization, "WHO International Prostate Symptom Score," in Nickel, C.; and Norman, R., in association with the Canadian Medical Association, *A Prostate Problem: Benign Prostatic Hyperplasia: A Physician's Guide to Care and Counselling*, Disease Management Counselling Series (Toronto: Grosvenor House, 1993): 41.

5. Nickel, C.; and Norman, R., in association with the Canadian Medical Association, *A Prostate Problem: Benign Prostatic Hypertrophy: A Physician's Guide to Care and Counselling*.

6. Cardario, B., "Replace Misinformation with Facts about Herbal Medicine," *Patient Care Canada* 9, no. 1 (January 1998): 64–89.

7. Bergess, R.; Windeler, J.; Senge, T.; and Trampisch, H. J., "Randomized, Placebo Controlled, Double-Blind Clinical Trial of Beta Sitosterol in Patients with BPH," *Lancet* 345 no. 8,964 (June 17, 1995): 1,529–32.

8. Helweck, C., "Patients Pick Placebo for Prostate," *Medical Post* 33, no. 17 (May 6, 1997).
9. Goldenberg, S. L.; Ramsay, E.; and Trachtenberg, J., "Alpha-Blocker Therapy for Benign Prostatic Hyperplasia: A Comparative Review," *Canadian Journal of Urology* 5, no. 2 (June 1998): 551–53.
10. Boyd, P.; Gould, A. L.; and Roehrborn, C. G., "Prostate Volume Predicts Outcome in Treatment of BPH with Finasteride: Meta-Analysis of Randomized Clinical Trials," *Urology* 48 (1996): 398–405.
11. Nickel, C.; and Norman, R., *A Prostate Problem*.
12. Wasson, J.; Reda, D.; Bruskewitz, R.; et al., "A Comparison of Transurethral Surgery with Watchful Waiting for Moderate Symptoms of Benign Prostatic Hyperplasia," *New England Journal of Medicine* 332 (1995): 75–79.
13. Editors, "PSA Test: How Well Does It Detect Prostate Cancer?" *UC at Berkeley Wellness Letter* 9 no. 11 (August 1993): 1–2.
14. Ellison, L.; Stokes, J.; Gilbens, L.; et al., *Monograph Series on Age-Related Diseases: Prostate Cancer*. Ottawa: Health Canada, 1998.
15. Catton, P. A., Chapter 1, "Demographics and Epidemiology" in *Managing Prostate Cancer*, ed. Klotz, L. (Toronto: Grosvenor House and the Canadian Urologic Oncology Group, 1992), pp. 13–16.
16. Canadian Journal of Oncology, "Recommendations from the Canadian Workshop on Screening for Prostate Cancer," reprinted in *Informed*, March 1, 1995.
17. Mahoney, J.; and Bora, B., "The Pros and Cons of PSA Testing," *The Canadian Journal of Diagnosis* 13, no. 11 (November 1996): 111–15.
18. Gamma Dynacare Laboratories, *Diagnostic Value of the Free PSA/Total PSA Ratio*, information flyer, December 1997.
19. Vallely, J. F., "What Are You Asking about Prostate Disease?" *CMAJ* (August 1997): 18–29.
20. Pearsall, K., "Chemoprevention: A Role for Vitamins," *Urology Times of Canada* 6, no. 4 (August 1998): 1, 13.
21. Gallagher, R. P.; and Fleshner, N., "Prostate Cancer: 3. Individual Risk Factors," *CMAJ* 159, no. 7 (October 6, 1998): 807–11.
22. Ibid.
23. Morganstern, S.; and Abrahams, A., *The Prostate Sourcebook* (Chicago: Contemporary Books, 1993), p. 35.

Chapter 19: Breast Health

1. Susan Love and Karen Lindsey, *Dr. Susan Love's Breast Book* (Reading, MA: Perseus Books, 1995), xxviii.
2. Kuusk, U., "Breast Lumps: Practical Office Workup," *CMAJ* (September 1997): 39–48.

3. Borins, M.; McCready, D.; and Eskin, B., "When Breasts Are Lumpy and Painful," *Patient Care Canada* 7, no. 2 (February 1996).

4. Canadian Cancer Society, Ontario Division, "Breast Cancer: Understanding Your Risk," fact sheet based on an article in the CMAJ 150 (1994): 211–16.

5. Editors, "Clear Thinking on Tamoxifen," *Health After 50* (July 1998): 1, 2.

6. National Cancer Institute of Canada, *Canadian Cancer Statistics, 1999* (Toronto, 1999).

7. Warner, E.; Carroll, J.; Heisey, R.; and McCready, D., "Hereditary Breast Cancer," *Canadian Family Physician* 45 (January 1999): 104–12.

8. Shafir, S., "Editorial: Genes Run in the Family," *Canadian Family Physician* 45 (January 1999): p. 13.

9. Thorne, S., "Exercise Lowers Breast Cancer Risk," World Conference on Breast Cancer. *Family Practice* 9, no. 21 (August 18, 1998): 20.

10. Editors, UC at Berkeley Wellness Letter 13, no. 11 (August 1997): 1.

11. Sergeant Brown, K., "The Latest News on Detecting Breast Cancer," *Living Fit* 4, no. 1 (October 1997).

12. Runowicz, C.; Petreck, J.; Gansler, T. (American Cancer Society), *Women and Cancer* (New York: Villard Books), pp. 48–49.

13. Warner, E., "Breast Cancer: Who Is at Risk?" *Patient Care Canada* 10, no. 6 (June 1999): 38–52.

14. Knekt, P.; Jarvinon, R.; Seppanen, R.; et al., "Intake of Dietary Products and the Risk of Breast Cancer," *British Journal of Cancer* 73, no. 5 (March 1996): 687–91.

15. Smith-Warner, S. A.; Spiegelman, D.; Yaun, S. S.; et al., "Alcohol and Breast Cancer in Women: A Pooled Analysis of Cohort Studies," JAMA 279 (1998): 535–40.

16. Fisher, B.; Constantine, J.; Wicherham, D.; et al., "Tamoxifen for Prevention of Breast Cancer: Report of the National Surgical Adjuvant Breast and Bowel Project P-1 Study," *Journal of National Cancer Institute* 90, no. 18 (September 16, 1998): 1,371–88.

17. Goel, V., "Tamoxifen and Breast Cancer Prevention: What Should You Tell Your Patients?" CMAJ 158, no. 12 (June 16, 1998).

18. Richardson, K., "SERM: Old Drug Part of New Concept," *Obstetrics and Gynaecology 2000* 12, no. 6 (September 1998): 1.

19. Northrup, C., *Women's Bodies, Women's Wisdom* (New York: Bantam Books, 1994), p. 290.

20. Baines, C.; and Miller, A. B., "Mammography versus Clinical Examination of the Breast," *Journal National Cancer Institute* (monograph) 22 (1997): 125–29.

21. Logan, D. M.; Aitken, E.; and Evans, W. K., "Breast Screening," *Journal SOCG* 21, no. 8 (July 1999): 780–85.

22. Swift, O., "It's a Go – Annual Mammography for Those Over Forty," *Medical Post* (April 8, 1997): 6.

23. The Canadian Cancer Society (CCS), *Facts on Breast Cancer* (Toronto: CCC, 1998), p. 1.
24. Baines, C., "Breast Cancer Screening: Will the Controversy Never End?" *Canadian Journal of Diagnosis* 151, no. 3 (March 1998): 65–71.

Chapter 20: You Gotta Have Heart!

1. Statistics Canada, Health Statistics Division, *Health Indicators*. Ottawa: Statistics Canada, 1996.
2. Editors, *Health After 50* 9, no. 6 (August 1997): 1.
3. Hayes, O., Laboratory Centre for Disease Control, Health Canada, "Fact Sheet: Cardiovascular Disease and Women," *Chronic Diseases in Canada* 17, no. 1 (winter 1996): 28–30.
4. Heart and Stroke Foundation of Canada, *Heart Disease and Stroke in Canada*. Ottawa, June 1995. (Fact sheet.)
5. Heart and Stroke Foundation of Canada, *Heart Disease and Stroke in Women*. Ottawa, 1996. (Fact sheet.)
6. Naylor, C.; and Levington, C., "Sex-Related Differences in Coronary Revascularization Practices," *CMAJ* 149, no. 7 (1993): 965–73.
7. Wenger, N.; Speroff, L.; and Packard, B., "Cardiovascular Health and Disease in Women," *New England Journal of Medicine* 329 (1993): 247–56.
8. Canadian Cardiovascular Society, "Canadian Guidelines for the Management of Lipid Disorders," developed at the Canadian Cardiovascular Society Annual Meeting, Winnipeg, MB, October 5 to 9, 1997. (Insert in the *Medical Post*, 1997.)
9. Heart and Stroke Foundation of Canada, *Heart Disease and Stroke in Canada*.
10. Coroll, A.; May, L.; and Malley, A., *Primary Care Medicine: Office Evaluation and Management of Adult Patient*, 3rd ed. (Philadelphia: Lippincott, 1995), pp. 69–71.
11. Blumenfeld, J., "Renal and Cardiac Complications of Hypertension," *Clinical Symposia* 2, no. 46 (1995).
12. Chockalingham, A.; Abbott, D.; Bass, M.; et al., "Recommendations of the Canadian Consensus Conference on Nonpharmacological Approaches to the Management of High Blood Pressure," *CMAJ* 142 (1990): 1,397–409.
13. National Institutes of Health, National Heart, Lung and Blood Institute, *National High Blood Pressure Educational Program: Sixth Report of the Joint National Committee on Prevention, Detection, Evaluation, and Treatment of High Blood Pressure*. Washington, DC: NIH, #98–4080, November 1997.
14. Appel, L. J.; Moore, T. J.; Obarzanek, E.; et al., "A Clinical Trial of the Effect of Dietary Patterns on Blood Pressure," *New England Journal of Medicine* 336 (1997): 1,117–24.
15. Messerli, F. H.; Schmeider, R. E.; Weir, M. R.; et al., "Salt: A Perpetrator of Hypertensive Target-Organ Disease?" *Annals of Internal Medicine* 157 (1997): 2,449–52.

16. Heart and Stroke Foundation of Canada, *Women, Heart Disease, and Stroke in Canada: Issues and Options*. Ottawa, 1997, p. 6. (Fact sheet.)

17. LaRosa, J. C.; Hunningshake, D.; Bush, D.; et al., "The Cholesterol Facts: A Summary of the Evidence Relating to Dietary Facts, Serum Cholesterol, and CHD: A Joint Statement by the American Heart Association and the National Heart, Lung and Blood Institute," *Circulation* 81 (1990): 1,721–33.

18. Canadian Cardiovascular Society, "Canadian Guidelines for the Management of Lipid Disorders," 1997.

19. Expert Panel on Detection, Evaluation and Treatment of High Blood Cholesterol in Adults (Canada), *Second Report on the National Cholesterol Education Program* 89 (1993): 1,329–445.

20. Hegele, R.; Bazanski, A.; Josse, R.; and Fodor, G., "Forum on Dyslipidemias," *Medical Post* (July 15, 1997, and October 21, 1997).

21. Heart and Stroke Foundation of Canada, *The Woman's Heart Disease and Stroke Test*. Ottawa, 1997. (Fact Sheet.)

22. Blair, S.; Brill, P.; and Barlow, C., "Physical Activity and Disease Prevention," in eds. Quinney, A.; Gauvin, L.; and Wall, T., *Toward Active Living: Proceedings of the International Conference on Physical Activity, Fitness, and Health*. Champaign, IL: Human Kinetics, 1994.

23. Editors, "Cardiovascular Disease and HRT," Canadian Consensus Conference on Menopause and Osteoporosis. *Journal SOGC* 16, no. 5 (May 1994): 12–14.

24. Glassman, A. H.; and Shapiro, P. A., "Depression and the Course of CHD," *American Journal of Psychiatry* 155 (1998): 4–11.

25. Ibid.

26. Heart and Stroke Foundation of Canada, *Women, Heart Disease, and Stroke in Canada: Issues and Options*, p. 8.

27. Marmot, M.; and Mustard, F., "Coronary Heart Disease from a Population Perspective," *Why Are Some People Healthy and Others Not?* eds. Evans, R.; Barer, M.; and Marmor, T. (New York: Aldine de Gruyter, 1994).

28. Boushey, C. J.; Beresford, S. A.; Omenn, G.; and Motulsky, A., "A Quantitative Assessment of Plasma Homocysteine as a Risk Factor for Vascular Disease," *JAMA* 274, no. 13 (1995): 1,049.

29. Nygård, O.; et al., "Plasma Homocysteine Levels and Mortality in Patients with Coronary Artery Disease," *New England Journal of Medicine* 337 (1997): 230–36.

30. Ornish, D., *Love and Survival: Eight Pathways to Intimacy and Health* (New York: HarperPerennial, 1998), p. 15.

31. Ford, D. E.; et al., "Depression Is a Risk Factor for Coronary Artery Disease in Men: The Precursors Study," *Archives of Internal Medicine* 158 (July 13, 1998): 1,422–26, in *Journal Watch* (Boston: Massachusetts Medical Society) 18, no. 15 (August 1, 1998): 3–4.

32. Lesperance, F.; and Frasure-Smith, N., "Depression Following Myocardial Infarction: Impact on Six–Month Survival," *JAMA* 270, no. 15 (October 20, 1993): 1,819–24.

33. Williams, R., *The Trusting Heart: Great News about Type A Behaviour* (New York: Times Books, 1989); cited in Kabat-Zinn, J., *Full Catastrophe Living: Using the Wisdom of Your Body and Mind to Face Stress, Pain, and Illness.* (New York: Delta Books, 1990), p. 212.

34. Kabat-Zinn, J., *Full Catastrophe Living*, p. 210.

35. Editors, "Cardiology Update," *Family Practice* 1, no. 8 (December 4, 1995): 47–48.

36. Borysenko, J., *Minding the Body, Mending the Mind* (Reading, MA: Addison Wesley, 1987), p. 25.

37. Russek, L. G.; and Schwartz, G. E., "Perceptions of Parental Caring Predict Health Status in Midlife: A 35-Year Follow-Up of the Harvard Mastery of Stress Study," *Psychosomatic Medicine* 59, no. 2 (1997): 144–49; cited in Ornish, D., *Love and Survival: Eight Pathways to Intimacy and Health* (New York: HarperPerennial, 1998), pp. 32–33.

Chapter 21: Hormone Replacement Therapy (HRT): The Big Decision

1. O'Leary Cobb, J., "The Perplexing Question of Long-Term Hormone Use," *A Friend Indeed* XII, no. 4 (September 1995): 2.

2. Furgate Wood, N.; Saver, B.; and Taylor, T., "Attitudes Towards Menopause and HRT among Women with Access to Health Care," *Menopause: Journal of NAMS* 5, no. 3 (1998): 178–88.

3. Rowbotham, M., "The Number One Reason for HRT?: Relief of Physical Symptoms," *Medical Post* 33, no. 7 (February 18, 1997): 25.

4. Hutchinson, S.; and Leong-Poi, H., "After HERS: What Is the Role of HRT in the Prevention of CAD in Women?" *Cardiology Rounds* (University of Toronto) III, no. 2 (August/September 1998): 1–6.

5. Grady, D.; Rubin, S.; Petitti, D.; et al., "Hormone Therapy to Prevent Disease and Prolong Life in Postmenopausal Women," *Annals of Internal Medicine* 117, no. 12 (December 15, 1992): 1,016–37.

6. Cagnaci, A.; Volpe, A.; Arangino, S.; et al., "Depression and Anxiety in Climacteric Women: Role of HRT," *Menopause: Journal of NAMS* 4, no. 4 (1997): 206–11.

7. Carroll, L., "Hormones May Prevent Alzheimer's Disease in Women," *The Chronicle of Neurology and Psychiatry* (autumn 1996): 5.

8. Editors, Chapter 8, "Estrogen and the Brain," *The Canadian Consensus Conference on Menopause and Osteoporosis* (Part II): 1,360–61.

9. Editors, "Estrogen Replacement Therapy Alleviates Symptoms of Rheumatoid Arthritis," *Family Practice* (May 10, 1995): 33–35.

10. Jeffrey, S., "HRT Helps Parkinson's Disease," *Medical Post* 34, no. 18 (November 12, 1998): 1, 71.

11. Calle, E., "Estrogen Replacement Therapy and Risk of Fatal Colon Cancer in Prospective Cohort: American Cancer Prevention Study," *Family Practice* (May 8, 1995): 35.

12. Maheux, R.; et al., "A Randomized, Double Blind, Placebo Controlled Study on the Effects of Conjugated Estrogen on Skin Thickness," *American Journal of Obstetrics and Gynecology* 170 (1994): 642–49.

13. Editors, Chapter 7, "Special Considerations," *The Canadian Consensus Conference on Menopause and Osteoporosis* (Part II).

14. Editors, "Canadian Consensus Conference on Menopause and Osteoporosis Statement," *Journal SOGC* 16 (1994): 1,647–49.

15. Editor, "Tailor HRT to the Individual," *Medical Post* 31, no. 35 (October 10, 1995): 1, 68.

16. Richardson, K., "Managing Migraines during Menopause," *Obstetrics and Gynaecology 2000* 3, no. 2 (1999): 5.

17. Colditz, G.; Hankinson, S.; Hunter, D.; et al., "The Use of Estrogens and Progestins and the Risk of Breast Cancer in Postmenopausal Women," *New England Journal of Medicine* 332 (1995): 1,589–93.

18. Schairer, C.; Byrne, C.; Keyl, P.; et al., "Menopausal Estrogen and Estrogen-Progesterone Replacement Therapy and the Risk of Breast Cancer (United States)," *Cancer Causes and Controls* 5 (1994): 491–500.

19. Stanford, J.; Weiss, N.; Voigt, L.; et al., "Combined Estrogen and Progestin Hormone Replacement Therapy in Relation to Risk of Breast Cancer in Middle-Aged Women," *JAMA* 274 (1995): 137–42.

20. Colditz, G.; et al., "The Use of Estrogens and Progestins and the Risk of Breast Cancer in Postmenopausal Women."

21. Colditz, G.; et al., "The Use of Estrogens and Progestins and the Risk of Breast Cancer in Postmenopausal Women."

22. Federal, Provincial, Territorial Advisory Committee on Population Health, *Report on the Health of Canadians, Statistical Report* (Ottawa: Health Canada, 1999).

23. Colditz, G.; Egan, K.; and Stampfer, M., "Hormone Replacement Therapy and Risk of Breast Cancer: Results from Epidemiologic Studies," *American Journal of Obstetrics and Gynecology* 168 (1993): 1,473–80.

24. Sherwin, B., "Androgen Enhances Sexual Motivation in Females: A Prospective Cross-Over Study of Sex Steroid Administration in the Surgical Menopause," *Psychosomatic Medicine* 47 (1985): 339.

25. *Harvard Women's Health Watch* (March 1996), cited in O'Leary Cobb, J., *A Friend Indeed* XIII, no. 7 (December 1996/January 1997): 3.

26. Blauer, A., "Why You Should Include Androgen in Your HRT Protocol," *Obstetrics and Gynaecology 2000* 1, no. 1 (February 1997): 8.

27. Fukuoka, M., "Growth Inhibition of MCF-7 Human Breast Cancer Cells by Aromatase Inhibitors," *Acta Obstetrics and Gynaecology Japonica* 51 (1991): 2,572;

cited in Greenwood, S., "Testosterone Supplements for Women: A Mixed Blessing," *A Friend Indeed* XI, no. 5 (1994): 1–2.

28. Blauer, A., "Why You Should Include Androgen in Your HRT Protocol."

29. Michael, E.; and Reid, R., "Non-Contraceptive Benefits of Oral Contraceptives in the Perimenopausal Woman," *JSOG* (supplement) 16, no. 5 (1994): 1–7.

30. NAMS, "Life After HERS: A Menopause Management Q and A Report," *Menopause Management* 7, no. 6 (November/December 1998).

31. MacLusky, N., "New Concepts in Hormone Management: Selective Estrogen Receptor Modulators (SERMs)," *Journal SOGC* (supplement) (November 1997): 1–56.

32. Editors, "The Estrogen Question," *Informed* 2, no. 2 (March 1996): 6–9.

Chapter 22: Complementary and Alternative Medicine Is Coming on Strong

1. Woodman, A., *Health Education Authority Guide to Complementary Medicines and Therapies* (London: Hamilton House, 1994), p. vii.

2. Editor, "Choosing and Using Complementary Therapies," *Women's Health Matters* (Health Letter of Women's College Hospital, Toronto) (December 1996/January 1997): 4–5.

3. Millar, W., "Use of Alternative Health Care by Canadians," *Journal of Canadian Public Health* 88, no. 3 (May/June 1997): 154–62.

4. Ibid.

5. Cadario, B., "Replace Misinformation with Facts about Herbal Medicine," *Patient Care* 9, no. 1 (January 1998): 64–87.

6. NAMS, *The NAMS 1997 Menopause Survey*, released at the Eighth Annual Conference of NAMS, Boston, 1997. On-line.

7. Davis, T., "Homeopathy at Menopause," *A Friend Indeed* XI, no. 7 (December 1994).

8. Editors, "Alternative Systems of Medical Practice–Homeopathic Medicine," National Center for Complementary and Alternative Medicine, NIH (1999). On-line.

9. Ibid.

10. Ibid.

11. Ibid.

12. Cadario, B., "Replace Misinformation with Facts about Herbal Medicine."

13. *The Complete Book of Natural Medicinal Cures*, by *Prevention Magazine* Health Books, Rodale Press, p. 94.

14. Cadario, B., "Replace Misinformation with Facts about Herbal Medicine."

15. Morreale, P.; et al., "Chondroitin Sulphate versus NSAIDS," *Journal of Rheumatology* 23, no. 8 (1996): 1,385–91.

16. DerMarderosian, A. (ed.), *The Review of Natural Products* (Philadelphia: Facts and Comparisons), July 1997.

17. Gieler, U.; von der Veth, A.; Haeger, J., "Mahonia Aquifolium: A New Type of Topical Treatment for Psoriasis," *J. Dermatol Treat* 6 (1995): 31–34.

18. DerMarderosian, A. (ed.), *Review of Natural Products*, November 1997.

Chapter 23: Body, Mind, and Soul

1. Grof, S., LSD *Psychotherapy* (Pamona, CA: Hunter House, 1980), p. 263.

2. Jung, C., *Modern Man in Search of a Soul* (New York: Harcourt Brace, 1933), cited in Leder, D., *Spiritual Passages* (New York: Jeremy P. Tarcher/Putnam, 1997).

3. Gallagher, W., *Working on God* (New York: Random House, 1999), p. xvi.

4. Clark Roof, W., *A Generation of Seekers: The Spiritual Journeys of the Baby Boom Generation* (San Francisco: HarperCollins, 1993), quoted in Gallagher, p. xxi.

5. Emberley, P., "Essays on the Millennium: Searching," *Maclean's* (December 28, 1998/January 4, 1999): 103–5.

6. Stern, L., "Living Proof of God's Existence," *Ottawa Citizen* (Saturday, September 6, 1997): 84.

7. Ibid.

8. Wilber, K. *The Marriage of Sense and Soul: Integrating Science and Religion* (New York: Broadway Books, 1998).

9. Dreher, H., "Recite Your Mantra and Call Me in the Morning," *New York* (May 11, 1998): 25–31.

10. Northrup, C. "How to Use the Healing Power of Prayer," *Dr. Christiane Northrup's Health Wisdom for Women* (March 1998): 6–8.

11. Dossey, L., *Healing Words* (San Francisco: HarperCollins, 1993).

12. Moore, T., *Care of the Soul: A Guide for Cultivating Depth and Sacredness in Everyday Life* (New York: HarperPerennial, 1992).

Conclusion: The Time of Your Life

1. Joseph, J., "Warning," from *Selected Poems* (London: Bloodaxe Dufour, 1992).

2. Buber, M., *Tales of the Hasidim: Early Masters* (New York: Schocken Books, 1947), quoted in Leder, D. *Spiritual Passages* (New York: Jeremy P. Tarcher/Putnam, 1997), p. 82.

Index